WOMEN'S GROWTH IN CONNECTION

WOMEN'S GROWTH IN CONNECTION

Writings from the Stone Center

Judith V. Jordan, Alexandra G. Kaplan
Jean Baker Miller, Irene P. Stiver
Janet L. Surrey

THE GUILFORD PRESS
New York   London

Last digit is print number   9 8 7 6 5

Library of Congress Cataloging-in-Publication Data

Women's growth in connection : writings from the Stone Center / by
   Judith Jordan et al. . . . [et al.].
      p.   cm.
   Includes bibliographical references and index.
   ISBN 0-89862-562-9. —ISBN 0-89862-465-7 (pbk.)
   1. Women—Psychology. 2. Self-actualization. 3. Self.
I. Jordan, Judith V.
HQ1206.W879   1991
305.42—dc20   91-12093
                                                                            CIP

The poem reprinted on page 213 is from THE COMPLETE POEMS OF EMILY
DICKINSON edited by Thomas H. Johnson. Copyright 1929 by Martha Dickinson
Bianchi. Copyright © renewed 1957 by Mary L. Hampson. By permission of Little,
Brown and Company. Reprinted by permission of the publishers and the Trustees of
Amherst College from THE COMPLETE POEMS OF EMILY DICKINSON edited by
Thomas H. Johnson, Cambridge, Mass.: The Belknap Press of Harvard University
Press, Copyright 1951, © 1955, 1979, 1983 by the President and Fellows of Harvard
College.

Preface

The ideas represented in this book have evolved over a period of years, as the authors have worked to articulate a perspective on women's development that more accurately reflects women's experience. We initially came together in a group to explore issues in the clinical treament of women. We realized that through years of supervision and then working in traditional clinical settings we had often developed a sense that what we were doing in the privacy of our therapeutic sessions did not match what colleagues and books were propounding about the ideal conduct of therapy. As we discussed clinical dilemmas together, we were energized and excited. We began to let go of more and more of the strictures of our traditional psychodynamic training.

We were troubled not only by the obvious misunderstandings such as "penis envy," but also by the more pervasive and insidious application to women of models of development inspired by a male culture; these theories consistently mislabeled women as deficient. Thus theories of "human development" which espoused increasing capacity for separation, autonomy, mastery, independence, and self-sufficiency as indications of health and maturity consistently portrayed women as too emotional, too dependent, lacking clear boundaries, and so forth.

Supported, emboldened, and encouraged, we began to take this message to others, initially in conventions of mental health professionals and most importantly through the Stone Center Colloquia series initiated when Jean Baker Miller was appointed the first director of the Stone Center for Developmental Services and Studies at Wellesley College.

These ideas have grown from and feed back into a nourishing process of group exchange. It has not always been clear where the ideas came from and in some way the question of authorship of these papers mirrors the very perspective we are exploring: there are individual ways of organizing the thoughts, and individual effort, time and sometimes "angst" has gone into making each chapter, but the generation of ideas, the expansion of the work has sprung from the group.

As Miller (1987) puts it in the introduction to the second edition of

Toward a New Psychology of Women, "At times, our ideas flow from the interactions among us, so that it would be inappropriate to say that an idea 'belonged' to any one person. The idea becomes enlarged and transformed in interchange so that it is not what it was when it began and it is truly everyone's creation. On other points we do not all think alike and we keep struggling to honor these differences" (p. xxiii). The shared creation of ideas is especially true of the central concepts that will reappear in slightly different articulations throughout the book. In some cases this group origin is identified and in other cases it is not. Some of our central concepts are similar to concepts developed by other groups of women, and we have tried to acknowledge these connections as well. Differing versions of basic points will be present from one chapter to another. Although we have been working on our perspective for ten years, we are not yet ready to reify concepts or definitions. Thus, the fluidity of ideas from chapter to chapter represents the kind of thinking which has gone into these conceptions. We are still questioning, still refining, still growing . . . in connection! But although we work together, it is important to emphasize that our work is not taking place in isolation and other groups of women are working along similar lines.

The chapters in this book are "works in progress," part of the beginnings of an evolving, everchanging picture of women's patterns of development. These papers represent the early formulations of what some of us initially called "self-in-relation theory," the "relational self," or the "Stone Center model" of development. We now believe that it can be seen better as part of the general "relational approach to psychological understanding"; this conveys that concepts which are central to our work—women's relational sense of self, the relational path of women's development, and the importance of empathy or responsiveness in relationships—are ideas that are central in the work of other women as well, most notably in Carol Gilligan's work on psychological theory and women's development and the approach which she and her colleagues have been developing over the years.

There is little that feels "settled" or final about these thoughts. Even the title "Growth in Connection" represents an attempt to convey the emerging, moving quality of these concepts about women's development. This book is not meant to be "an answer" but an invitation to join us in our questions, in an inquiry into all of our "truths." The papers included here were selected to convey some basic framing of this perspective. We look forward to subsequent collections which will reflect further elaborations of the work and also the changes and development of these formulations by minority women and lesbian women.

About the Authors

Judith V. Jordan, Ph.D. is Director of Women's Studies at McLean Hospital and Lecturer in Psychology at Harvard University. She is also a Visiting Scholar at the Stone Center for Developmental Services and Studies at Wellesley College and an Instructor in Psychology in the Department of Psychiatry at Harvard Medical School.

Alexandra G. Kaplan, Ph.D. is Director of Counseling and Program Director for Consulting at the Stone Center, Wellesley College, and Lecturer in Psychiatry at the Cambridge Hospital, Harvard Medical School.

Jean Baker Miller, M.D. is a Clinical Professor of Psychiatry at Boston University of Medicine, a Lecturer at Harvard Medical School, and Director of Education at the Stone Center, Wellesley College.

Irene P. Stiver, Ph.D. is Director of the Psychology Department at McLean Hospital, Belmont, Massachusetts. She is also on the faculties of the Harvard Medical School and Harvard University, and is a Visiting Scholar at the Stone Center, Wellesley College.

Janet L. Surrey, Ph.D. is Director of Psychological Services, Adult Outpatient Department, McLean Hospital, Belmont, Massachusetts. She is also Project Consultant and Research Associate at the Stone Center, Wellesley College, Instructor in Psychology, Department of Psychiatry, Harvard Medical School, and the on adjunct faculty at the Episcopal Divinity School, Cambridge, Massachusetts.

Contents

Introduction

This book is intended as a sampling of some provocative ideas about women's meaning systems, values, passions, organization of experience, and ways of being in the world. We believe the organizing factor in women's lives is "relational growth" and we have tried to portray that in a number of different ways: in Part I some of the beginning principles are presented and in Part II these formulations are applied to such topics as work inhibitions, depression, eating disorders, and therapeutic implications of this model.

Much of the initial work centered on our reexamination of existing theory. We did not so much seek to discard these theories as to sharpen and articulate what is useful from them and to develop new concepts and models that better represent women's lives. One of our and other women's central critiques of existing developmental theory concerns the common notion that development evolves through stages of ever increasing levels of separation and spheres of mastery and personal independence. This theory emphasizes "the separate self," an autonomous, self-sufficient, contained entity. A Western bias of individualism and a "Lone Ranger" ethic of meeting challenges underlie most psychological theories of the self.

Freudian theory, built on the primacy of instinctual drives and suggesting that relationships are secondary to drive, did little to further our understanding of either primary relatedness or women's special psychological development. Object relations theorists came closer to acknowledging the power of relationship; but they retained the language of drive (the other is an "object" of the drive) and guilt over destructive impulses is often seen to be at the core of concern and love (Klein, 1975; Winnicott, 1963; Jordan, Chapter 17, this volume). Fairbairn (1946) and Guntrip (1973), less widely read in this country than Klein and Winnicott, actually moved farther away from the Freudian drive model.

Sullivan (1953) radically reframed existing theories of development and treatment in his model of interpersonal psychiatry: "A personality can never be isolated from the complex of interpersonal relations in which the person lives and has his being" (p. 10). His system departed from the traditional preoccupation with drive theory. His theory, however, still focused on the endpoint of "the self," albeit as made up of "reflected appraisals"; and the mutuality of connection was not a feature of his thinking.

Kohut's emphasis on empathy in the analytic setting led toward a renewed interest in the relationship in therapy; his notion that selfobjects are needed throughout life also lessens the press for the independent, internally structuralized adult (Kohut, 1983). But his description of the self, using the selfobject to maintain narcissistic equilibrium, suggests a need-determined relationship. The idea of mutuality, of fullness of contact, of connection is also not represented in this theory.

Daniel Stern, a psychoanalyst and infant researcher, has made a stunning contribution to altering our image of the passive, dependent infant being shaped toward engagement in relationship and then ultimately to independence and mastery (Stern, 1986). In microscopic analyses of mother–infant interactions, he reveals the active interest and involvement of the infant in the relationship. He rejects the language of other as "object" and begins to provide us a vocabulary for speaking about self-other experience from very early infancy.

Several feminist theorists and writers have provided the most compelling impetus for us to question and rethink existing theories. Jean Baker Miller, in *Toward a New Psychology of Women* (1976), helped us move from a deficiency model of women to a position where we saw, named, and valued women's strengths. Empathic relating is at the heart of this new understanding of women. But we have moved from earlier framing of our thinking as a "self-in-relation model" to looking at the importance of relational development; we question and are cautious about the setting up of a new theory of "Self," even if altered with the attachment of hyphens.

As we were elaborating the basic ideas in Jean's book, writings of other women enriched us. Chodorow (1978) provided an analysis of how women become mothers, as understood through object relations theory, and helped free many women from the hold of traditional explanations of the Oedipus complex and other psychoanalytic notions. But her analysis in some ways remained true to its object relations origins, seeing relationships as secondary to drive satisfaction and frustration.

Most importantly, Gilligan's (1977, 1982) work on women's development reframes developmental models and brings women's and girls' voices into the center of a new psychology. Gilligan's analysis of the centrality of connection in women's sense of self shows how profoundly this basic experience of connection affects women's ways of approaching relational conflicts and crises. Her careful listening to women's and men's voices reveals the primacy of responsive relationships as a powerful determinant of women's psychological reality. Her work has enabled many people to listen more fully to themselves and to others and to understand and value voices that previously were dismissed, misunderstood or not listened to. Gilligan and her colleagues, in articulating the dissonance between women's voices and previous psychological theories, have made it easier to follow the misunderstandings which accrue when women's (and men's) development is measured primarily in terms of separation and autonomy, as was the case with previous models of self and moral development. The studies with girls as well as with women which Gilligan and women working with her have undertaken (Gilligan, Brown, & Rogers, 1989; Gilligan, Lyons, & Hanmer, 1989; Gilligan, 1990) and the continuing attention of this group to voice and language as integral to the understanding of psychological processes make their work centrally important to our understandings of women's development and to the development of a relational psychology.

Similarly, Belenky et al. (1986) gave us a picture of different modes of knowing which has enhanced our understanding of women's' special and different ways of knowing, in particular "connected knowing." In addition to enlarging us in many ways, Adrienne Rich's work (1983) helped us focus attention on cultural imperatives toward heterosexuality. One of our foremost tasks for the future is to better understand the specifics of women's experience based on class, race, age, ethnicity, and sexual preference. We have learned from many more women than we can cite in this brief account.

Many of our most difficult challenges have centered around the use of language and the attempt to find the words that best capture what we want to communicate. As we look back over these chapters, we find language used in ways with which we are no longer comfortable, but as part of the representation of the evolution of the ideas, this old and awkward language must at times remain.

The authors are all clinicians, clinical supervisors, and teachers.

While we have seen deeply into many lives, the data that form the basis of these ideas are not based on research in the traditional sense. But there is a long tradition of clinical data forming the core for theory building and at this time our work rests on this beginning point.

A new understanding of psychological development in women leads to a different definition of "psychopathology" which ultimately necessitates a new psychotherapy. While our original ideas arose in the context of the practice of psychotherapy, we are beginning only now to clarify the implications of this approach for doing psychotherapy; we are looking at the ways in which we diverge from traditional practice, the ways in which we use empathy, the place that mutuality has in therapy, and many more factors which are just beginning to come into focus.

Parts I and II of this book move from theoretical statements about women's relational development to applications of this perspective. Most of the chapters were originally Working Papers of the Stone Center for Developmental Services and Studies at Wellesley College; a few papers were published elsewhere. Each was chosen because it represented a particular early aspect of the work.

It is appropriate that the book begins with a chapter by Jean Baker Miller, " The Development of Women's Sense of Self," because Jean's work *Toward a New Psychology of Women* is the single most significant influence on all our work. In this chapter Miller notes that definitions of self in Western psychology emphasize separation and individuation but neglect the intricacies of human interconnection.

"Women and Empathy" is an example of a topic in evolution. It was the first paper that three of the authors presented at the Stone Center Colloquium Series; it dealt with certain basic formulations and opened the way for further exploration but many of the concepts put forth there have grown and changed. Since this is true for several of the papers, we have included the date they were originally presented to give the reader a sense of the historical development of the ideas.

Janet Surrey's "Self-in-Relation" highlights the relational view of growth through connection and describes the two-directional processes of the mother–daughter relationship as an early model of relational development. It is the first paper in which the perspective is named "self-in-relation," a name which has stuck despite our ambivalence about its aptness.

In "Empathy and Self Boundaries" Jordan explores empathy as a complex cognitive and affective process central to the development of relational capacities and therefore to the sense of self in women. The idea of "self-empathy" is introduced as a useful therapeutic construct. In "The Meaning of Mutuality" the shift from a psychology of separate self to relational self is furthered in the discussion of intersubjectivity. In addition, the destructive consequences of imbalances in mutuality in relationships are examined.

Stiver's "Beyond the Oedipus" notes the deficiencies of the traditional oedipal theory as applied to women and its failure to explain the complexities of the strong connections and the strong conflicts between mothers and daughters. The relational model offers a context to reconcile these seemingly contradictory observations.

Alexandra Kaplan's, Rona Klein's, and Nancy Gleason's chapter, "Women's Self Development in Late Adolescence," suggests that within a relational frame, late-adolescent women's development is characterized by relational change and conflict, but not distance or lessening of the relational bond. The eruption of difference from or conflict with parents can be motivated by the adolescent's wish to be known and valued, even as she changes. If this process occurs, it can lead to a greater sense of mutual understanding and mutual empowerment.

Part II consists of applications of the relational model to particular life problems and, to a lesser extent, therapy. Irene Stiver's early paper on the meanings of dependency in female–male relationships notes that "dependency" as a relational term has taken on pejorative connotations because of its longstanding identification with feminine characteristics. Both women and men struggle with this need to depend on each other, but their struggles emerge from different life experiences and different cultural expectations.

Janet Surrey's chapter on "Relationship and Empowerment" describes psychological empowerment as arising from interaction within mutually empathic and mutually empowering relationships; clinical and political applications of this model are also explored.

In "The Construction of Anger in Women and Men," Jean Baker Miller notes that anger as we know it is "constructed" by our culture, and not traceable to an inherent "drive." The restraints placed on women's expression of anger are different from those placed on men. Thus cultural concepts of "femininity" lead to characterization of women's expressions of anger as pathological. The next chapter, "Women And Power," traces the differences between the notion of "power over" and "empowerment." Jean Baker Miller notes that empowering other people does not fit accepted conceptualizations and definitions of power. Further, when women contemplate the use of power on their own behalf and for their own interests, many of them equate the prospect with destructiveness and selfishness—characteristics that they cannot reconcile with a sense of feminine identity.

Alexandra Kaplan's chapter, "The Self-in-Relation: Implications for Depression in Women," posits that the high incidence of depression in women is related to the overlap between key dynamics of depression and central features of the psychological development enforced on women. Specifically, a relational perspective highlights how women's felt responsibility for relationship, when thwarted or deflected, can generate major depressive features of vulnerability to loss, inhibition of action and assertion, inhibition of anger, and low self esteem.

In "Work Inhibitions in Women," Stiver points out that although work is an important source of identity and self esteem for women, it is not easily integrated into women's lives in our current social setting. Women's experience with work-related issues differs quantitatively and qualitatively from that of men. Our cultural definitions of job success reflect a male model in most work environments, and are typically not congruent with qualities that women value. Women often need validation of their standards and beliefs.

Surrey's work on "Eating Patterns" examines the widespread disturbances in eating patterns, dieting, and body image among women today within a sociocultural context which devalues, pathologizes, and misunderstands women's relational yearnings and sense of "self-in-relation."

In "Female or Male Therapists for Women: New Formulations," Kaplan discusses the psychotherapy research which suggests that therapeutic gain comes from a positive client–therapist relationship. Women's relational self-structure attunes them to affective connection and the primacy of mutually enhancing connection—two crucial elements in a positive therapy relationship. Men's upbringing may not as readily prepare them for clinical work within a relational frame.

Stiver looks at therapy in "The Meaning of Care." Here the traditional model of therapy, which stresses "objectivity," "neutrality," and distancing, is explored. This model reflects a style more congenial to men than to women, since it emphasizes unemotional and impersonal attitudes. Although various therapeutic strategies contribute to distancing in therapy, the formal and informal language which is used in diagnosing is examined with particular emphasis on the ways in which women are more victimized than men by these processes.

Jordan continues the examination of a relational perspective in the conduct of therapy in "Empathy, Mutuality, and Therapeutic Change." She begins a tentative outline for the applications of a relational perspective to the practice of psychotherapy, noting in particular the centrality of empathy and mutual development to the therapeutic enterprise.

This book, then, is very much a compilation of works still in progress. Although the papers are ordered topically rather than by date of original publication, the reader will note a gradual development of ideas. We hope that readers will engage with the work through their own dialogues. We encourage you, then, to journey with us in the process of discovery and reformulation in much the same way that we have engaged with each other.

We are also just beginning to think about the use of this perspective to better understand men; we know that the shift we are suggesting from a psychology of "The Self" to one emphasizing relationships does not apply to women's psychology only. It points to the need for a rethinking of our study of all people. Further we need to extend our thinking to specific groups who are not yet adequately represented in some of this work: lesbians, racial and ethnic minority women, and other marginalized groups.

Psychological theory, like any other cultural institution, reflects the larger Western patriarchal culture in the unexamined assumption that the white, middle class, heterosexual "paradigm man" defines not just his own reality but human reality. Thus, without a critique of patriarchal bias in existing approaches to "human development," the experience of the "paradigm man" will be reified as "truth" while that of others will be distorted for not conforming to patriarchal dictates.

Similarly, we recognize that what we—five white middle-class well-educated women—are putting forth as a perspective of women's development is clearly limited by our own life experiences, by the nature of the work we do and the people with whom we work. Clearly we could have had a more complex, more encompassing perspective if we had begun with a broader realm of experience from which to draw. It is especially important, in carving out a perspective on relational empowerment, to incorporate the patterns of relationship that exist with those who are marginalized by the dominant culture. Without this, there is no way that we can speak for all women. We do not want to repeat the error of other theoreticians: speaking as if there is one voice, one reality for humans, for women, when in fact we recognize the exquisite contextuality of human life. We regret the limits of our model-building at this time and we have taken steps to include more minority women and lesbian women in the development of these ideas. We are trying to expand our understandings through more frequent dialogue with those who can teach us about other "realities" and points of view.

I

A DEVELOPMENTAL PERSPECTIVE

1

The Development of Women's Sense of Self

JEAN BAKER MILLER

The concept of the self has been prominent in psychological theory, perhaps because it has been one of the central ideas in Western thought. While various writers use different definitions, the essential idea of a "self" seems to underlie the historical development of many Western notions about such vast issues as the "good life," justice, and freedom. Indeed, it seems entwined in the roots of several delineations of fundamental human motives or the highest form of existence, as in Maslow's self-actualizing character.

As we have inherited it, the notion of a "self" does not appear to fit women's experience. Several recent writers have spoken to this point, for example, literary critic Carolyn Heilbrun (1979) and psychologist Carol Gilligan (1982). A question then arises: Do only men, and not women, have a self? In working with women the question is quite puzzling, but an examination of the very puzzle itself may cast new light on certain long-standing assumptions. Modern American theorists of early psychological development and, indeed, of the entire life span, from Erik Erikson (1950) to Daniel Levinson (1978), tend to see all of development as a process of separating oneself out from the matrix of others—"becoming one's own man," in Levinson's words. Development of the self presumably is attained via a series of painful crises by which the individual accomplishes a sequence of allegedly essential separations from others, thereby achieving an inner sense of separated individuation. Few men ever attain such self-sufficiency, as every woman knows. They are usually supported by wives, mistresses, mothers, daughters, secretaries, nurses, and other women (as well as other men who are lower than they in the socioeconomic hierarchy). Thus, there is reason to question whether this model accurately reflects men's lives. Its goals, however, are held out for all, and are seen as the preconditions for mental health.

Almost every modern theorist who has tried to fit women into the prevalent models has had much more obvious difficulty, beginning with Freud and extending through Erikson and others. Some have not even tried. In Erikson's scheme, for example, after the first stage, in which the aim is the development of basic trust, the aim of every other stage, until young adulthood, is some form of increased separation or self-development. I am not referring at this point to the process by which each aim is attained (although that is an intimately related point that will be discussed below), but to the aim itself, the goal. It is important to note that the aim is not something like development of greater capacity for emotional connection to others; or for contributing to an interchange between people; or for playing a part in the growth of others as well as one's self. When the individual arrives at the stage called "intimacy," he is supposed to be able to be intimate with another person—having spent all of his prior development striving for something very different.

Much recent writing deploring men's inability to engage in intimacy has come from the women's movement. But men, too, have been making the same point. Almost all of modern literature, philosophy, and commentary in other forms portrays men's lack of a sense of community—indeed, it denies even the possibility of communicating with others.

Thus, the prevailing models may not describe well what occurs in men; in addition, there is a question about the value of these models even if it were possible to fulfill their requirements. These two questions are related, as I will try to suggest. It is very important to note, however, that the prevalent models are powerful because they have become prescriptions about what *should* happen. They affect men; they determine the actions of mental health professionals. They have affected women adversely in one way in the past. They are affecting women in another way now, if women seek "equal access" to them. Therefore, we need to examine them carefully. It is important not to embrace them because they are the only models available.

THE BEGINNINGS

What are some of the questions that arise when we try to bring women's experience into the picture? We can take Erikson's theories as a starting point, not to attempt a thorough examination of them, but to use them as a framework for consideration of a few of the many features in women's development.

In the first stage of life, according to Erikson, the central goal is the infant's development of a sense of basic trust. Another important dimension, however, is also involved. Even at that early stage in all infants, but encouraged much more in girls, the young child begins to be like and act like the main caretaker, who, up until now, has usually been a woman—not to "identify" with that person as some static figure described only by gender, but with what that person *actually* is doing. I think that the infant begins to develop an internal representation of itself as a kind of being that, for the moment, I will call by a hyphenated term—a "being-in-relationship." This is the beginning of a sense of "self" that reflects what is happening *between* people. The infant picks up the feelings of the other person, that is, it has an early sense that "I feel what is going on in the other as well as what is going on in myself." It is more complex because it involves "knowing"—feeling—what is going on in that emotional field between us. The child experiences a sense of comfort only as the other is also comfortable, or, more precisely, only as they are both engaged in an emotional relationship that is moving toward greater well-being, rather than toward the opposite--that is, only as the interactions in the emotional field between the infant and the adult are moving toward a "better" progression of events.* In this sense, the infant, actively exerting an effect on the relationship, begins to develop an internal sense of itself as one who changes the emotional interplay for both participants—for good or ill.

The beginnings of a mental construction of self are much more complicated than those suggested by such commonly used terms as *fusion* or *merger* for the mental constructions of the first stages of infancy, as drawn from Mahler (1975), object relations theorists, and others. New research on infant–caretaker interactions also indicates the inappropriateness of those terms (see, for example, Stern, 1980, Stechler and Kaplan, 1980; Klein, 1976). This research suggests that these constructs are not likely to describe adequately the complex internal representations of the self and the "other," or, rather, the

---

* This point has been made in various ways by many theorists, such as M. Klein, H. S. Sullivan, and several others. The features that they emphasize, however, are different.

internal self–other relational patterns that the infant is likely to create even from the earliest age.

When we talk about a sense of self in this field, we have been referring to a "man-made" construct meant to describe an internal mental representation. The suggestion here is that from the moment of birth this internal representation is of a self that is in active interchange with other selves. Moreover, this interaction has one central character- istic, and that is that people are attending to the infant—most importantly, attending to the infant's core of being, which means the infant's emotions—and the infant is responding in the same way, that is, to the other person's emotions. The earliest mental representation of the self, then, is of a self whose core—which is emotional—is attended to by the other(s) and in turn, begins to attend to the emotions of the other(s). Part of this internal image of oneself includes feeling the other's emotions and *acting on* them as they are in interplay with one's own emotions. This means that the beginnings of the concept of self are not those of a static and lone self being ministered to by another (incidentally, this construct has a strong male flavor), but rather of a self inseparable from dynamic interaction. And the central character of that interaction involves attending to each other's mental states and emotions.

This early "interacting sense of self" is present for infants of both sexes, but the culturally induced beliefs of the caretakers about girls and boys play a role from the moment of birth. These beliefs are, of course, internalized even in the woman caretaker, although more so in fathers, according to suggestions from some studies (e.g., Rubin et al., 1974; Block, 1978). Girls are encouraged to augment their abilities to "feel as the other feels" and to practice "learning about" the other(s). Boys are systematically diverted from it—to their deprivation and detriment, in my opinion. (In my opinion, this redounds, too, to the detriment of the whole construction of our societal structure and of our models of thinking.)

Out of this interplay of experience one certainly develops a sense of one's self, that is, an internal or mental representation of one's self. Moreover, one develops a sense of one's self as a person who attends to and responds to what is going on in the relationships between two or more people.

Much of the literature tends to suggest that because she is the same sex as the caretaker, the girl cannot develop an internal sense of self; that is, that boys develop a sense of self because they separate themselves from the female caretaker. This is truly an incredible notion. First, it ignores all of the complexity of the interaction between caretaker and infant. It is as if there were no interaction because mother and child are both of the same sex—an amazing negation of the very idea of girls and women.

Second, the literature has generally ignored the extraordinarily important character of the interaction—that of attending to and responding to the other. This is the essential feature of what comes to be called "caretaking." It is also the basis of all continuing psychological growth; that is, all growth occurs within emotional connections, not separate from them. Current theories ignore, too, the likelihood that the early self is built on the model of this very process—as opposed to the very different kinds of interaction that exist in the current world. The very notion of true caretaking precludes anything that would lead the infant to feel submerged, fused, or merged with the other. These words may describe some of the phenomena observed after *distortions* in caretaking have occurred, but they are unlikely to characterize the infant's prototypic sense of self.

Third, current notions tend to ignore the likelihood that the only possibility of having any sense of self at all is built on the core process I have described. As suggested above, it begins to be discouraged early on in boys. For girls, it is encouraged, but complications are added at this and at each succeeding phase of development.

Surrey has suggested that this early mental representation of the self in girls can be described as a more *encompassing* sense of self, in contrast with the more boundaried, or limited, self that is encouraged in boys from a very young age. She suggests, too, the term "oscillating" sense of self as compared to the current, more linear model, with the "oscillation" following from the ongoing growth of empathy in the child as well as in the mother (see Surrey, Chapter 3, this volume; Jordan, Surrey, & Kaplan, Chapter 2, this volume). Many implications follow. To begin with, certain events in later life that other models see as detracting from the self are instead seen as satisfying, motivating and empowering. For example, to feel "more related to another person" means to feel one's self enhanced, not threatened. It does not feel like a loss of part of one's self; instead it becomes a step toward more pleasure and effectiveness—because it is the way the girl and woman feel "things should be," the way she wants them to be. Being in relationship, picking up the feelings of the other and attending to the "interaction between" becomes an accepted, "natural-seeming" way of being and acting. It is learned and assumed; not alien or threatening. Most important, it is desired; it is a *goal*, not a detraction or a means to some other end, such as one's own self-development. Thus, it forms a *motivation*.

We have come to think of this whole experience as so "foreign," I believe, because our cultural tradition has emphasized such a different direction. In the dominant and official culture, attending to the experience of others and to the relationships between people is not seen as a *requirement* of all of life. It has been relegated to the alien and mysterious world of mothers and infancy—and misunderstood. Sometimes, when I have tried to talk about this, psychiatrists have said, "Oh, I see what you mean. All right, I agree that women are more altruistic." That is not what I mean. That is attempting to slot this description into the old categories. It suggests a "sacrifice" of parts of a kind of self that has developed in a different fashion. To engage in the kind of interaction I am discussing is not a sacrifice; it is, in fact, a source of feeling better and more gratified, as well as more knowledgeable—about what is really happening. I believe it is closer to the elementary human necessities from which our dominant culture has become unnecessarily removed.

Another implication relates to self-esteem, or the sense of self-worth. The girl's sense of self-esteem is based in feeling that she is a part of relationships and is taking care of those relationships. This is very different from the components of self-esteem as usually described and, incidentally, as measured by most available scales. Another ramification involves the issue of competence or effectiveness. The girl and woman often feel a sense of effectiveness as arising out of emotional connections and as bound up with and feeding back into them. This is very different from a sense of effectiveness (or power) based in lone action and in acting against or over others. This sense of effectiveness can develop further in the next and all subsequent ages, but it grows upon this base.

AGENCY WITHIN COMMUNITY

To move quickly through the next ages of life, I will sketch a few suggestions about each of them, leading only as far as adolescence. Erikson speaks about the second stage of childhood as one in which the goal is autonomy; others have spoken about separation and individuation. I would suggest, instead, that we could think of this as a period when the child has more abilities, more possibilities "to do," and more physical and mental resources to use. The child also has an enlarged "point of view" on all events, as it were, that is, a more developed sense of how she or he sees things. There is not, however, nor need there be, any increased separation. Instead, there are new configurations and new "understandings" *in the relationship*. Maintaining the relationship(s) with the main people in her or his life is still *the* most important thing.

We might think of this as something like a phase called "agency-in-community." These words are borrowed from Bakan (1966) but not used with his definitions. Instead, by "agency" I am searching for a word again, a word that means being active, using all of one's resources, but without the connotations of aggression--another large topic, but one that cannot be developed here (see Miller, Chapter 10, this volume). Here, again, the "doing" is different from what has been described in the past. Often for little girls, it means doing *for* following the model of what the mother is doing (see Jordan, Surrey, & Kaplan, Chapter 2, this volume; Surrey, Chapter 3, this volume). What the mother is still doing with little children is attending to their feelings and "*doing for*" them, although not totally. So the action, again, has a different character—it is doing for other(s) within a relationship, with the little girl using increased powers, an increased number of "opinions" about how and what she wants "to do," and an increased assertion of what she can do.

In her internal representation of herself, I suggest, the girl is developing not a sense of separation, but a more developed sense of her own capacities and her greater ability to put her "views" into effect. That is, she has a sense of a larger scope of action—but still with an inner representation of a self that is doing this in relation to other selves. A larger scope of action is not equivalent to separation; it requires a *change* in her internal configuration of her sense of self and other, but not a separation.

The child can move on to a larger, but a more articulated sense of herself *only because of* her actions and feelings *in* the relationship. These actions and feelings are inevitably different from the other person's. They are obviously not identical. The point is that she is attuned to the feelings of the other person; and just as her feelings are influenced by other's feelings, so too, do they influence the other's feelings. She has a wide range of feelings and actions, and they vary at different times, with one or another in ascendancy, but they occur within the relational context.

Of course, the character of the relationship differs from that of infancy; new qualities come in. But this does not lead to a "separate" sense of self. It leads to a more complex sense of self in more complex relationships to other selves.

The whole notion of describing human interaction in geographic or spatial terms, along a scale of close or distant (i.e., separated), seems questionable. Surely it is the *quality* of the interaction that is the question—the interplay of "conceptualized feelings" (i.e., feelings *cum* concepts), the doing of good or bad to the other—in relation to the nature of each's needs. A growing child has the potential to do more that he or she could do before. The caretaker who recognizes and supports this enlarged ability does not become more distant. The caretaker becomes *more caring* in one more way—that is, *more related*—and the child does, too.

CHILDHOOD

When we move to the next stage, which is based on the oedipal stage, we may ask whether one reason that people, beginning with Freud, have had such trouble delineating this stage in girls is that it may not exist. There is no major crisis of "cutting off" anything, and especially relationships. And there is no need to fulfill the goal of "identifying with an aggressor," that is, the threatening and dominant male figure. (Several theorists believe that all of society, culture, and thought is built on this oedipal moment of identification with the aggressive father. It is interesting to think about the possibility that society need not be built on this base.) However, there is a message that may come in to play more forcefully at this time (though it begins earlier and it continues later)--that the girl should now focus all her energies on the well-being, growth, and development of men. Nonetheless, the relationship to the mother and to other women continues. A pronounced turning away from the mother and toward the father may occur because of particular conditions in particular families, especially when the mother herself encourages and models this way of being. Western culture has dictated that mothers should uphold the superior importance and power of the man. These forces begin to affect deeply the girl's sense of herself and her relationship to her mother and to complicate the relationship in many ways. However, the relationship to the mother and to other women continues, although it may be less obvious and it may be made to seem less important. There are ethnic, class, and historical variations in the degree of influence of the mother or father within the family, but, in general, the greater importance, value, and power of the father—and the devaluation of the mother—seems to come through psychologically.

In latency, or the period that, according to Erikson, has "industry" as its goal, there is increasing evidence that girls are not very latent. What girls may do is learn to hide more, if we are talking about sexuality, as Freud was when he initiated the use of the term. But if we are talking about relationships, this is certainly the time when the girls are very intensely involved in all of their relationships, especially with other girls. Many girls are very interested in men and boys, too, but the boys are often either not interested or actively deprecating and destructive to girls. The boys are out learning "industry," which others have talked about as "learning the rules of the game and how to play it" (Gilligan, 1982). Most of these rules, incidentally, seem directly traceable to war games. In a study of this period, Luria (1981) describes the events in a grade school playground. She talks about the boys' learning not only how to be "warlike" and to win out over others, but how to cheat and get away with it. When she asked the girls what they were doing, they often said, "Nothing." The girls are hanging around the edges of the playground "just talking." What are they talking about? They are talking about the issues in their families and how to solve them. In discussing their families, the girls are, of course, very involved in an emotional interaction with one another. Surrey (Chapter 3, this volume) has pointed out that the vast amount of psychological development that occurs within the relationships between girls at this time has been one of the major neglected areas in psychological study.

ADOLESCENCE

Adolescence has been seen as a time when the individual has greatly increased capacities. Traditionally, psychologists have *divided* them in several ways: for example, sexual capacities; aggressive capacities—which I will call, for the moment, agentic (the ability to act); and cognitive capacities, with the development of formal thought that greatly expands the universe. However, many studies still indicate that this is a time when girls begin to "contract" rather than expand. Clara Thompson (1942) noted this long ago. She said that for boys, adolescence is seen as a period of opening up, but for girls it is a time for shutting down. In different terms, Freud said this, too. Freud believed that girls now had to learn that they were not actively to use all of themselves and all of their life forces from a base centered in their own bodies and in their own psychological constructions. For Freud, this meant, of course, the derivatives of their sexual drive. Instead, these forces are now to be turned to the use of others—men, in the first instance, and to the service of the next generation, via childbearing. That is, girls had to resolve their psychological issues by becoming passive and masochistic—to accomplish the necessary submission to the man and to "sacrifice" themselves for children.

Freud's observations may have reflected much of what hap-pened—and still happens. That is, in regard to sexuality, most girls still learn that their own sexual perceptions, sensations, and impulses are not supposed to arise from themselves, but are to be brought forth by and for men. Thus girls still tend to experience their physical and sexual stirrings as wrong, bad, evil, dirty, and the like. This is to say that part of what has been going on in the girl's earlier internal representations of herself has included several problematic parts. One of these involves bodily and sexual experience. This situation can lead to an attempt to deal with this experience by turning to passivity and submission. The girl picks up the strong message that her own perceptions about her bodily and sexual feelings are not acceptable. They acquire connotations of badness and evil. They become parts of her self that are shameful and wrong. She has sought to bring these parts of herself into relationships with others all along, but has had difficulty in doing so. She still seeks to act on these desires within relationships with others. But she meets opposition. In the face of this, the solution of "doing it for others" can seem to offer a ready answer. The problem is that this solution is one that attempts to leave her--and her sense of herself, with all of her own psychological constructions--out of the relationship.

In heterosexual relationships, if the girl or young woman tries to have her own perceptions, to follow her own desires, and to bring them into sexual experience with boys, she still is destined for conflict. Despite all of the recent talk, the girl's attempt to act on the basis of her own sexuality still leads to conflict with her potential male partners. It will also lead to internal conflict with certain components of her sense of self. One is the part that says she should—and that she wants to—be attuned to others, which leads to a conflict if the other is behaving in ways that are excluding her perceptions and desires from the relationship. Another is the part that has made sexuality an unaccept-able aspect of her internal sense of self and therefore prevents her from bringing a large part of herself into the relationship.

A similar dynamic exists in regard to "agency," that is, the girl's capacity to perceive and to use her powers in all ways. Women are not supposed to do this, and they have incorporated the idea that to do so is wrong and shameful. The girl has learned and done many things, until now, within a relationship. However, because of societal influences, she has also incorporated a sense—again, to varying degrees—that she is not fully and freely to use all of her powers. During adolescence, however, she receives this as a much stronger message.

Thus her sense of self as an active agent—in the context of acting within a relationship and for the relationship—has been altered to some degree all along by a sense of a self who must defer to others' needs or desires. However, at adolescence she experiences a much more intense pressure to do so. Her sense of self as developed so far now faces a more serious conflict with the external forces she confronts.

The question is how she will deal with this conflict. As with sexuality, I believe that the major tendency is for the girl to opt for the relationship both in her overt actions and in an alteration of her internal sense of self. She will tend to want most to retain the self that wants to be a "being-in-relationship" but she will begin to lose touch with the definition of herself as a more active "being-within-relationship." If one part has to go, and until now it did, most girls lose more of the sense that they can bring their agency and sexuality, as they experience it, into the relationship.

To restate some of these points, at adolescence the girl is seeking fulfillment of two very important needs: to use all of her capacities, including her sexual capacity, but seeking to do so within a context that will fulfill her great desire to be a "being-in-relationship." This wish to do so has developed all through earlier ages. She wishes that the other person will be able to enter into a relationship in this fashion. I believe that the boy really has the same needs, at bottom. However, he has been much more preoccupied with trying to develop "himself" and a sense of his independent identity. The culture has made the very heavy demand that he be so preoccupied. It has been doing so all along, but it does so at adolescence in an even more forceful way. He has also picked up the idea that the girl should adapt to him, and he has not been encouraged to continue the development of the sense that he is primarily a boy-in-relationship with a primary responsibility for others and a desire to concentrate on the relationship between himself and others.

Thus girls are not seeking the *kind* of identity that has been prescribed for boys, but a different kind, one in which one is a "being-in-relation," which means developing all of one's self in increasingly complex ways, in increasingly complex relationships.

The model of a "being-in-relationship" that women are seeking is not easy to attain in present conditions. As I have tried to suggest, it is a very valuable model and, I believe, a model more related to reality--the reality of the human condition. In the current situation, however, it still tends to mean for women the old kind of relationship, with the suppression of the full participation of the woman's way of seeing and acting. This has been the historical pattern, certainly. For most women it is still the case. Even so, the woman's struggle continues into later life; but many more factors now complicate it.

PRACTICAL IMPLICATIONS

The practical implications are many. To suggest just a few, women probably do talk about relationships more often, and this is often misinterpreted as dependency. It is very important to listen carefully to what women are saying. Often it is not about wanting or needing to be dependent *or* independent, but about wanting to be in relationship with others and, again, to really comprehend the other; wanting to understand the other's feelings; wanting to contribute to the other; wanting the *nature* of the relationship to be one in which the other person(s) is engaged in this way (see Stiver, Chapter 8, this volume; Surrey, Chapter 3, this volume; Jordan, Surrey, & Kaplan, Chapter 2, this volume). Thus, very often I have heard described as dependent women who are taking care of (and still developing psychologically from taking care of) about six other people. Sometimes they were doing so within a framework that contained many factors of realistic dependency, such as economic dependency or social dependency. Sometimes they had to adopt the psychological framework of the other because that is what their partners expected or demanded. But that is better described as the condition of a subordinate (Miller, 1976), which is still the social condition. This distinction is important.

It is not because of relationships per se that women are suppressed or oppressed. The issue is the *nature* of the relationships. In fact, without the recognition of the importance of relationships to women, we do not help women to find a path that leads them to growth and development. Some psychologists fall into a tendency to encourage "independence" or "separation," which is not what many women want. In the past, mental health professionals encouraged dependency with submission. The point is that the construction of concepts on that axis is inappropriate and misleading.

Perhaps I can illustrate these points by referring briefly to parts of the therapeutic work with one young woman, Ms. D. Ms. D., a 23-year-old woman, had been depressed and had felt worthless in an extreme way since about the age of 13. She was clearly very intelligent and also had a profound quality of thought. She was exceptionally physically attractive.

She did not know where all of the troubles were coming from and could not connect their onset with any specific events. She saw her father as a sort of nice guy; he was light, humorous, and the parent she liked. By contrast, she perceived her mother as a difficult, agitated, "screaming" person, someone no one would want to be like or even to be around. This is one description of parents that therapists hear frequently.

There was one thing that seemed related to the trouble beginning at age 13, although Ms. D. did not make this connection initially. The main part of her relationship with her father appeared to center around her tagging along with him in what seemed his major interest, football.

From the time she was about 12 or 13, he did not let her tag along anymore, nor did he let her play with him, her brothers, and the other neighborhood boys. This also is one fairly common occurrence.

She had two brothers, 2 and 4 years younger, to whom she felt very devoted. From young childhood, she had always been very sympathetic to them, felt she understood them, and did a great many things for them.

Something else began around age 13: Many boys began to pursue her. Some were clearly making a straightforward dash for sex; others seemed to seek her ability to hear their needs, to understand them, to be responsive, to be sympathetic, to help them--all of which she did. In neither case, however, were the boys interested in her feelings and concerns if she tried to bring these into the relationship. By the time of therapy, she had lost much of her ability to do so.

I will highlight in abbreviated fashion some of the features that emerged in therapy. Ms. D. came to see that she had developed in many ways, even with all that was bad and lacking in her life. She had related to others in a way that fostered their development. She did this and did it with pleasure and willingness, but she herself was not given much sense of self-worth and self-validation for doing so. No one recognized it fully, or gave her much affirmation for it. Thus, for one thing, she lacked a huge portion of the basis for self-esteem that she could and should have had. Second, almost no one reciprocated, that is, wanted to know and to respond to her needs and desires as she perceived and felt them.

Only after some time in therapy did she see that she had worked at bolstering her father (which she felt was her task) and her brothers; most important, she connected some of this to the "life's work" that had preoccupied her mother all along. She could see, for instance, that a great part of her mother's "ranting and raving," as she called it, resulted from the attempt to "shore up" her father and help her more valued brothers. Her father always had been shaky in his work, and there was a lot to do in the effort to help him "succeed." Her mother had been trying to do that. A large part of her mother's behavior was, however, both a cry for help at her felt obligation to accomplish an impossibility and a "protest" against having to accomplish that impossibility. Late in therapy, Ms. D. could begin to feel a sense of connection to her mother in the recognition that they both had been engaged in that task. Both had gained little sense of value from it. Simultaneously, her mother had not been able to value her daughter, as she had not been able to value herself.

After this recognition, Ms. D. was able to alter some of her resentment toward her mother, although acknowledging the ways that her mother had failed her. Later, too, she came to see her father as someone who had never been prepared or able to hear her concerns or to be responsive to her. She was able to perceive this only after she had finally become able even to *think* of seeking this kind of interaction with him. When she tried to bring her own needs into discussions with him, she perceived his inability to relate to her in this way. It was not like football.

Ms. D. had to confront her anger. She had a large amount of anger at both her father and her mother, for different reasons. It took a long time, but she became more able to allow herself her anger, as she also became able to see how much she had really contributed to others' development. That is, she had first to feel some sense of value before she could tolerate a view of herself as a person with anger (see Miller, Chapter 10, this volume). Then, the understanding and redirection of her anger further relieved her sense of worthlessness. Very importantly, she came to see that she would not have had a large amount of anger if she had not had her own set of perceptions, expectations, wishes, desires, and judgments, that is, the sense of self that she had thought she never had. She was angry because of the violation of the self she really had. She, like many people, particularly women, had said originally that she had no sense of self at all; she was able to discover one and then to go on to build on it.

Her biggest problem in a way remains: how to be the kind of self she wants to be, a being-in-relationship, now able to value the very valuable parts of herself, along with her own perceptions and desires—and to find others who will be with her in that way. She still encounters situations, particularly but not only with men, in which she feels annihilated as a person. I think she is experiencing situations that are common to all of us.

RICHER MODELS

To generalize from this example, then, the model of self-development as it has been defined so far does not help us to understand or to help women well. Many women perceive the prospects held out by this model as threatening, for good reason. I think their perception reflects at bottom a fear of forfeiting relationships. By contrast, men's fears occur in different forms. Indeed, most men see the prospect of self-development not only as desirable but also as a basic definition of what they must do in life. Moreover, seeking to understand women opens paths to enlargement of a model of a "self" to one that

encompasses more fully the range of human necessities and possibilities.

For Ms. D. there had been problems in relationships, especially in
having directed a large portion of her life to relationships that
primarily benefited others. However, to have overlooked their value,
and her value in them, would have robbed Ms. D. of the major source
of her strength and her potential for greater strengths.

The features I have suggested are present even in many highly
accomplished women and women who do not care for families in the
concrete sense. There is a small group of women today who seek a
sense of self similar to that which has been advocated for men. But even
many of these women express many of the same themes. They are often
the relatively advantaged women who feel very pressured to advance
in careers. They often find that their desire to live and work in a context
of mutually enhancing relationships conflicts with male norms. There
is pressure to believe that the latter are better and to devalue the
relational desires in themselves.

Important evidence is emerging from other parts of the psychological field. Notably, Gilligan's (1982) work in developmental psychology
suggests that women's sense of self and of morality revolves around
issues of responsibility for, care of, and inclusion of other people. It is
embedded in a compelling appreciation of context and an insistent
unwillingness to construct abstractions that violate their grasp of the
complexities of the connections between people. Women were
previously seen as deficient or at a low level of development as a
consequence of their encompassing these realms of context and of
psychological connection. These features are found even in as
accomplished a group as current women Harvard students. In other
studies, McClelland (1979) finds that women tend to define power as
having the strength to care for and give to others, which is very
different from the way men have defined power.

As always, the artists have said it long ago. It is interesting to note
that in much of literature the man has been in search of his self, as in
David Copperfield, Portrait of the Artist as a Young Man, and many other
novels. Women express desires, but they have tended to cast them in
the overarching terms of wanting to make deep connection with
another (others) and usually to enhance another, as in George Eliot's
Middlemarch or Charlotte Brontë's *Villette.*

Overall, then, the concept of a "self" as it has come down to us has
encouraged a complex series of processes leading to a sense of
psychological separation from others. From this there would follow a
quest for power over others and power over natural forces, including
one's own body. This would seem to be inevitable if one cannot be

grounded in *faith* in the kind of interconnections I have tried to suggest. Have such definitions of a separated self become conceivable *only* because half of the species has been assigned to the realms of life that involve such necessities as attending to the complex particularities of building the day-to-day emotional connections with others? This means, in effect, giving primary attention to participating in and fostering the development of other people—and even direct concentration on sustaining of the sheer physical life of others. Simultaneously, these realms delegated to women have been granted inferior value. They have not been incorporated into our perceptions as sources of growth, satisfaction, and empowerment. It then becomes difficult to conceive of them as the wellsprings of true inner motivation and development. But they are.

Another way to put this is to say that women's actual practice in the real world and the complex processes that those practices entail have not been drawn upon, nor elaborated on, as a basis of culture, knowledge, theory, or public policy. They then come to sound almost unreal or idealistic, but they are real; they are going on every day. If they were not, none of us would have lived and developed at all. But they have been split off from official definitions of reality.

An underlying question may be: Has our tradition made it difficult to conceive of the possibility that freedom and maximum use of our resources—our initiative, our intellect, our powers—can occur within a context that requires simultaneous responsibility for the care and growth of others and of the natural world? We cannot hope that such a sense of responsibility will develop *after* the person develops first as a separated "self," as currently defined. I believe that the search for the more appropriate study of women in women's own terms can not only lead to understanding women, certainly a valid goal in itself, but can also provide clues to a deeper grasp of the *necessities* for all human development and, simultaneously, to a greater realization of the realities of the vast, untapped human capacities. This is not an easy thing to do, because our whole system of thought, our categories, the eyes with which we see and the ears with which we hear have been trained in a system removed from this activity.

We have all been laboring under only one implicit model of the nature of human nature and of human development. Much richer models are possible. Glimpses of them have always been struggling to emerge, through the artists and the poets, and in some of the hopes and dreams of all of us. Now, perhaps, we can work at learning about them in this field.

An earlier version of this paper was presented at The Stone Center Dedication Conference in October 1981.

2

Women and Empathy: Implications for Psychological Development and Psychotherapy

JUDITH V. JORDAN
JANET L. SURREY
ALEXANDRA G. KAPLAN

As described by object relation theorists and self psychologists, empathy is an affective intuitive process involving a temporary breach of ego boundaries and regressive, symbiotic merger. The quality of this empathic bond is likened to the quality of the empathic connection between infant and mother. In both contexts, empathy appears to have mysterious, hidden qualities and to be associated with a temporary loss of a more mature functioning.

The purpose of these papers is to begin an alternative description of the experience of empathy based on new theoretical understandings of women's development. Our concept challenges the assumed link between affective processes and loss of identity. Instead, we propose that empathy involves both affective *and* cognitive functioning and is a far more complex, developmentally advanced and interactive process than is implied by those theories which associate empathy with regression, symbiosis, and merger of ego boundaries.

In the spirit of this working paper series, we would like to share these ideas while they are evolving. Judith Jordan began a reexamination of the concept of empathy. Her work stimulated the other authors to expand topics on which they had been working—Janet Surrey's examination of the mother–daughter relationship as the primary model of psychological development and Alexandra Kaplan's examination of the therapeutic process. Thus the papers offer formulations on these major topics in addition to empathy itself.

We do not all agree on certain points, even on some fundamental assumptions. These differences extend to our use of terminology. We are struggling to find words which will more adequately describe the phenomena we are studying.

Our differences are part of an ongoing interchange. We hope that they capture some of the quality of our continuing dialogue, and, in doing so, carry forward the intent of these working papers.

Empathy and the Mother–Daughter Relationship

JUDITH V. JORDAN

Most clinical and developmental theory reflects concepts of ego strength that emphasize capacity for delay, objectivity, and firm ego boundaries. Individuation, separation, and objectivity generally are considered indicators of increasing maturity and development (Gilligan, 1977). In fact, these may be potentially adaptive qualities for a typical male milieu, but not necessarily for a typical female milieu. The "average expectable environment" seems to differ for males and females, presenting different interpersonal demands and leading to different adaptive capacities (Carson, 1971). In David Bakan's (1966) terms, our society tends to overemphasize the *agentic* ethic (self-protective, assertive, individualistic, pushing toward achievement) at the expense of the *communal* ethic (being at one with other organisms, characterized by contact or union). The study of empathy may provide one means for examining the relative development of agentic and communal qualities in an individual such that any action for the self would contain a consideration of the effect of this action on others.

DESCRIBING EMPATHY

Schafer (1959) defines empathy as "the inner experience of sharing in and comprehending the momentary psychological state of another person." Empathy often has been construed as a mysterious, contagion-like, and primitive phenomenon or has been dismissed as a vague and unknowable subjective state. Empathy, however, is a complex process, relying on a high level of psychological development and ego strength. (Indeed, it may provide a good index of both, and a developmental study using empathy as an indicator of ego strength would be most interesting.) In order to empathize, one must have a well-differentiated sense of self in addition to an appreciation of and sensitivity to the differentness as well as the sameness of another person.

Empathy always involves affective surrender and cognitive structuring, and, in order for empathy to occur, ego boundaries must be flexible. Experientially, empathy begins with the basic capacity and motivation for human relatedness that allows perception of the other's affective cues, verbal and nonverbal. This is followed by a surrender to affective arousal in oneself—as if the perceived affective cues were one's own—thus producing a temporary identification with the other's emotional state. Finally, there occurs a resolution period in which one regains a sense of separate self that understands what has just happened. For empathy to be effective, there must be a balance of the affective and cognitive, the subjective and objective. Ego boundary flexibility is important, since there is an "as if," trying-out quality to the experience in which one places oneself in the other's shoes or looks through the other's eyes. There is a momentary overlap of self and other representations as distinctions blur experientially. If either relaxation or restructuring of ego boundaries is impaired, empathy will suffer.

Given the balance between affect and cognition that must exist for accurate empathy to develop, one might expect differential patterns of strengths and weaknesses in empathic ability for males and females. On the one hand, if self boundaries are too rigid, the other's affective state will have little impact on one's own self. In that case any attempt at understanding the other will be a distanced, intellectual effort to reconstruct what is going on, or a projection of one's own state onto the other. On the other hand, if self boundaries are excessively diffuse, the self–other differentiation may be lost, opening the way for uncontained merging or use of the other as a narcissistic extension of self. In both cases the opportunity for a genuine sense of understanding and being understood—that is, of essential human connectedness—is sacrificed.

MALE–FEMALE DIFFERENCES

In general, it has been found that females are more empathic than males (Hoffman, 1977). Males tend to have more difficulty with the essential and necessary surrender to affect and momentary joining with the other, since it implies for them passivity, loss of objectivity, and loss of control. This may lead to widespread constriction of empathic responsiveness in men. Problems with empathy for females, however, typically involve difficulty reinstating a sense of self and cognitively structuring the experience. Women also have trouble bringing an empathic attitude to bear on themselves (something I call self-empathy, which Schafer has referred to as "intrapsychic empathy"). Many women do not develop dependable self-empathy because the pull of empathy for the other is so strong, because females are conditioned to attend to the needs of others first, and because women often experience so much guilt about claiming attention *for* the self, even *from* the self.

A clinical example may shed some light on this difficulty: A bright and creative artist whom I see in treatment reports that when her husband returns home from work—no matter what her own struggles or accomplishments of the day—she finds herself feeling for him in his fatigue, not wanting to bother him with her concerns. Knowing he likes to talk with her about his day, she encourages him to share with her. She later feels angry, however, that he does not do the same for her; she also fears it is because he does not value her work or her feelings. This woman's empathic response to her husband is caring and important, but as an unvarying pattern, she begins to feel her internal state is not valued as much as her husband's. Because she is so tuned in to her husband's affective state, she sometimes does not feel she has a choice *not* to respond. His pain is her pain. Empathy, then, can lead to the other always coming first at the expense of valuing one's own experience. Therapists can play an important role in helping these people (usually women) bring an empathic attitude to bear on themselves as well as on others.

SOCIALIZATION

The different roles toward which the members of each sex are socialized obviously play a part in the quality of empathy that evolves in each. Looking at conscious and unconscious standards for sex role socialization, we see that characteristics which are most adaptive for the mothering/nurturing role are encouraged in females, while in males there may be selective and active discouragement of those very same traits. As Winnicott (1971) notes, the "good enough mother," "the mother who mirrors the infant," "starts off with an almost complete adaptation to her infant's needs." Motherhood relies on a careful tuning to the other, a sensitive empathy to the subtle or unarticulated internal states of the infant, and any traits that would enhance these abilities are likely to be developed in females. Young girls, therefore, are encouraged to attend to others' affective states and to maintain proximity to others; they also are allowed significant affective expression, particularly when the expression is nonaggressive and prosocial. Girls are urged to develop perceptual acuity in reading others' reactions to themselves.

For boys, on the other hand, socialized to be good soldiers or effective competitors in a largely alienated work world, highly developed empathy might be seen as most unadaptive. Young boys, then, are encouraged to pursue individual "mastery" of tasks and to contain affect, particularly if it suggests to them need of another, fear, or inability to act on one's own. Traits such as autonomy and self-reliance are encouraged and valued for males.

Early Childhood Identification

One important factor in the development of empathy in females is the nature of the early mother–daughter relationship. Chodorow (1978) speculates, drawing on object relations theory, that societal values which encourage and support the early attachment of mother and daughter, as well as the nature of the identification with the maternal figure, allow for self–other boundary flexibility in girls. Boys, in contrast, are socially supported to curtail the primary identification with the mother, forcing them to create less flexible self–other differentiation.

If we look at the model of mother as mirror of the infant around which self feelings develop, we will immediately notice some differences in mother–daughter versus mother–son relationships. I will speculate a bit about some of these differences. The mother, identifying more with the daughter (an identification based in part on body sameness and supported by cultural norms), may experience affectively tuned empathy more directly and readily with a daughter than with a son. Further, the mother may feel more comfortable about encouraging a daughter to feel more connected with her at an affective level. It is likely that this difference is more striking with a clearly sex-typed 3- or 4-year-old than with an infant, but it may be there to some extent from the beginning. One study which supports the notion that mirroring may evolve differently between mother–son and mother–daughter pairs was done by Moss (1967). He reported in observations of early mother–infant interaction that already at 3 weeks, and again at 3 months, mothers imitate female babies more than male babies and that there is greater responsiveness on the part of the female infant to the mother's ministrations. While the acknowledged greater neurological maturity of the female infant may contribute to this difference in responsiveness, it is not within the scope of this presentation to fully review the relevant infant research. Also, studies of early sex differences often yield conflicting results about mother–infant interactions. With boys, the process of understanding on the mother's part may be more "intellectual" and less immediate. Further, the experience of looking to the mother for mirroring and confirming becomes questionable at some point for the boy, as he recognizes and often ultimately devalues her differentness. It is likely that these differences in the experience of being mirrored may give the boy a diminished sense of being in contact with and understanding another person in a directly affective way.

The factors shaping sex-role differences in childhood are extremely complex. The assumption of broad similarity between mother and daughter based first on the mother's perception of body sameness and gender assignment profoundly shapes the way the mother interacts with the girl. However, society also exerts a powerful influence on the mother, and there are pressures against viewing boys as "like her." There are clear expectations that boys be raised to be like their fathers, like men, in very important ways, particularly in the expression and management of affect. Fathers are even more concerned and typically more assiduous in encouraging a "masculine" pattern of affective expression in their sons. Further, it is clear that the sex differences in empathy which have their roots in the early mother–infant relationship undergo major changes in the course of development. Boys are encouraged to model themselves after fathers, are actively encouraged to suppress certain relational sensitivities (e.g., feeling pain or crying when saddened or hurt by another or when seeing someone else in pain), and are taught to accept peer standards of "toughness" and invulnerability. All of this amplifies disconnection and lessens empathic responsiveness.

It is striking that in the sex differences found in empathy, the major difference is the lower amount of vicarious affective arousal in males when responding to another's affective state (Hoffman, 1977). In other words, males and females are equally good at labeling and noticing different affective states in others when they are motivated to attend to them. The motivational difference, generally overlooked in research, may in fact be crucial—that is, females typically are more motivated to attend to affect in others. This difference disappears in research settings that direct participants to attend to affective signals. In these studies, nevertheless, females demonstrate more emotional attunement and responsiveness to the other's feelings—more feeling *with* the other. In interplay between infant/child and mother, it is likely that the child also mirrors the mother. Again, the daughter may be experienced by the mother as providing a closer reflection of the mother than does the son, who represents masculine differentness. Chodorow (1978) suggests the girl may at times be experienced by the mother as an extension of herself, while the boy may become an object for her. She notes the possible pathological ramifications for children of each sex—for example, narcissistic projection of the mother onto the daughter, more frequent "false empathy" with the daughter (which really amounts to projection), and seductive behavior with the son. It is also possible that this early interplay can lead to a girl's sense of being understood and connected at a more direct emotional level and to a boy's more distance-mediated sense of relatedness.

SEX-ROLE IDENTIFICATION

Sex-role identification differs for boys and girls. Based on an early, dimly experienced sense of the other, both boys and girls form a primary identification with the major caretaking person, usually the mother. With cognitive development, however, boys experience a growing awareness of the differentness of the mother from them. Along with the cognitive label "I am a boy" and recognition that the father is a man, it becomes necessary for a boy to switch his primary identification to the father (Chodorow, 1978). Due to greater father absence—both physical and psychological—the child's identification with the father is apt to be mediated by abstract or role-defined factors. Taking the role of the other for the boy, then, may be less particular, less affectively specific, and more generalized. Such a development would lessen empathic presence and capacity for immediate, affective interpersonal involvement. But the girl's relationship with the mother Is allowed to be immediate and particular, with identification arising in the context of intense affect. Consequently, boys and girls develop quite different modes of personal interaction. For example, it is interesting to note sex differences in a study of play behavior of 10-year-olds cited by Gilligan (1977): Boys tended to form larger groups, had more formal rules, got involved in more adjudication of disputes, and related as if to a "generalized other." Girls' play was more dyadic, private, and cooperative. If disputes arose between girls, the game ended, as preservation of the relationship was far more valuable than the game itself.

SUMMARY

Having a same-gender nurturing figure has a great impact on the quality of empathy that develops. In our culture the special quality of the early attachment and identification between mother and daughter profoundly affects the way the self is defined in women as well as the nature of their interpersonal relatedness. The more frequent mirroring, mutual identification, and more accurate empathy may all strengthen the girl's sense of relatedness, connection, and a feeling of being directly, emotionally understood. Further, such an interactional pattern would enhance the development of empathic skills. Research data have indicated this is the case—females do tend to be more empathic than males, with the important exception of self-empathy. Because accurate empathy rests upon a foundation of affective sensitivity and responsiveness, flexible ego boundaries, and cognitive capacity to understand clearly, it may be an important (although overlooked) indicator of ego strength and development. The centrality of this process cannot be overstated, yet it has received relatively little attention until recently. Unfortunately, traditional notions of ego strength have overemphasized separateness, objectivity, and autonomy. The careful study of the psychological development of girls and women, then, promises a better understanding of the important process of empathy and ultimately offers an opportunity to expand our appreciation of the crucial and necessary interplay of affective and cognitive, self and other, "agentic" and "communal."

I shall close with several quotes from Kohut (1978) that capture the experience and importance of empathy: He writes, "Empathy is a fundamental mode of human relatedness," "the recognition of the self in the other," "it is the accepting, confirming and understanding human echo," "the resonance of essential human alikeness," "a psychological nutriment without which human life as we know and cherish it could not be sustained."

The Relational Self in Women:
Clinical Implications

JANET L. SURREY

Dr. Jordan has given us a powerful statement illuminating the central importance of empathy in human development. She challenges us to describe the complex developmental processes that underlie its emergence and that may hamper or inhibit its development. I shall continue her discussion of the significance of the mother–daughter relationship in establishing the early precursors of adult women's greater capacity for relatedness, emotional closeness, and boundary flexibility—all of which are crucial to the development of empathy. Further, I will propose some aspects of a new model of self-development based on this capacity for relationship—defining the basic core self structure in women as "self-in-relation" and describing its origin within the mother–daughter relationship. I believe that describing women's development in this way will contribute to a more realistic theory of the psychology of women. Such a theory should be genuinely relevant to understanding and describing our own lives, it should offer practical help to us as teachers and clinicians in our work with women, and, perhaps most importantly, it should be a significant step toward a more comprehensive understanding of human development for both men and women.

Indeed, it is critically important for us to work on describing women's development, not just to understand women, but to add new dimensions to our total understanding of both male and female psychology. As Jean Baker Miller (1976) has pointed out, women in our culture are the "carriers" of certain aspects of the human experience—for example, emotionality, vulnerability, and, most of all, the fostering of growth and development of others. Only through describing women's experience can we begin to map out a theory of full human development. Further, women need to find what Carol Gilligan (1982) has called their own "voice," not only as individuals, but to contribute to the expansion of our current developmental theory, a theory that has clearly been written of the men, by the men, and for the men (the "phallocentric model," if you will). Where women's development has been seen as parallel or mirroring men's development—for example, in the work of Freud, Erikson, Sullivan, Kohlberg, and Piaget—it has led

So de constructing
re constructing

to what Jean Baker Miller describes as the "deficiency" model of female psychology. That is, women, using male models, begin to define themselves as *lacking* something critical—whether it be a penis or a firm, "separate" sense of self. Our theoretical work, therefore, is based on reexamining this negative identification and illuminating the more unique or central aspects of women's development.

A NEW VIEW OF HUMAN DEVELOPMENT

Let us examine the way self-development has been defined in our current theory. The whole notion of "separation-individuation" as the basis of human development implies that the person must first disconnect from relationship in order to form a separate, articulated, firm sense of self or personhood. The process of male development is clearly defined as the disconnection and differentiation from the mother early in childhood. Only much later in the life cycle, according to Erikson, do intimacy and generativity become "tasks" to be "mastered competently." Thus intimacy, empathy, and relatedness can be experienced as threats to autonomy, agency, and self-determination. New interest in the importance of "object" relationships and empathy is appearing in the current psychoanalytic and developmental literature. Even in using these newer theories, however, it is critically important for women to think through the centrality of relationships in organizing and fostering self-development.

To see beyond the limits of the model of *separation-individuation*, I would like to propose a new construction: *relationship-differentiation*. it is difficult to find the right language to describe such a developmental growth process, and we have debated about the right word. By differentiation, I do not mean to suggest as a developmental goal the assertion of difference and separateness; rather I mean a dynamic process that encompasses increasing levels of complexity, structure, and articulation within the context of human bonds and attachments. Such a process needs to be traced from the origins in early childhood relationships through its extensions into all later growth and development.

THE MOTHER–DAUGHTER EXPERIENCE

To begin a discussion of the "self-in-relation" model, consider again Dr. Jordan's description of the mother–daughter relationship. The *identification* process between mothers and daughters is crucially important. The ease and fluidity of *mutual* identification appears to be significantly different from what is acceptable between mothers and sons. (It is important to note that what is acceptable can also change with changing cultural beliefs.) The connections based on feeling states and identification develop over time into a *mutual reciprocal* process in which mother and daughter become highly responsive to the feelings of each other. Both are energized to "care for," "respond to," or "attend to" the well-being of the other. Through this mutual sensitivity and mutual caretaking, mothers already are teaching "mothering" or "caring" practices to girl children. By "mothering" I do not necessarily mean what has been traditionally labeled as "one-directional" mothering, but attentiveness and emotional responsivity to the other as an intrinsic, ongoing aspect of one's own experience. Incidentally, another critical area for further study is the whole notion of what constitutes "mothering." Winnicott's (1965) idea of the "good-enough mother" who is capable of "fusing" in such a way as to be responsive to the feeling states and needs of the infant, needs to be carefully critiqued and explored, and further attention needs to be paid to the awesome complexity and skill involved in "mothering behaviors" (Ruddick, 1980). We can at least say that within this early mother–daughter relationship—certainly as it grows over the life cycle—we can begin to see the precursors of women's capacity and pleasure in relatedness, that is, the ability to identify with the other, the sense of connectedness through feeling states, and the *activation* and *energizing* based on complex cognitive operations involving the awareness of the needs and/or "reality" of another person as well as one's own.

I am not diminishing the significance of other lines of self-development (e.g., competence, agency, or initiative). I am implying that these other capacities are developed for women in the *context* of important relationships. It is probable that, for women at all life stages, relational needs are primary and that healthy, dynamic relationships are the motivating force that propels psychological growth.

We have suggested some of the early developmental precursors of women's relational self structure and have sketched a preliminary model for tracing development of the capacity for empathy over the life cycle. In adult women, we see the same factors developed with further elaboration: First, we see that women experience a heightened, enhanced sense of their personal identity and personal powers in the context of relationships. Second, we see this early emotional sensitivity develop into complex cognitive and affective interactions that we later identify as empathy. Third, we see this connectedness and the capacity for identification as the basis for the later feeling that to "understand" and to "be understood" are crucial for self-acceptance and are fundamental to the feeling of existing as part of a unit or network larger than the individual.

Kohut (1971) emphasizes the importance of empathy in a more one-directional parent-to-child phenomenon. I am broadening this to a more two-way *interactional* model, where it becomes as important to understand as to be understood. All of us probably feel the need to feel understood or "recognized" by others. It is equally paramount, but not yet emphasized, that women all through their lives feel the need to "understand" the other—indeed, desire this as an essential part of their own motivating force. I am speaking here about the more usual and typical form of self-development; I will later discuss some problems that can follow in development based on such a model—at least in our own cultural context.

but must be age - app ?!!

plus need to consider intersectionality.

ELEMENTS OF A NEW THEORY

Now take a moment to develop the image of what a *relationship-differentiation* theory of self-development would be like: (1) Critical relationships would be seen as evolving throughout the life cycle in a real, rather than intrapsychic, form. As we know, one of the hardest developmental tasks is the challenge to grow into psychological adulthood in relationship with one's own parents, especially one's mother. (2) We would have to account for the capacity to maintain relationships with tolerance, consideration, and mutual adaptation to the growth and development of each person. Such a system would validate developmental movement in many directions, recognizing the reality of the "child" and the "adult" in each human being, or perhaps recognizing periods of greater and lesser need and varying forms of need. All fruitful relationships need to accommodate to this cyclical and multifaceted movement, and this is a critical foundation for acceptance of such movement within ourselves. (3) We would account for the ability to move closer to and further away from other people at different moments, depending on the needs of the particular individuals and the situational context. (4) We would explore the capacity for developing additional relationships based on broader, more diversified new identifications and corresponding patterns of expanding relational networks—including relationships with father, triangular relationships, preadolescent and adolescent friendship patterns, sexual relationships, marriage, mothering and family networks, teaching relationships, role modeling, women in work groups, and still broader reference groups. Such a female-centered theory would, therefore, trace the development of identity through specific relationships and relational networks. Such a theory would need to examine the nature of the cognitive and emotional internal capacities necessary for such growth as well as the availability of appropriate relational networks to foster the development of such capacities, especially at critical developmental milestones. Here I think of how important was the emergence of consciousness-raising groups in facilitating the women's movement of the 1960s and 1970s. (5) We would examine the potential problems and vicissitudes inherent in the development of these relational capacities. Our new theory would probably *not* talk about "fixed" states, developmental "crises," or one-dimensional, undirectional goals of development.

In her well-known book *The Reproduction of Mothering*, Nancy Chodorow (1978) has discussed the development of the capacity for mothering. She has highlighted some of these aspects of female development. Yet she still talks about "preoedipal development" in women persisting longer into adult life and leaving women with more permeable, less definitive ego boundaries. I genuinely believe we need new models, new language, and new visions—visions which include a broader view of both the gains and losses for women of more flexible and inclusive ego boundaries.

Maybe there is no such thing as "oedipal resolution" for women. Maybe the real question with which we need to begin is this: What are the implications of a theory of healthy male development that posits disconnection from the mother and affirmation of difference between men and women (symbolized by "resolving the oedipal situation") as the foundation of healthy development?

LEARNING FROM CLINICAL EXPERIENCE

Much of the model just outlined has been developed in the context of our work as therapists. Clinical material allows us access to some of the vicissitudes and obstacles to development that may shed light on "normal development." Now, I do not know what "normal development" means for women, or for any human being. Clearly, there are external circumstances that may hamper the healthy unfolding of all human beings; for women, I have some sense of what profound obstacles are inherent in the power relations within our culture. With this in mind, I will use some clinical material to illustrate how the "self-in-relation" model may be useful in illuminating some common problems in women's development.

In clinical practice we see many adult women who experience difficulty in delineating, articulating, and acting directly on their own needs and perceptions. We see women who are unable to experience the sense of self necessary for self-determined motivation outside the context of a primary dyadic relationship and who become anxious and severely depressed at the real or perceived loss of an important relationship. Such a model helps us to understand the experience of existential anxiety, confusion, and depression in the face of loss, separation, or isolation. I will cite a clinical example:

Difficulty Attending to Oneself

Penny is a 32-year-old, single social worker; she is bright, an ardent feminist, and competent in her work with disturbed children. She is seen as powerful and assertive and can be quite aggressive in fighting for the needs of her clients. She is strongly identified with her own agency and is vocal and active in organizing her colleagues to press for professional status, better working conditions, and salary increases. In her private life, however, she has extreme difficulty mobilizing herself for her own interests. She constantly overdraws her bank account, has her phone turned off for nonpayment of bills, and cannot do her professional writing. Sitting at home at night, she felt so anxious about not being able to do her own work that she had started smoking marijuana regularly to treat her increasing depression and feelings of low self-esteem. Therapy has helped her to see that she can be mobilized by the needs of others or when she is part of a collective unit, but that it is painfully difficult for her to act for herself. She is more functional when her boundaries are extended, but has difficulty drawing them closer, placing her own needs in a more primary focus. Understanding this has at least alleviated some of the anxiety, shame, and confusion associated with her paralysis and has allowed her to take somewhat greater control in her own personal life. Also, sustained validation of Penny's positive capacities in her therapy has helped her to recognize and use her own strengths for herself. Penny often tended to present herself in therapy as an empty, depressed person and needed help acknowledging and valuing the "hidden" parts of her life where she was functioning extremely well.

The Problem of Separating

A second common theme that emerges in clinical practice has to do with the difficulties some women may experience in separating or distancing from ungratifying or destructive relationships with either men or women. Often this problem can best be understood not as a problem of masochism or low self-esteem, but as a problem related to early self-definition as a "mothering" person. As we have said, it is probably true that even in the early relationship between mothers and daughters, mothers teach "mothering" behavior by allowing or at times expecting empathy and caretaking from their daughters. Thus it is the girl's mothering relationship *with her mother*, then, that forms her most basic primary self-definition. Each mother identifies with and reinforces those qualities in her little girl that reflect back her own personal definition of qualities that represent "good" mothering. The mother may subtly reinforce gentleness, concern for others, and nonaggressiveness—those qualities in herself that she positively values; at the same time, she may be disturbed by qualities she sees in her daughter that she devalues in herself. Thus the little girl is deeply affected by her mother's unconscious identification with her as a "good" or "bad" mother and takes on the characteristics of her own mother in an unconscious process of identification.

A patient of mine told me how she watched her young daughter playing with dolls, and in spite of the fact that the mother, who saw herself as "liberated," preferred that her daughter play "Doctor," she felt enormously pleased when the daughter played "good" mother to her dolls and horribly threatened when she played "bad" mother— that is, unloving, inattentive, or punitive. This is a powerful message when the mother consciously may be hoping that the little girl will be different than she, or grow up to be more assertive and self-determining. The mother herself may even be that way in her professional life, but, in relation to her daughter, she is primarily mother. The girl's most basic sense of self, therefore, is formed in identification with the primary caretaker of the preadolescent period, and those qualities that the mother values and devalues in herself as a "mother" are transmitted in a powerful, unconscious manner. Through the process of mutual identification the daughter learns to be "the mother," that is, a caretaker and nurturer of others. This probably accounts for the persistence of this primary sense of identity as the "caretaker of others" and a profound sense of "badness" associated with acting as the "bad" mother. Thus self-enhancing, self-determining behavior may elicit this negative "bad mother" introject for the woman, causing her, even in adulthood, to feel "selfish" when she acts on her own needs.

A common problem for women can be seen in the context of what I call "stepping out of the mother–daughter relationship." A girl's primary relationship with her mother may not move on sufficiently from the early form of the mother–child relationship to a more complex, articulated pattern of relationship. The mutual caretaking and identification, often largely unconscious, remain as the core structure a woman feels, making it extremely problematic for her to act in ways that deviate from this form of intense interpersonal connectedness. In such cases, whatever the expense to herself, it becomes intensely difficult for the woman to act in a way that might hurt another person. This often explains the difficulty some women have in separating from self-destructive or ungratifying relationships with men or women—they cannot tolerate being an "agent of abandonment" and continue to feel totally responsible for the other person's feelings.

Maryanne, another patient, is a 38-year-old single woman who has been unable to separate from a 10-year relationship with a married man who had been her boss. The relationship was harmful and painful, but every time Maryanne tried to separate she not only felt terrified of aloneness but also felt a terrible sense of guilt and self-disapproval for hurting and abandoning this man. Her mother had been in an unhappy marriage with an abusive alcoholic, and Maryanne could not understand how she could be so aware of the disaster of her mother's martyrdom and still be repeating it in her own life. This left her feeling crazy and confused about her own behavior. As we looked closely at the situation, she began to see how much she had identified with the qualities of her mother that she consciously despised; consequently, whatever the personal expense, she could not tolerate behavior in herself that might conceivably hurt another person. Interestingly, her mother would reinforce this by continuing to sympathize and identify with her daughter's victimization but never speak to the daughter's complicity in this destructive relationship.

The Price of Change

Another issue involved in "stepping out of the mother–daughter relationship" involves the complex process of differentiation. The girl may unconsciously experience the process of differentiation—otherwise known as creating newly defined self-images—as an aggressive, destructive act toward her mother. Such differentiation from the mother may also leave the girl feeling totally alone, unsupported, and abandoned. Because of the nature of the mother–daughter relationship, the whole process of differentiation may become problematic. Often women present in therapy with a powerful, conscious disidentification with their mothers that covers a very profound and deep unconscious identification. Again, I will give a clinical example:

Karen is a 30-year-old, single woman with whom I have worked in therapy for 3 years. She is the second child and the only daughter in a family with four sons. Her father and brothers are all high achievers. As a child she was seen as nearly retarded and was thought to have a learning disability. Her mother was not well educated but valued education highly in her sons. Karen barely got through high school and achieved an associate degree from a community college. She then began working on her own and built up a small business that began to be quite successful. When I first saw her, she wanted to go to graduate school for an MBA. Psychological testing revealed an IQ of 138—a dramatic contrast to her family's label as dumb.

Karen also had been labeled as helpless. Her mother had treated Karen as through she was incapable of thinking for herself and had infantilized the daughter in order to maintain her own sense of herself as a needed mother.

During the course of treatment, Karen has been able to return to school and is currently in a prestigious MBA program. Nonetheless, she experiences tremendous anxiety accompanying exhilaration with her own success. Recently she has begun to have recurrent dreams of being at her mother's deathbed, of her mother having a terminal illness. Partially these dreams reflect her rage and concomitant guilt at feeling mislabeled and narcissistically used by the mother. I think another aspect of this anxiety is her own sense of being different from mother—not to mention different from the person she had been "seen" to be through her mother's eyes.

Karen's growing up and being self-sufficient and self-determining took away the essential part of her mother's primary self-identification. Her mother's primary sense of self-worth rested in caring for the dependent daughter, so Karen, by establishing a new identity, felt she was destroying her mother, or, in more theoretical language, disturbing the internalized preadolescent mother–daughter relationship.

I think this is a common problem for women, especially at this time in history when there is so much talk about opportunity for self-development and change in the lives of women. The dynamics of the process are often powerful and disturbing to women experiencing life changes, and they engender guilt, anxiety, and depression that must be explored and acknowledged, recognizing the strong, powerful bonds of the early mother–daughter relationship.

NEED FOR A NEW MODEL

A new developmental model such as the one I have suggested will help us in understanding some common psychological problems and in working with and developing ideas for facilitating and creating new growth-enhancing structures for women. It can also help us to explore ourselves and our work as female therapists and shed new light on the structure of the therapeutic relationship.

Empathic Communication in the Psychotherapy Relationship

ALEXANDRA G. KAPLAN

In speaking to the question of what makes for successful outcomes in psychotherapy, it must be remembered that not so long ago there was serious debate as to whether psychotherapy of any sort was more beneficial than no treatment at all. More recently, there has been an acceptance of the findings indicating that psychotherapy is of value, and the question has switched to *why* therapy works. Here there is great divergence in the results of studies of therapy outcome, depending on the theoretical orientations of the researchers, the source of their data (patient, therapist, outside observer, etc.), their definition of "success," and so on. However, within this divergence, a consensus is beginning to emerge—a consensus that seems to hold up whether one looks at theoretically based clinical writings or at findings from outcome studies. This consensus, simply put, is that to the extent that gains from therapy can be documented, the gains are most directly an outgrowth of the patient–therapist *relationship*. Guntrip (1973), for example, states that "the only true therapeutic factor is that of good personal relationships that combine caring with accurate understanding." Similarly, major reviews of psychotherapy research by Bergin and Lambert (1978), Dent (1978), Gurman (1977), and Orlinsky and Howard (1978) all conclude that the relational qualities between client and therapist are more closely related to outcome than are any particular clinical skills or specific techniques.

This is an extremely important recognition, although its implications have barely been explored. What it suggests is that, in any consideration of therapy training, clinical technique, or modalities of therapy, it may be necessary to ask: In what ways, and with whom, will the relational component of therapy be enhanced?

WOMEN AND MEN AS THERAPISTS

There are many implications in this question, only one of which will be dealt with here: Specifically, when relational concerns are at issue, in our culture women and men are differentially reared for those relational qualities that facilitate therapy. As Judith Jordan and Janet Surrey have made clear, over the years women live out their lives attuned to relationships, thereby gaining daily experience with the nuances of interpersonal space and empathic understanding; men, by contrast, do not give nearly this much attention to relationships. This does not mean, in itself, that women by definition have the "edge" over men as therapists. Men bring to therapy experience and training in the authority component of their role; they typically have a sense of competence and confidence that, when used well and not abused, can facilitate management of the therapy hour. This is one reflection of men's greater comfort with the direct use of their own resources and abilities (as discussed by Miller, 1976).

It does seem a logical assumption, however, that to the extent that women are more at home with and adept at the relational component of the therapy role, they will function more successfully as therapists than will men. In fact, this has been borne out by at least some research. Orlinsky and Howard (1980), for example, in a study of therapy outcome with female patients and female and male therapists, found that in general the patients did better with female than with male therapists, but not strikingly so. However, when they looked at experience level of therapists, they found that experience was unrelated to outcome for female therapists, but highly related to outcome for male therapists. That is, the highly experienced male therapists were as good as any female therapist, but the less experienced male therapists had at least twice the others' rate of worse and unimproved patients. Orlinsky and Howard consider the distinct possibility that experience functions to increase male competence in precisely those relational skills with which women are embued throughout their lives.

What, then, is the nature of the empathic mode that is more highly developed in women and that seems to facilitate therapeutic work? In the current literature there are differences of opinion as to the nature of empathy in therapy. The differences center on one basic question: How connected must therapist and patient be for the relationship to be considered empathic? Ehrenberg (1974) discusses the therapeutic benefits that accrue from working on the "intimate edge," defined as the "maximum contact possible without fusion or violation of the separateness and integrity of each participant." However, writers such as Searles (1975) and Giovacchini (1976) argue that for true empathic interaction in therapy, there must be a temporary breaching of ego boundaries—a symbiotic fusion between patient and therapist.

THE SELF AND EMPATHY

The controversy over the ideal degree of connectedness for an empathic relationship derives from traditional developmental theories that Surrey just described: The self evolves and matures as it grows *away* from relationships, via self–other differentiation, increasingly firm ego boundaries, and the capacity for separation. In other words, there is one continuum, with fusion and merger at one end and differentiation and separation at the other end. (And we all know which is the good end, of course.) So when you consider therapy in that model, the closer therapist and client become, the more they move toward fusion and away from differentiation.

By contrast, I submit that such a model is *not* appropriate for understanding empathy within the therapeutic process—or anywhere.

THE DUAL NATURE OF EMPATHY

Let me begin by returning to the crucial point raised by Jordan that empathy has two components, the affective and the cognitive. The affective component comprises feelings of emotional connectedness, a capacity to fully take in and contain the feelings of the other person. The cognitive component rests essentially on one's integral sense of self and the capacity to act on the basis of that sense of self. The "old model" that I just mentioned says that they vary together, that both are either fused or separate.

I suggest that not only do the affective and cognitive components of empathy *not* vary together but for effective empathy they *cannot*—that this is an impossible condition for effective empathy. They are separate, but coexisting.

The Affective Part

Consider the affective component: It is on this dimension that the intense contact is made, and there is a deep connectedness, an interpenetration, of *feelings* between two people. This is difficult to put into words, so as the three of us met to plan this presentation we tried to describe the cues that we use to identify genuinely empathic moments. In part they have a physiological quality in which our posture, our teary eyes, our tense muscles unconsciously reflect the state of the patient, thereby transmitting to us a kind of visceral experience of the patient's emotional state. Another quality is a kind of associative empathy, in which the therapist takes on the client's emotional state and transfers it to something in her or his own experience. For example, as a patient described a dream, the dream image—the room in which the person in the dream was walking—temporarily became the room of the therapist's youth, the locus perhaps of feelings that were evoked by the dreamer/patient.

In terms of affect, then, we are indeed talking about qualities of intensity and interconnectedness. But you will notice that I did not use words such as *symbiotic fusion, enmeshment,* and *merger.* I think such words are inappropriate, because they imply not only an interpenetration of feeling but also a loss of identity; ego boundaries as well as affect are implicated in those terms.

The Cognitive Part

According to the position I am putting forth, the cognitive component of empathy follows a different, essentially contradictory, course from that of the affective. Specifically, while there may be an interpenetration of affect, identity remains differentiated. The therapist, throughout, never loses sight of herself as a distinct being; at the same time she is emotionally joined with another.

It is the capacity to maintain a sense of self that permits the therapist, while being deeply affectively connected, to make the complex clinical judgments that must be made. For example: What is the source of the patient's reactions? How do they fit into other dynamics of the therapy? Is this a point at which I should intervene, and, if so, how? This kind of self-integrity, then, in tandem with the affective experience, permits the therapist also to make the important assessment of whether the feelings that she seems to be sharing with the patient truly reflect an empathic response, or are a part of her own defensive or countertransferential reaction to what the patient is expressing. (Not all feelings evoked by our patients are empathic feelings!) In truly fused emotional situations, such processing of one's own reaction, distinct from that of the patient, would be impossible.

AFFECT AND COGNITION—SIMULTANEOUS BUT CONTRADICTORY?

It is legitimate to question at this point whether these seemingly contradictory experiences can truly coexist. Can one be affectively connected and cognitively differentiated at the same time? One possible model for understanding this can be found in the work of Rothenberg (1979) on the topic of creativity. Rothenberg did intensive interview studies of highly creative poets and scientists in order to discern the processes by which their creativity emerged. Creative states have been described by some as marked by regressed primary processes and looseness of association that might even be close to schizophrenia. But Rothenberg found quite the opposite. Creativity consists of complex cognitive formations, several of which he identified. The one which is of particular interest here is what he called "Janusian thinking." (This is named after the mythical figure with two heads facing in opposite directions.) Janusian thinking, in Rothenberg's description, means simultaneously using opposite or antithetical concepts that are equally operative and equally true. This idea reflects the situation that I believe to be true regarding empathy. The therapist is both intimately connected with the other person and yet, without losing that connectedness, is in touch with her own individuality.

Now I will take that one step further: If Rothenberg's model of Janusian thinking is indeed appropriately applied to empathy, can empathy then be thought of as a creative process? This notion has important implications when considered in contrast to the portrayal of empathy as fusion and merger—terms which imply a regressive and somewhat magical, mysterious process. This contrast is not just a chance phenomenon. It reflects basic differences in perception and theory. Given that women are schooled in empathy throughout their lives, including this coexistence of seemingly contradictory positions, it could be that for the less experienced men the coexistence is harder to achieve, and maybe is not achieved, in what they call empathy. While object relations theory speaks of the need for both "fusion" and "separation" in the empathic process, most writers approach it sequentially, so that they describe temporary "fusion followed by separation." However, I would argue that if a sense of differentiation does not *coincide with* affective connectedness, there is a risk that cognitive controls—informed by the affective experiences that are essential for effective therapy—will be lost. In other words, the very process of affective closeness, if one does not have sustained experience with it, can momentarily impair one's judgment and one's sense of self. I would even speculate that this might be one of the causes (certainly not the only cause) of the incidence of intercourse between some male therapists and female patients. That is, the male therapist, trying to connect emotionally to the woman, could be flooded by his affective response to her, which he then acts out rather than monitors because he is lacking enough differentiation and practice in these emotional realms to process his feelings.

EMPATHIC UNDERSTANDING AND MOTHERING

We can now turn more precisely to those aspects of experience that prepare women for the empathic relationship in therapy. As Surrey and Jordan have stressed, much of this centers on preparation of women for the caretaking role. We have heard about how that evolves between mother and daughter, but I think we can take it even further, to consider that these higher socialization processes prepare women more generally for the caretaking and relational work of our society—whether that work be in the home or in paid employment. Because the intensity of caretaking involved in parenting, especially of an infant, and the intensity of therapy are similar, we can consider similarities in those two processes.

The link between empathic understanding as a therapist and as a mother is not a new idea. Direct parallels between modes of communication in mothering and therapy have been eloquently noted by many writers on psychotherapy. Winnicott (1965), for example, draws a direct parallel between the fundamental characteristics of the "holding environment" as created by the mother and the analyst. Modell (1976) has elaborated on this position:

> There are actual elements in the analyst's technique that are reminiscent of an idealized maternal holding environment. The analyst is constant and reliable, he (*sic*) responds to the patient's affects, he accepts the patient, and his judgment is less critical and more benign: he is there primarily for the patient's needs and not for his own; he does not retaliate; and he does at times have a better grasp of the patient's inner psychic reality than does the patient himself and therefore may clarify what is bewildering and confusing. (p. 261)

Kestenberg and Buelte (1977) have also recognized features of therapy that resemble those of the early "holding environment." They note some of the similarities in nonverbal communication of empathy through mirroring, in which a smile, a sigh, or the rate of breathing is reflected back to the infant or patient. Similarly, they point out that nonverbal empathy may be expressed by both mother and therapist by shaping in space—that is, the awareness of and adjustment to the infant's or patient's bodily postures.

Apart from being somewhat idealized pictures of the roles of therapist and mother, these two descriptions do capture the essential elements of the parallel qualities of empathic communication in both situations. Consequently, they form a useful starting point in understanding the relationships between empathy in therapy and in mothering. However, when we look more closely at the *means whereby* this maternal empathy is achieved (according to the object relations theorists), the same problems arise that were apparent in their conceptualizations of empathy in therapy.

In other words, just as Winnicott talked about "merger" and "fusion" in the creation of therapeutic empathy, so too does he talk about a primary state of mother/infant merger. "The infant and the maternal care form a unit," according to Winnicott; "at the earliest stages the infant and the maternal care belong to each other and cannot be disentangled." It is during this stage of merger that the mother relies on empathy for understanding, using her identification with the infant as the means for knowing what the infant feels like and therefore what it needs. Likewise, Kestenberg and Buelte talk about the "regression in the service of empathy" as the maternal route to the fullest understanding of the infant's needs.

As in the discussion on empathy in therapy, I would argue that terms like *regression, merger, fusion,* and *symbiosis* belie the mother's sense of a mature self coexisting with this intense affective connectedness and minimize the complexity of decision making and processing that also occur.

So here too we have coexisting yet seemingly contradictory qualities of intimate attachment—not at the expense of, but along with, differentiation. And again, theories which fail to recognize this distinction cast mothering into an infantalizing and magical light, missing the complicated intellectual and emotional process that it is. Certainly women are trained for the empathic qualities of mothering— qualities which demand a creative merger of affective closeness and also a very high level of cognitive activity.

In sum, empathy in therapy is essential to the successful facilitation of the patient's growth. It is not, however, some mysterious quality that some people "just somehow" seem to have more than others. It is a quality that is learned in relationships and over time, in the course of development, and—for therapists—in the process of training for and doing therapy.

This paper was presented at a Stone Center Colloquium in December 1981.

3

The Self-in-Relation: A Theory of Women's Development

JANET L. SURREY

For the past two years in these Stone Center Colloquia we have been discussing important aspects of women's psychological development, covering such diverse topics as women and power, empathy, work, anger, incest, and eating patterns, among others. Throughout many of these papers, there have been references to the idea that the "self" in women may be experienced in a way that is not addressed by current psychoanalytic and developmental theories. The construct of the "self-in-relation" has played an important part in our understanding of these diverse topics and has proved helpful in suggesting innovative programs and therapeutic interventions. I would like to focus more specifically on the central organizing construct of the "self-in-relation," to reflect on the ongoing exploration of this idea, and to elaborate on further aspects of it. I hope this will help lay the groundwork for further discussion during the current series. We at the Stone Center and this year's colloquia speakers hope that you will participate with us in exploring, advancing, and critiquing our theoretical formulations throughout the series.

The idea of self is prominent in current psychological theories describing childhood and adult development. The inquiry into the nature of the self as an organizing principle in human development has been a fundamental aspect of psychological, philosophical, and spiritual investigation. Since it is beyond the scope of this paper to attempt to review this extensive literature, for present purposes I will propose a working definition of self: a construct useful in describing the organization of a person's experience and construction of reality that illuminates the purpose and directionality of her or his behavior.

Recently several authors have proposed that there are important sex differences in the experience and construction of the self. A central theme of *Toward a New Psychology of Women* (Miller, 1976) is that "women's sense of self becomes very much organized around being able to make and then to maintain affiliation and relationships" (p. 83). Miller discusses the necessity of developing new language and new concepts to describe women's unique experiences and points to the problems that arise when the principles of male development are cast as universal principles of human development. Carol Gilligan (1982) has written further of the importance of women finding their own voice in order to describe "ourselves to ourselves" and has indicated that women's experiences of connectedness to others leads to enlarged conceptions of self, morality, and visions of relationship. It is essential to point out that the inquiry into the nature of women's development is a step in the evolution of understanding human development. Women in Western society have been "carriers" of certain aspects of the human experience (Miller, 1976), and a full understanding of human development can be derived only from a thorough elucidation of both female and male experience.

Our conception of the self-in-relation involves the recognition that, for women, the primary experience of self is relational, that is, the self is organized and developed in the context of important relationships. To understand this basic assumption, it is helpful to use as a contrast some current assumptions about male (often generalized to human) development. Currently, developmental theory stresses the importance of separation from the mother at early stages of childhood development (Mahler, 1975), from the family at adolescence (Erikson, 1963), and from teachers and mentors in adulthood (Levinson, 1978) in order for the individual to form a distinct, separate identity. High value is placed on autonomy, self-reliance, independence, self-actualization, "listening to and following" one's own unique dream, destiny, and fulfillment. Intimacy and generativity in adulthood (in Erikson's terms) are seen as possible only after the "closure" of identity. In his theoretical framework, relational "trust" is established in early infancy and does not reemerge as central until the end of adolescence. Our theory suggests, instead, that for women a different—and relational— pathway is primary and continuous, although its centrality may have been "hidden" and unacknowledged.

The values of individuation have permeated our cultural ideals as well as our clinical theories and practice. In psychological theory the concepts and descriptions of relationship appear to be cast in this model, and much of current theory wrestles with the problem of developing a model of "object relations" from a basic assumption of narcissism and human separateness. The notion of the self-in-relation involves an important shift in emphasis from separation to relationship as the basis for self-experience and development. Further, relationship is seen as the basic goal of development: that is, the deepening capacity for relationship and relational competence. The self-in-relation model assumes that other aspects of self (e.g., creativity, autonomy, assertion) develop within this primary context. That is, other aspects of self-development emerge in the context of relationship, and there is no inherent need to disconnect or to sacrifice relationship for self-development. This formulation implies that we must develop an adequate description of relational development in order to understand self-development.

EMPATHY AS A CRUCIAL FEATURE

Recent theories on the early development of the self have emphasized the importance of empathy (Kohut, 1971; Winnicott, 1971). However, the interest in connections with others is much more prominent at all stages of life for women. Research and clinical observation show that most women have a greater ability for relatedness, emotional closeness, and emotional flexibility than do most men. The capacity for empathy, consistently found to be more developed in women, can be seen as the central organizing concept in women's relational experience. Before discussing the development of the capacity for empathy, I want to emphasize that our definition of relationship involves an experience of mutual empathy. The ability to be in relationship appears to rest on the development of the capacity for empathy in both or all persons involved. Kohut (1971) has emphasized the importance of parental empathy and mirroring in the child's early self-development, but almost no attention has been devoted to the topic of *teaching* and *learning* empathy. The "good enough mother" (Winnicott, 1971), capable of providing an empathic facilitating environment for the growing child, does not suddenly appear with the birth of an infant. Much unrecognized learning must have taken place to allow the complex capacities for mothering to emerge in response to the changes of the growing child (Miller, 1976). The development of the capacity for empathy needs to be studied and elaborated carefully. For the present, we are postulating that the best realm available in which to study its origin is in the early mother–daughter relationship. Jordan (see

Chapter 2, this volume) has reexamined the concept of empathy in this light. She has shown that the ability to experience, comprehend, and respond to the inner state of another person is a highly complex process, relying on a high level of psychological development and learning. Accurate empathy involves a balancing of affective arousal and cognitive structuring. It requires an ability to build on the experience of identification with the other person to form a cognitive assimilation of this experience as a basis for response. Such capacities imply highly developed emotional and cognitive operations requiring practice, modeling, and feedback in relationships.

Kohut (1971) has emphasized the profound importance to the developing child of the experience of empathy from the early parental figures and has also described the role of empathy in reconstructive therapy. However, he does not describe the *origins* of the capacity for empathy, leaving it to be construed by many as a highly subjective, intuitive, perhaps innate phenomenon.

The concept of the relational self, however, relies heavily on a new definition of empathy that stresses the growth of this capacity as primary in women's development (Jordan, Chapter 2, this volume). The self-in-relation theory begins to sketch a developmental model to account for the development of empathic competencies in women, beginning with the early mother–daughter relationship. The assumption is that the self is organized and developed through practice in relationships where the goal is the increasing development of mutually empathic relationships. It is important, however, to put this enlarged definition of empathy within the context of the other key structural elements that are important in the development of the self-in-relation.

THE MOTHER–DAUGHTER RELATIONSHIP AS THE MODEL OF RELATIONSHIPS

The model of self-in-relation assumes a developmental pathway. We can explore the mother–daughter relationship as the earliest model of this kind of relationship, that is, the foundation of the core self-structure necessary for empathic development. The model presented here is not necessarily totally specific to the nuclear mother–daughter relationship of early childhood. It is not limited to this relationship only. Indeed, we believe any fruitful relationship must include the fundamental elements presented here—at least to some degree. However, we will use this mother–daughter relationship as the relationship that is probably nearest to the "purest" example. As Freud recognized, this aspect of women's psychology has not been well understood, although it has been receiving more attention in recent years (Chodorow, 1978). The mother–daughter relationship represents only the beginning of a process that can be developed through important relationships with other significant people in childhood, and throughout life if relational contexts are available.

I will focus here on three crucial structural aspects of the mother–daughter relationship. The first is the girl's ongoing interest in and emotional desire to be connected to her mother. All children have a deep fascination with early adult figures in their lives. The attention to and interest in people is a primary part of their construction of reality. However, the attention to the exploration of the feeling states of the parent, especially the mother, is probably reinforced more in girls. A patient of mine described her 3-year-old daughter's frequent questioning of her: "What are you feeling, Mommy?" She would respond very carefully and thoughtfully to this question and would also examine in therapy why the daughter might be asking. She was puzzled that she hardly recalled such an interaction with her 5-year-old son. This early attentiveness to feeling states and the mother's corresponding ease with and interest in emotional sharing may form the basic sense of "learning to listen," to orient and attune to the other person through feelings, the origin of the capacity for empathy and the beginning practice of relational development. A male colleague of mine described his childhood experience as "learning not to listen, to shut out my mother's voice so that I would not be distracted from pursuing my own interests." For boys, then, "separation" means not only a simple physical but an emotional disconnection, often with the goal of not being bound or "controlled" by mother's feeling states or needs.

For girls, "being present with" psychologically is experienced as self-enhancing, whereas for boys it may come to be experienced as invasive, engulfing, or threatening. "Being with" means "being seen" and "feeling seen" by the other and "seeing the other" and sensing the other "feeling seen," which is the experience of mutual empathy. Usually this open connection is not only allowed but encouraged between mothers and daughters. This may be the origin of the process of "seeing through the eyes of the other." In clinical situations, we may see partial failures to differentiate or develop in this process, which can leave the girl feeling unclear about "whose feelings belong to whom" and with a tendency to experience the feelings of the other as her own, especially if she does not have adequate opportunities for exploration and clarification. However, when these opportunities are available, it is through this process of describing and exploring feelings that one begins to "know the other" and the "self."

The ability of the mother to listen and respond, empathize or "mirror" the child's feelings has been well described by Winnicott (1971), Kohut (1971), and others; it has also been seen as the beginning of the development of the experience of the self. Here we are describing the girl's open relationship with the mother and the mother's open relationship with the daughter as the beginning stage for the development of self-in-relation. The second key aspect of this relationship is the child's increasing capacity for mutual empathy, developed in a matrix of emotional connectedness. The mother's easier emotional openness with the daughter than with the son, along with her sense of identification with this style of personal learning and exploration, probably leave the daughter feeling more emotionally connected, understood, and recognized. This sense of connection forms the framework necessary for the process of differentiation and clarification that will follow. The key factor here is the idea that the mutual sharing process fosters a sense of mutual understanding and connection. For boys, the emphasis on early emotional separation and the forming of an identity through the assertion of difference foster a basic relational stance of disconnection and disidentification. Girls, then, develop the expectation that they can facilitate the growth of a sense of self through psychological connection and expect that the mutual sharing of experience will lead to psychological growth.

Again, mothers are likely to appreciate the enhancement of their own self-awareness through this process of mutual empathy because it complements their own relational stance. Mothers often report a profound deepening of self-awareness in their ongoing experience of relating to a growing child. They report learning in tandem about themselves and their daughters through their relational connection in infancy and all through life. I am impressed with the number of mothers who are finally able to allow themselves to seek therapy after their daughters have begun therapy.

Related to this last example is the last key formative factor, which can be called "mutual empowerment." The emotional and cognitive connections based on shared understanding develop over time into a mutual process in which both mothers and daughters become highly responsive to the feeling states of each other. Through the girl's awareness and identification with her mother as the "mothering one" and through the mother's interest in being understood and cared for, the daughter as well as the mother becomes mobilized to care for, respond to, or attend to the well-being and development of the other. Moreover, they care for and *take care of the relationship* between them. This is the motivational dynamic of mutual empowerment, the inherent energizing force of real relationship. It becomes important for the girl to experience validation of her own developing empathic competence. Thus mothers help to empower their daughters by allowing them to feel successful at understanding and giving support at whatever level is appropriate at a particular period of development. In fact, part of learning to be a "good enough" daughter involves learning to be a "good enough" mother or "empathic relator" to one's mother and later to other important people. This ongoing process begins to allow for experience and practice in "mothering" and "relational caretaking."

The development of a positive sense of knowing how to perceive, respond, and relate to the needs and feelings of the other person is an important aspect of woman's self-development. The sense of mutual empowerment leaves both mother and daughter feeling effective and motivated to respond to the other. Each can feel pleasure in her own as well as the other's competence. Thus each can be empowered in the relationship, and this sense of competence begins to be transferred to other relationships. Out of this empowerment as a "relator" comes the empowerment to act in general—and to act as a "related being." Thus, through this mutual sensitivity, caring, and empowerment, mothers are already teaching "mothering, caring, relational practices" to girl children. By mothering, of course, I do not mean what has been seen traditionally as one-dimensional mothering but rather a mode in which all of life activity is carried on in a context of attentiveness and responsivity to the other as an intrinsic ongoing aspect of one's own experience, what we call the self-in-relation. We can postulate that as the early mother–daughter relationship grows over the life cycle, it forms the precursors of women's style of learning, of pleasure, and of self-enhancement in relatedness.

Another way to view this reciprocity is to see it as the source of mutual self-esteem. A good relationship is highly valued by both mother and daughter and becomes a fundamental component of women's sense of self-worth. This, too, continues to evolve through other relationships throughout the life cycle. Self-esteem, then, is related to the degree of emotional sharing, openness, and shared sense of understanding and regard. This sense may be nearly impossible to achieve totally, especially in a culture that stresses separation as an ideal and in which validation of the need for relationship may become distorted and hidden. For women, guilt and shame often become tied to the experience of failure in mutual empathy. That is, women suffer if they feel they have not participated in relationships in this way—with their mothers and/or with other people later. However, if other growth-promoting situations can be made available, these failures can become the challenges to further relational growth. A sense

of self-worth becomes intricately involved in "good enough" understanding and caring for the other and in a sense of mutual concern for
the well-being of each other. This is a key factor in women's
self-esteem, though it is often overlooked. It is rarely mentioned as a
component of self-esteem in men. Accordingly, very few clinical or
research indices of self-esteem deal with this significant aspect. It is
important to note that the dimensions of the mother–daughter
relationship have been so clinically cast in problematic and negative
terms that it becomes difficult to suspend judgment and to see the
underlying structures with clarity. It seems easier to focus on the
clinical problems rather than on the growth-promoting structures of
the relationship.

The basic elements of the core self in women can be summarized
as: (1) an interest in and attention to the other person(s), which form the
Another important aspect to emphasize is that the development of
accurate empathy involves a complex process of interactive validation
of the differences between the self and other. It includes, too, the
recognition of the other as a growing individual with changing needs
and newly developing competencies. Within the early mother–
daughter relationship, the daughter is encouraged to learn to take the
role of the mother (or, we could say, the "provider," the "listener," or
"surround") as well as the daughter (the "receiver," the "speaker," or
the "figure"), depending on the needs of the situation or the individual
at any given time. We have called this the "oscillating mother–
daughter introject."

Through this process, the capacity to learn to "see" the other and
to "make oneself known" to the other highlights one's own self-
knowledge and fosters growth in the other and in the self. Thus mutual
"care taking" is a fundamental aspect of learning. Moreover, it is
directly related to energizing and mobilizing in response to one's new
understanding, which is the basis of empowerment. Clearly, in
problematic situations both the mother and the daughter can become
overinvolved in feeling responsible and overprotective toward the
other. However, this model suggests that healthy degrees of reciprocity
and role flexibility are essential for women's growth. The dynamics of
such reciprocity establish in women the capacity to move from one
perspective to another as the needs of a relational situation arise. This
can more generally be termed the "oscillating self-structure." If
empathy implies the ability to become "ground" to the "figure" of the
other, mutual empathy involves alternations and fluctuations of
figure–ground experiences basic to relational growth and learning. It is
essential to note that learning takes place through these alternations
and fluctuations.

base for the emotional connection and the ability to empathize with the other(s); (2) the expectation of a mutual empathic process where the sharing of experience leads to a heightened development of self and other; and (3) the expectation of interaction and relationship as a process of mutual sensitivity and mutual responsibility that provides the stimulus for the growth of empowerment and self-knowledge. Thus the self develops in the context of relationships, rather than as an isolated or separated autonomous individual. We are emphasizing the importance of a two-way interactional model, where it becomes as important to understand as to be understood, to empower as well as to be empowered.

To put it another way, all of us probably feel the need to feel understood or "recognized" by others. It is equally paramount, but not yet emphasized, that women all through their lives feel the need to "understand" the other—indeed desire this as an essential part of their own growth and development, as an essential part of self-worth and the ability to act.

Thus the hyphenated expression "self-in-relation" implies an evolutionary process of development through relationship. Such language is used to differentiate this notion from a static self construct and to describe an experiential process implying openness, flexibility, and change.

Perhaps this is like evolving from a language of three-dimensional space and Newtonian physics to four-dimensional space and relativity theory. It is important to maintain the vision that although the sex differences we are describing may at times be quite subtle, and individually and culturally relative, they may represent a difference that results in enormous consequences in areas of critical human interactions.

The idea of the self-in-relation does not in any way idealize women's altruism or relational capacities. In fact, the vicissitudes of such development in this culture need to be elaborated carefully in order truly to understand the problems women encounter. This theory is an attempt to develop a model that better fits our experience and to create more relevant and realistic self-images so that we can be more constructive in developing clinical, educational, and social strategies for fostering women's development by focusing and building on women's specific strengths.

PATHWAYS OF DEVELOPMENT

While it is difficult to find appropriate words to describe the pathway of relational development, we have used the construction "relation-

ship-differentiation" as a contrast to the idea of separation-individuation. By differentiation we do not mean to suggest as a developmental
goal the assertion of difference or separateness. The word is used here
to describe a process more like embryological development. By
differentiation we are referring to a process that encompasses
increasing levels of complexity, choice, fluidity, and articulation within
the context of human relationship. What this new model emphasizes is
that the direction of growth is not toward greater degrees of autonomy
or individuation and the breaking of early emotional ties, but toward a
process of growth within relationship, where both or all people
involved are encouraged and challenged to maintain connection and to
foster, adapt to, and change with the growth of the other. This is the
basic model inherent in parenting, but we are broadening it to include
a more generalized dynamic of mutual interactional growth within
relationship. It is not through separation but through more highly
articulated and expanded relational experience that individual development takes place. For example, the adolescent does not necessarily
want to "separate" from her parents, but rather to change the form and
content of the relationship in a way that affirms her own developmental changes and allows new relationships to develop and take priority.
If this important need to continue the relationship but also to change in
relationship is not honored, both daughters and mothers will feel
shame and diminished self-worth. Many common societal and clinical
descriptions make them feel "unable to separate" when that is not
what they want or need. The ability to move and change in relationship
clearly depends on the capacities and willingness of all people
involved to change and grow, that is, not just the child. Since this
growth is interactional, it is often difficult to see who "leads" or
"initiates" the process.

What may distinguish the human species from other animals in
this regard is the interconnection of generations over the life cycle,
rather than the complete separation of the young from the parents. The
mother–daughter relationship has been seen to represent this cyclic
involvement of each generation in caring for the other (for example, in
the myth of Ceres and Persephone). Clearly, continuity of relationship
necessitates mutual growth, commitment, and responsiveness to the
changing and evolving needs of all persons involved. It is likely that
the problems of adolescence, for example, may have as much to do
with parental difficulties in changing as with the adolescent herself.

One more notion I would like to propose at present to describe this
line of development is "relationship-authenticity." This describes the
ongoing challenge to feel emotionally "real," connected, vital, clear,
and purposeful in relationship. It necessitates risk; conflict; expression

of a full range of affect, including anger and other difficult emotions; and the willingness to challenge old images, levels of closeness and distance, and patterns of relationship. This is the challenge of relationship that provides the energy for growth—the need to be seen and recognized for who one is and the need to see and understand the other with ongoing authenticity.

DEFINITION OF RELATIONSHIP

Finally, I would like to offer a working definition of *relationship*, especially to distinguish it from other common terms, such as *attachment*. By relationship I mean an experience of emotional and cognitive *intersubjectivity*: the ongoing, intrinsic inner awareness and responsiveness to the continuous existence of the other or others and the expectation of mutuality in this regard. We might term this "subject relations theory" to distinguish it from "object relations theory," where the "object," based on the construction of the separate self, may not be experienced fully as a subject with his or her own comprehensive personal construction of continuous reality. Nor is this definition of relationship equivalent to other concepts, such as "extension of ego boundaries" or "mutuality" defined as "separate but equal coexistence," where the needs and satisfactions of the other become as important as one's own (as defined by Sullivan and Freud). Being in relationship also involves the capacity to identify with a unit larger than the single self and a sense of motivation to care for this new unit. This is the real problem for "separate self" theorists: to define how separate selves interact and coexist. "Attachment" implies a state of emotional connection where the presence of the "object" becomes related to a sense of well-being, security, and need gratification. "Separation" implies a process of "internalizing" the attachment and lessening the "need" for the other or the relationship. Our definition of relationship does not imply continuous physical or emotional contact, nor does it imply a contractual, externally defined pattern of relationship or a lessening of the importance of relationships as the child grows. One way of looking at this developmental differentiation is to say that while the infant has its own characteristics that influence the quality of its relationships, it also has less flexibility and a more limited way of relating initially; for example, the infant cannot be left alone physically for too long a period. But the infant grows toward a much greater range and flexibility in relating. The caretaker is not only an "object" to which an infant attaches, but a subject with her or his own qualities that immediately begin to influence the relationship and determine its course. They *both* will proceed to become further defined as people as they change *because of* the relationship. Optimally, they both will grow toward more relatedness, not less; toward better relatedness, not separation. And better relatedness means more flexibility, scope, and choice for all individuals and for the relationship itself.

Our definition of relationship implies a sense of knowing oneself and others through a process of mutual relational interaction and continuity of "emotional-cognitive dialogue" over time and space. It connotes also a way of being in the world as part of a unit larger than the individual, where the "whole" is experienced as greater than the sum of the parts. The relationship or the new relational unit (e.g., couple, family, friendship, network, or work groups) comes to have a unique existence beyond the individuals, to be attended to, cared about, and nurtured. In this model the self gains vitality and enhancement in relationship and is not reduced or threatened by connections. Thus the ongoing process of intersubjective relationship obviously does not involve continuous physical connection but does involve a continuous psychological connection. It is important to stress that the emotional-cognitive presence of the other forms a basic component of one's "self-experiences." The process and dialogue of relationship—the interaction, interconnection, and readiness to re-spond—are maintained on a psychological level. This sense of continuity is a basic aspect of the mother–child relationship. For example, mothers often report this as a major difference between them and their husbands in child care. Although the man may be highly committed to caring for the child, it is the woman who experiences the unceasing continuity of awareness. I am postulating here this experience of continuity—the holding of the other as part of the self—as a component of all real relationships.

Communication in this model becomes interaction and dialogue rather than debate. In working with a particular couple I was struck by the difference between the man and the woman in their description of the communication process. When she spoke of her own needs and perceptions, she wanted him to listen actively, playing a part in the developing movement of ideas to a stage of increased focus and clarity. He was ready for *debate*. "When I argue and debate with her, it is because I treat her like an equal who knows what she feels and can *argue* effectively on her own position." She found that his position created confusion, disorganization, and a feeling of disconnection rather than *fostering* her idea of communication. She was asking from him what she feels she does for him—going "with him" on his line of thinking at that time, temporarily taking herself "out of the picture."

Each had much difficulty understanding the other's model of relationship.

The relational line of development, then, suggests that relationship *and* identity develop in *synchrony*. For the growing child, the direction of such relational development might be described as moving from an early emotional responsivity to conscious adult responsibility. As Gilligan (1982) has suggested, the morality of responsibility in women involves the growing development of a mature and thoughtful consideration of the interests of all persons involved in any moral choice. A new concept and term— "response/ability"—seems to apply more aptly to women's self-development and form of action and empowerment than does "agency" or "autonomy."

Inherent in this model is the vision of women's development as moving from a relationship of caretaking to one of consideration, caring, and empowering; that is, moving from the early definition of the mother–daughter relationship toward more comprehensive and flexible adult forms of relationship. The pathway of development includes both the outer, "real" relationship and the inner sense of relationship. The capacity to "become one's own mother,"—that is, the internalizing of the attentive, listening, caring relationship to oneself (as illustrated in what Jordan (Chapter 2, this volume) calls self-empathy)—does not occur in isolation but within relationship. Much of our work in therapy involves the relational process of helping the woman client to make known her own experience and to bring her experience into her own relational context. This also means encouraging the woman to seek out new models and to develop and explore new forms of relationships, networks, and community. The development of new and diverse forms of relationship (beyond the nuclear mother–daughter dyad or the immediate family) is essential for woman's full development, especially in arenas such as the workplace and the larger social, economic, and political scene. Moreover, the presence of women who value and model relational growth can bring new energy and structure into these arenas.

I would like to conclude by illustrating the usefulness of this model in clinical practice. For purposes of brevity and also to illustrate the earlier discussion, these examples will focus primarily on the mother–daughter relationship in adult women. I will not detail all of the other relationships that also play a role.

The Relational Self: Stages of Growth

A 33-year-old woman (I will call her Elizabeth), whom I have been seeing for 5 years in therapy, had originally come for help in choosing a career. At that time she was involved in a highly parentified sexual relationship with her boss, a man 20 years older. She was his administrative assistant. Seeing herself as extremely inadequate intellectually, she had never completed college. The first two years of our work involved her return to college, then entrance into graduate school in a prestigious MBA program. This accomplishment involved a shift in her self-image to one that was very different from her mother's image of her as dependent and intellectually limited. Relinquishing this internalized self-image produced anxiety because it felt like the abandonment of her mother. In fact, it did lead to a temporary dislocation in the relationship with her mother, since her mother could not accommodate psychologically to her daughter's enormous growth and increasing success in the business world.

Here we see how significant changes in self and in self-image create the need for shifts in both the inner and the outer relationship to the mother. In this instance, in order to change during this first period of therapy, Elizabeth had to focus her primary sense of herself in other relationships. At this time, the main relationship that allowed for growth was the relationship with the therapist, and her development proceeded in this new relational context. Further, she began to develop mutually empathic and supportive relationships with women friends in graduate school. This was the first time in her life she had had healthy, growth-enhancing peer relationships with women, and much time in therapy was spent encouraging the development of these relational ties and helping Elizabeth to grow in her relational capacities with peers.

Following graduation from business school, Elizabeth ended her relationship with her former lover, who was unable to adapt to and encourage her new sense of self. She quickly became quite successful in her work and focused intensely on developing her business career. She then became sexually involved with a man who ostensibly did not want to be in a "serious, committed relationship." This began a new era of relational development. She began to experience herself as split into two selves. The first was assertive, active, and confident in her work, where she felt great satisfaction with her working relationships with colleagues and clients. As soon as she came home and was with her lover, she experienced herself as "another person," weak, passive, stupid, and childlike, wanting constant affection and reassurance. She kept trying to end the relationship and was continually terminating and then reinvolving herself in it. During this period of therapy, we again worked on developing new images and models of self-in-relationship.

It appeared that this new relationship elicited the fear of

reexperiencing her early relationship with her mother. This pattern was reinvoked by the intense dyadic intimacy of this sexual relationship. She needed the relational context and support from the therapist to grow and develop into new modes of dyadic relationship beyond that which had been possible for her and her mother when she was a child. Elizabeth struggled with learning to bring her more highly developed relational skills to this intense sexual relationship, and now has been able to reclaim this aspect of her relational self in a more mature way. She is able to value and act appropriately on her own relational needs. This has meant a clear, steady, open, and active description of her needs for more commitment and mutuality in the relationship. It has meant relinquishing her need to be in constant control of her feelings, learning to ride with and accept her own frustrations, and negotiating over time to reach mutually acceptable compromises. The relationship has become very satisfactory to both, and they have married.

During this period of reestablishing herself in an intimate, heterosexual relationship, Elizabeth's relationship with her mother has changed. Having recently accepted her daughter's new career status with great pride, her mother has now been helpful in discussing Elizabeth's developing relationship with her husband. Elizabeth has come to feel that she can learn from her mother in this area, and her mother, also, has begun to work toward changes in her own marriage, based on her interactions with her daughter. The relationship has never been more enjoyable to each, and both are experiencing greater satisfaction in their marital relationships. It is important to note the corresponding growth and mutuality in the relationship with her mother as Elizabeth has grown to establish a new form of relationship with her husband.

There is often this back-and-forth transfer process, where new learning in current relationships leads to development, whenever possible, in older, more long-standing parental or sibling relationships (which are even more challenging to the maintenance of adult self-images). What is important to note is the emphasis on encouraging development in new relationships based on the new self-images that emerge in the therapeutic relationship. There is a focus on relational learning and an attention to the transfer process, as inner development is revealed through growth in relationship.

Fostering Growth in Relationship: Allowing New Self-Images

Another example of working in this model involves helping the woman client to accept new self-images derived from new relationships including, but not exclusively so, her relationship with the therapist. Judith, a 35-year-old, extremely attractive, vital, and spirited single woman, originally sought help because she was unable to develop a "good relationship" with a man, which she thought she desperately wanted. Although she had a wide circle of good female and male friends, played the flute professionally, taught music to young children, and was spunky and independent, she felt extremely depressed and guilty over her "selfishness" (defined as "liking things her way") and her "sexuality" (she was quite interested and enthusiastic about sex). She showed me letters from her southern Presbyterian mother that emphasized the need for her to be less selfish, independent, and emotionally intense so that a man would want to marry her. In a deep sense, Judith felt her mother was right, although she also felt quite angry and rebellious. A great deal of time in therapy was spent allowing Judith to be able to admit that she enjoyed her life, although she missed having an ongoing steady relationship with a man. She felt that to admit to feeling good about herself or to accept her own life meant that she would forever forfeit the possibility of marriage. She literally had a massive anxiety attack following a session during which she expressed a positive feeling about herself.

Part of the therapy has involved an active effort on Judith's part to develop relationships with women who are also trying to establish new life styles. I encouraged Judith to seek out older women with whom she could identify, including some of her musician friends. In this particular instance, Judith's mother was unable to "change with" or accommodate to the daughter's changing self-image. We worked in therapy on the sense of disconnection, despair, and anger at the mother, and Judith has experienced much anxiety, sadness, and grief over this felt loss. However, when Judith finally was able to state that she enjoyed her life, and accepted the possibility of a single life style, she soon developed an intense relationship with a man with whom she is currently involved. Now a new phase of relational development has begun.

This paper was presented at a Stone Center Colloquium in November 1983.

4

Empathy and Self Boundaries

JUDITH V. JORDAN

Developmental and clinical theory have generally emphasized the growth of the autonomous, individuated self in such a way that early developmental milestones are typically characterized by greater separation from mother, increasing sense of boundedness, self-control, self as origin of action and intention, and increasing use of logical, abstract thought. This particular bias, if we can call it that, likely derives from several influences: (1) The modeling of psychology as a science on Newtonian physics, which emphasized notions of discrete, separate entities acting on each other in measurable ways; (2) the emphasis in Western, democratic countries on the sanctity and freedom of the individual; (3) a culture that perceives its task as a weaning of the helpless, dependent infant toward greater self-sufficiency and independence (unlike Japanese culture, which views the infant as initially independent, in need of shaping toward dependency); and (4) a study of the psyche that grew from an understanding of pathology in which the ego was seen as needing to protect itself from assaults by both internal impulses and external demands. Freud commented that "protection against stimuli is an almost more important function for the living organism than reception of stimuli" (Freud, S., 1920, p. 27). In traditional psychoanalytic theory, the individual is seen as growing from an undifferentiated, then embedded and symbiotic phase into an individuated, separate state. Mahler's (Mahler, Pine, & Bergman, 1975) theory of separation-individuation details the hypothetical normal development of an increasingly individuated and separate self. Early studies of schizophrenia (Freeman, Cameron, & McKhie, 1958), which emphasized the pathological disruption of boundaries between self and other in psychotic decompensations, reinforced the notion that healthier, more mature modes of functioning were predicated on greater separation of self and other. Landis points out in his review of ego boundary research that "in most discussion in the literature, firmer boundaries, even extremely impermeable ones, are seen as positive and adaptive, and 'open,' 'weak' boundaries are usually viewed as indications of serious defect" (Landis, 1970, p. 17).

George Klein (1976) was one of the first analytic theorists to point to an imbalance in much of self theory. He posited two major lines of development of the self: "One is an autonomous unit, distinct from others as a locus of action and decision. The second aspect is one's self construed as a necessary part of a unit transcending one's autonomous actions. 'We' identities are also part of the self. Like any biological 'organ' or 'part,' the organism is . . . and must feel itself to be . . . both separate and a part of an entity beyond itself" (Klein, 1976, p. 178). More recently, systems theorists have applied the ideas of "a set of interacting units with relationships among them" to development (Miller, 1978, p. 16). Stern (1980) has referred to the "self with the other," Stechler and Kaplan (1980) have written about the coexistence of affiliative and autonomous tendencies, Pollack (1982) has studied "we-ness" in children and their parents, Kohut (1982), Miller (1976), and Surrey (1983) have posited the special importance of what might be called a "relational self" in women. Concomitantly, Newtonian physics has given way to the "new physics" and quantum theory, which emphasizes flow, waves, and interconnections. Instead of emphasis on static structure and discrete, bounded objects existing separately in space, then, we are seeing a growing appreciation of process, relationship, and interaction. In developmental and clinical theory, this is mirrored in growing emphasis on the development of interpersonal connection and relationship rather than on the self as developing away from, or independent of, relationship. Too often, however, relational issues have been phrased in regressive terms, such as *merged, symbiotic,* or *undifferentiated,* suggesting that intense interpersonal connection involves a movement into more primitive functioning. If there is not appreciation for the development of more complex, differentiated patterns of connection and intimacy, then the relational aspect of the definition of self will continue to be inadequately understood and devalued.

It is against this backdrop of developmental bias that I find the study of empathy most stimulating and relevant. Empathy is central to an understanding of that aspect of the self which involves we-ness, transcendence of the separate, disconnected self. It is, in fact, the process through which one's experienced sense of basic connection and similarity to other humans is established. Heinz Kohut has described empathy as "a fundamental mode of human relatedness, the recognition of the self in the other; it is the accepting, confirming and understanding human echo" (Kohut, 1978, pp. 704–705). Without empathy, there is no intimacy, no real attainment of an appreciation of the paradox of separateness within connection.

Perhaps in part because of the tendency to see less autonomous functioning as regressive, or merely because of the relative lack of attention to the developmental line of the relational self, empathy has often been construed as a mysterious, contagion-like, and primitive phenomenon or dismissed as a vague and unknowable subjective state. Empathy, however, is a complex process, relying on a high level of ego development and ego strength and, in fact, may provide a good index of both of these. Kohut (1959) has referred to empathy as "vicarious introspection," and Schafer has spoken of generative empathy as" the inner experience of sharing in and comprehending the momentary psychological state of another person" (Schafer, 1959, p. 345). Schafer emphasizes the point that this knowing is approximate, "based to a great extent on remembered, corresponding, affective states of one's own" (1959, p. 347). Again, this points to the affective-cognitive integration. Greenson (1960, p. 418) refers to "emotional knowing," and Fliess (1942, p. 213) writes of "trial identification."

There are actually several components to empathy as I understand it. In order to empathize, one must have a well-differentiated sense of self in addition to an appreciation of and sensitivity to the differentness as well as sameness of the other. Empathy always involves surrender to feelings and active cognitive structuring; in order for empathy to occur, self boundaries must be flexible. Experientially, empathy begins with some general motivation for interpersonal relatedness that allows the perception of the other's affective cues (both verbal and nonverbal) followed by surrender to affective arousal in oneself. This involves temporary identification with the other's state, during which one is aware that the source of the affect is in the other. In the final resolution period, the affect subsides and one's self feels more separate; therapeutically, the final step involves making use of this experience to help the patient understand his or her inner world better.

For empathy to be effective, there must be a balance of affective and cognitive, subjective and objective, active and passive. Self boundary flexibility is important, since there is an "as if," trying-out quality to the experience, whereby one places one's self in the other's shoes or looks through the other's eyes. There is a momentary overlap between self and other representations as distinctions between self and other blur experientially.

Piaget's (1952) principles of assimilation and accommodation may provide one way to conceptualize what happens in the empathic process. In empathy there is likely a rapid oscillation of accommodation of images of the self to images of the other, and assimilation of the images of the other to the images of the self. As in Piaget's model, these two processes move toward equilibrium, which is never reached in a static, final way. There is a shifting balance, with momentary overlaps or congruence of self and other representations which then differentiate. When assimilation predominates, the self boundaries may be too rigid to allow the other's affective state to have any real impact, leading to lack of understanding of the other's inner state or projection of one's own affects onto the other. On the other hand, if self-representations are fluid or poorly articulated, the imbalance will be in the direction of overreliance on accommodation, in which case one could become lost in the other's experience, possibly causing difficulty in accurately observing or structuring the experience. Without an adequately articulated and relatively constant set of self-representations or self-images, any temporary identification might become a threat to the constancy of the self. On the other hand, self-images that do not allow for a sense of "we-ness" or affective joining with another would also contribute to a sense of self as endangered by the empathic process; for example, empathy would be experienced as a regressive loss of self-distinctiveness.

Because self-representations are not global, but cohere around specific affective experiences, it is possible that self boundaries vis-a-vis certain affects might be more rigid or loose than with others. Similarly, then, empathic attunement can be more highly developed with regard to certain experiences than others. When there is dissociation of affects or less richly developed affective awareness, there is less likelihood of development of both vicarious affective arousal and cognitive appreciation of certain affects in others. Thus empathy cannot be accurately spoken of as a global function. While there may be general factors that influence empathic attunement (e.g., certain interpersonal motivational dispositions, comfort with a wide range of affective arousal, self boundary flexibility), individuals will differ in their empathic responsiveness to different internal states of another. For example, one woman I see in treatment is tremendously empathic vis-a-vis most of her husband's psychological states. She is someone, however, who has never been allowed to know her own anger, using reaction formation to keep it from awareness. Similarly, when her husband is angry, even when not at her, she is relatively unresponsive, lacking in understanding and distant from his inner state. It is as if a generally empathic approach was lost in this area because of the defense against aggressive impulses that this woman has developed. In my work with couples, it is not an atypical complaint that when the wife gets tearful or particularly affectively charged, the husband either gets uncomfortable and wants to do something to change the situation, or wants to get his wife to do something, while the wife simply wants him to acknowledge her affect and to be with her while she experiences it. It may be that the husband's intolerance of his own tearfulness or sad affect makes it difficult for him to empathize with these feelings in his wife.

An interesting question in the study of the developmental line of empathy arises in the context of the above examples. In part, we may be concerned with the increasing complexity and differentiation of emotional attunement as the individual matures, but it may also be that certain aspects of empathic responsiveness are constricted or lost as the individual develops. McLean (1958) has suggested there is a neural basis in the limbic system for primitive empathic responses. Simner (1971) and Sagi and Hoffman (1976) have demonstrated that 1-to-2-day-old infants cry in response to the distress cry of another infant, clearly not something we could call empathy as we understand it, but a possible precursor to real empathy. According to Hoffman (1978), by 2 or 3 years of age, children are developing a sense that others may have inner states differing from their own and can recognize certain affects in others. Piaget (1928) suggests that conceptual role taking and the decline in egocentrism occur more clearly around 7 to 8 years of age. A study by Dymond, Hughes, and Raabe found that empathy, both social insight and ability to take the role of the other, increases from age 7 to 11; it was also suggested that older children "become more aware of which feelings are 'safe' to recognize and admit and which need 'defenses' "(Dymond, Hughes, & Raabe, 1952, p. 206). It is likely that this is where the sex differences found in empathic ability become salient as well; Hoffman's (1977) review of these studies indicates that males and females tend to be equally able to recognize and label the affective experiences of another person (cognitive awareness) but that females demonstrate generally more vicarious affective responsiveness to another's affect. Women tend to imagine themselves in the other's place more; this does not involve self–other diffusion, since females are as capable of knowing another's inner state even when it is different from their own. It is likely that this sex difference, already present in school-aged children, is augmented in adolescence, as males are taught to act or master rather than "merely feel" in response to affective arousal, while there is more latitude for affective arousal, particularly in the area of distress or vulnerable feelings, for females. A study by Lenrow (1965) found that children who express distress with tears are more apt to respond empathetically to others in distress than brave, noncrying children. Again, this suggests that the broader the range of affective arousal and tolerance of feelings in oneself, the more potential empathic responsiveness may occur to the other. As there is a narrowing of which affects are appropriate for the self, there also may be a curtailment of empathic responsiveness, a loss of the immediate, pressing reactivity to another's inner state.

When we think in terms of self-representations instead of "the self," it becomes clear that to think of self boundaries as a unitary phenomenon may also be misleading. Thus to speak of empathy as a regressive merging suggests that the empathizing individual undergoes a widespread loss of distinctness of self that runs counter to ordinary functioning in which the self is experienced as separate, contained. Even the modification that this is a "temporary identification" (Schafer, 1959) suggests a momentary total surrender; or, as Olden comments, in empathy "the subject temporarily gives up his own ego for that of the object" (Olden, 1953, pp. 112–113). While this points to the temporally limited and reversible quality of empathy, it also perpetuates the error in the sense of seeing the self as *either* distinct and autonomous *or* merged and embedded. Is it not possible to experience a sense of feeling connected and affectively joined and at the same time cognitively appreciate one's separateness (Kaplan, 1983)? Different self-representations coexist and can rapidly be activated, each contributing specially to the overall shape of the self, if you will. Klein (1976) points to the organizational function of the self as providing continuity, coherence, and integrity. For the 3-year-old dealing with separation as a physical act where one either steps toward or away from the mother, autonomous and affiliative motivations may appear mutually exclusive. To contain both motives, then, might threaten the sense of continuity, coherence, and integrity of the self. And even in adults, there may be occasions when these two functions are incompatible, leading to conflict. However, the two can and do coexist. Self-representations characterized by clear boundaries and appreciation of differentness from important others can exist alongside self-representations in which there is much self and other overlap. Self-representations are schemata that form through the processes of accommodation and assimilation. As such, they have a responsive, self-modifying quality as well as an active, shaping function. There is an ever-changing balance between separation and inclusion. We can look at one side or the other, but it is the overall process that best captures the ongoing nature of self-definition and awareness.

Just as it has been suggested that one is either connected or separate, merged or autonomous, there has been a tendency to view affective arousal as involving loss of effective cognitive functioning, that is, one is either emotional or rational. Empathy, as an affective experience of joining with the other, then, has been thought of as a more primitive mode of functioning or knowing the other. Several concrete examples of empathy elucidate some of the complexity of the empathic process. The first example involves a comparison of two mothers feeding a 1-1/2-year-old child. The first mother is watching TV as she sits by her child and mixes the cereal. She more or less shovels the food in, with little eye contact or attention to the child. Sometimes the baby's mouth is still full when the next spoonful comes at him; sometimes he has already swallowed. There is very little affective response to the baby's reactions on the mother's part. There is little or no accommodation of the mother to the infant, virtually no empathic involvement. The second mother sits across from her baby, with good eye contact and occasional physical contact. As she moves the spoon toward the baby's mouth, one can see her own head begin to lift slightly and her mouth will open in anticipation, often as the child's mouth opens, but sometimes before. If some of the food dribbles out, the mother lifts the food back toward the child's mouth and opens her own mouth again. It is possible that what we are seeing is motor mimicry, in which the mother unconsciously imitates the child's facial movements, or a complicated interactional process in which the mother actually provides cues to the baby to engage in a mirroring interaction. The mother is perfectly aware she is not eating, but she is also experiencing some identification with the eating child; she is cognitively, affectively, and motorically aroused and interacting with the child at a level that involves some overlap of boundaries. She is simultaneously aware of separateness and joined with her child. Her identification with the child in part allows greater accommodation to the special needs of the child. In this case, then, greater overlap of self–other representations and identification lead to a clearer and sharper appreciation of the separate state of the other. This is the paradox of empathy; in the joining process one develops a more articulated and differentiated image of the other and hence responds in a more accurate and specific way, quite the opposite of what regressive merging would lead to.

A detailed examination of an empathic moment in a therapy session might shed further light on the quality of affect and self–other representations during this process. A patient is describing to me getting ready for her first prom; as she tells me about her preparations, I find myself feeling, with her, anticipation and excitement . . . a little anxiety. I am listening to the details of her experience, what her dress looks like, her date's name, but the images of her adolescent excitement are blurring now with memories of wearing my first pair of high heels, my first lipstick. In my mind, I see her walk down the stairs I walked down in my high-heeled shoes. There is an oscillation back and forth; she is now in her pink dress, now in my green one. As this occurs, I am also observing my affective state, aware of the process. I am not cognitively confused about who is who, but I feel deeply present and sharing, knowing what she is feeling. I do not get lost in my own reverie, and the images that I examine are a shifting mix of my own memories and the images I have built up over time in working with this patient. I am sensitive to the glow in her face, the expectancy in her posture. Again, using a Piagetian model, I am engaged in a process of assimilating the patient's story into my own memories and construc-tions, but I am constantly alert to the places where her images and affect become distorted by my own associations and I adjust, or accommodate, my affect and thought to match hers more clearly. It is important that I attend to my affect as well as my thoughts in this process. In an informal survey, therapists indicated they were aware of empathic moments most keenly in therapy because of their own compelling affective arousal ("I found myself feeling like crying," "I felt an urge to yell 'stop it' to the abusive parent being described to me"). To assume that affective arousal necessarily leads to cognitive confusion is to underestimate the capacity for integrated functioning; similarly, to assume that an experience of "we-ness," to borrow George Klein's term, necessarily disrupts the experience of "I-ness," is to fall into polarities of functioning that may not be accurate. Such dichotomizing suggests an overly concrete and rigid definition of boundaries rather than an appreciation of the ongoing adjustments and tensions inherent in the experience of self.

We have already touched on the possibility that the capacity for empathic functioning may be somewhat specific to the affective experience involved; for example, someone might be quite empathi-cally attuned to sadness but not to anger, to self-pride but not to shame. Realizing that empathic attunement is a relative rather than absolute potential, let us look at some broad problems that can arise in empathic capacity. In the renewed interest in empathy in the last decade we have tended to look primarily at the empathic ability of the therapist or at empathy as the psychoanalytic mode of understanding (Kohut, 1959). It is also very important, however, to address the quality of empathy in the people we see in treatment. Here, again, attention to the self boundaries enriches the picture of empathy.

Mr. R. is a 35-year-old architect who came to treatment at the urging of his wife; his rather vague complaint was that he was unhappy in his marriage and in his job. At first glance he is a very attractive, well-built man with finely chiseled features. But Mr. R's boyish good looks have little aliveness. Eye contact is rare, and there is little modulation in his voice; he ruminates a good deal with little affect. Mr. R. was the only child of elderly parents; mother was depressed and father quite obsessive. He grew up in an isolated, constricted household in which feelings were rarely shown and never discussed. Mr. R. has never felt close to anyone. He did not feel angry or sad when he came to therapy; he simply did not feel. In talking about people in his world, Mr. R. rarely appreciated the inner experience of others. In fact, at times he was puzzled greatly by his wife's emotional reactions. Mr. R. clearly lacked a rich affective repertoire, so that when others discussed feelings with him he often had no internal referent for comprehending their experience. Further, he had developed rigid self-definitions. In family therapy, which he attended in addition to individual therapy, he spent much of his time pointing out the ways he differed from others, particularly if they expressed strong feelings. In his marriage he frequently faced the complaint that his wife felt she had no impact on him. In the beginning of treatment Mr. R. was not overly unhappy about his isolation, but in his second year he has begun to speak of a deep sense of loneliness. On occasion he has cried about the sadness of his childhood; and he has expressed some understanding of others' feeling states; and eye contact has increased. His family therapist reports that although his difficulty in listening is still a source of frustration for other family members, Mr. R. is more tuned in to others and more accurate in his reading of their feeling states. In this man we can see the overly rigid self boundaries and the poor tolerance of affect of isolated individuals. Classically lacking in empathy, these individuals cannot relax self boundaries enough to allow the affective flow necessary for empathic connection.

Another source of empathic failure may be the individual who becomes overly stimulated by another's affect. For these individuals the self boundaries may be excessively permeable, and responsiveness to the other's affect may in fact diminish the sense of a separate self. Ms. S. is a 30-year-old housewife who came to therapy because she was in the midst of a divorce and was feeling increasingly depressed and anxious. Complicating the divorce was the fact that her husband was romantically involved with her best friend of the last 10 years. Earlier she had supported her husband's availability to this friend following the death of the friend's fiance, because she "felt so much for her pain and loneliness." Although very upset about the loss of both her husband and her best friend, Ms. S. began to recognize that she had become more aware of herself and her needs since her husband had left home. She notes that now when her husband returns to visit their children, she can identify what probably had been happening in the relationship all along:

"I get smaller and smaller when he's around. It's like his needs and feelings fill up the room. All I know is how he thinks about everything. He gets bigger and bigger and I start feeling his feelings and thoughts; I lose myself and get smaller. I can't hold on to myself or my feelings. The same with her [the friend] when she's around; it's always her thoughts or feelings that I notice. They're both so selfish and I can't even figure out what I feel or think. My whole life has been taking care of other people's feelings so I don't even know my own."

This is not a disturbed woman describing grossly impaired ego boundaries; this is a relatively well-functioning woman whose self boundaries at times may be too permeable in the sense of being too sensitive to the distress of others in such a way that she ceases to act in her own best interest. While Mr. R. initially could not, even with great cognitive elaboration, develop an appreciation of another's inner states so that he might feel less isolated, Ms. S. was unable to prevent herself from responding strongly to distressing affective cues in others. She was unable to maintain a sense of boundedness, and her language paints a vivid picture of the shrinking of the sense of self as she experienced a strong vulnerability to the other's affective state. In both cases we have what might be called faulty empathy related to self boundaries; with Mr. R. we see that overly rigid boundaries and fear of influence by the outside world interferes with empathic attunement, while in Ms. S.'s case self boundaries did not adequately protect her in the sense of helping her act on her own behalf. While at times the permeability of self boundaries was not adaptive for Ms. S. and in therapy she developed more control over her responsiveness to others' affective distress, it should also be noted that this woman had a vital, warm sensitivity to people and a genuine concern and involvement with others. She was someone to whom many friends turned when they sought understanding and astute advice. One change for her in therapy might be construed as an increase in empathy directed toward the self.

Self-empathy is a construct that many find troublesome. Schafer has referred to "intrapsychic empathy" (Schafer, 1964, p. 294), Kohut speaks of the "ability of empathizing with ourselves, i.e. with our own past mental organizations" (1959, p. 467), and Blanck and Blanck speak of "retrospective self-empathy" (1974, p. 251). If one takes Schafer's (1968) tripartite definition of self as "agent" (knower, doer), "object," and "locus," or if one thinks of the conventional division of ego into observing and experiencing ego, this construct may be of some use. The observing, often judging, self can then make empathic contact with some aspect of the self as object. This could occur in the form of having a memory of oneself in which the inner state at that time has not been fully integrated because it was not acceptable. To be able to observe and tolerate the affect of that state in a context of understanding becomes a kind of intrapsychic empathy that actually can lead to lasting structural change in self-representations. Unlike empathy with another, where the self boundaries undergo more temporary alteration and the final accommodation may be slight, with intrapsychic empathy there is more opportunity for enduring change in both the representation of self taken as object and in the observing self. The motivational and attitudinal state of nonjudgment and openness, taking an experience seriously, readiness to experience affect and cognitive understanding may contribute to important shifts in the inner experience of troublesome self-images. As a therapist, I have often been moved by seeing this experience of self-empathy.

One patient, who was quite identified with her critical, punitive father and spoke of herself in very derogatory terms, one day was giving an extremely unfavorable description of herself as she went off for her first day of school. Every comment seemed to come from the rejecting paternal introject: "I was such an obnoxious little kid. I wanted everyone to pay attention. No wonder my father got so mad." A therapeutic intervention indicating that of course she wanted to feel special as she went out into this new, maybe even scary, part of the world at first did not seem to have any impact. The self-condemnations rolled forth like armored tanks. Later in treatment, when we were looking at the same incident, however, this woman burst into tears and said, "Suddenly I saw myself as the little girl, so scared and uncertain. My heart just went out to her. I could see myself, that little girl, and really see what was happening inside. I feel it now for her . . . the pain. I feel it now for me. I couldn't feel it then. But I understand why I was acting that way." It was not simply that she became more accepting and less punitive vis-a-vis certain self-representations, although that was an important part of it. But she also actually connected with the affect that had been split off in the memory: both the self as object and the experiencing self as modified by this exchange. And the identification with the critical father was altered in the direction of being less punitive and harsh in her self-judgments. As Schafer points out, this is "an aspect of benevolent or loving superego function as well as attentive ego function" (Schafer, 1964, 294).

Another woman I see is in many ways characterized by a richly developed empathy. She came to therapy because of depression, fear of leaving her house, and lack of confidence in social situations. She was somewhat constricted in presenting herself at first and felt she had little of interest to say to anyone. As we explored her relationships, however, it became clear that she was actually quite close to many friends and to her husband. The descriptions of her interactions with her husband in particular suggested that she was very attuned to his inner world, listening in an accepting, nonjudgmental way to his thoughts and feelings and understanding a good deal about his feelings. She demonstrated the same responsiveness with her friends, who appeared to appreciate deeply her ability to listen, understand, and provide insight. The capacity to apply these skills (if we can call them that) to herself, however, was quite lacking. Until the therapy, she did not seem able to take her own inner experience as a serious object for interest and attention; she also was plagued by punitive introjects, so that rather than understanding certain affective experiences, she condemned them in herself. She later described the difference in the attitude she extended to others and the one she extended to herself by noting: "I care for others sometimes like a sheepherder. I watch and notice and pay attention to their distress. It isn't that I'm just totally accepting because sometimes I point out if I think they're off the mark or something, but I put myself in their place and I understand. With myself, though, I used to be like a lion tamer with a bull whip." In the course of therapy she experienced major shifts such that she could bring her very rich skills for empathy to bear on herself as well as on her friends; her depression has shifted dramatically. She has gone back to graduate school, and people have remarked on her confidence and social ease.

This resonates with some of the research and theory building Carol Gilligan has done in which she points to the morality of responsibility and of caretaking among women (Gilligan, 1982); a crucial, sometimes difficult component of this is the ability to bring the sense of responsibility and caring to bear on the self as well as on others. It involves a balance of autoplastic and alloplastic modification in which at times the self-representations are altered in the direction of accommodating to the demands of external reality, including other people, but at other times finding a way to assimilate the external to fit existing schema.

The relative paucity of research on empathy is troubling, although recent developmental studies by Sander (1980), Hoffman (1977, 1978), Demos (1982), and Stern (1980), among others, are beginning to provide us with a far more complex picture of early mother–infant interaction than we had envisioned before. Concurrently, Kohut's emphasis on empathy in the analytic situation has spurred a renewed interest in this topic among clinicians. Recent infant research has dispelled the old image of the infant as existing in a confused, disorganized state, the passive recipient of impinging internal and external stimuli (Stern, 1980; Sander, 1980). And clinical observations of patients and "normal" adults have suggested that the old notion of the autonomous, separate self may exist in epigenetic charts but not in reality. Thus in the infant we see autonomous, active structuring of experience from an early age and early evidence of differentiation, while in the adult we see ongoing need for selfobjects and definition of self in terms of "we-ness" as well as "I-ness." We are, then, beginning to construct new models of self that can encompass both the sense of coherent separateness and meaningful connection as emergent structures throughout the life span. The old lines of movement from fusion to separateness, from domination by drive to secondary process, and from undifferentiation to differentiation are presently being questioned. A major flaw in existing theory has been the lack of elaboration of the developmental lines of connection and relationship; there has been a tendency to resort to either the now questionable model of the fused mother—infant pair or heterosexual genital union to conceptualize intimacy and self—other connectedness. Clearly, a vast and rich array of what Stern would call "self with other" experiences are lost in this model. It has been noted, particularly in understanding female development, that this model is sadly lacking and even distorting; I think as we begin carefully to explore empathy and relational development we will see that the model misrepresents self-experiences of both males and females. We have further juxtaposed connection versus separateness as if they were mutually incompatible, and we have failed to trace the complicated evolution of autonomous functioning in the context of self in relationship. The study of empathy, depending on the balance of cognitive and affective processes, involving overlapping self–other representations, is crucial to the delineation of a developmental model that encompasses the self as separated and the self as part of a relationship structure.

Basch has noted that "reality lies in relationships, not in the elements that make the relationships possible"; "man is best studied as an activity, one delineated at any given time by the relationships in which he is active" (1983, pp. 52–53). Both researchers and clinicians must direct increased attention to the complexities of the self in relationship; this will necessarily involve a better understanding of how self boundaries are formed, maintained, and altered. Empathy, which Kohut called "the resonance of essential human alikeness" (Kohut, 1978, p. 713), is central to the growth of the emergent self as a structure of coherent separateness and meaningful connection.

In summary, this chapter points to the need for new models of self in which the developmental lines of connection and relationship are explored. Empathy, here described as a complex cognitive and affective process, is central to an understanding of the paradox of separateness within connection. Using Piaget's model of assimilation-accommodation, the importance of self boundary flexibility to empathic attunement is discussed. Self-representations, involving overlap of self–other images, are rarely characterized by absolute separation of self and other. In addition to a developmental outline of self boundaries and empathy, patients' problems with empathy are traced to overly rigid self boundaries or excessively permeable boundaries. Self-empathy is introduced as a useful therapeutic construct.

This paper was presented at a Stone Center Colloquium in January 1984.

5

The Meaning of Mutuality

JUDITH V. JORDAN

There are few psychological or clinical theories that do not acknowledge in some way the importance of relationships to individual development. Most theories, however, reserve the relational emphasis for the earliest years of life, particularly the mother–infant bond, and view autonomy, separation, and independence as hallmarks of maturity. The individual is separated out from context, studied as a self-contained being; internalization of structure, which renders the individual more independent, is seen as the desired endpoint of development.

As the limitations of this model are being examined (Miller, 1976; Gilligan, 1982; the work of the Stone Center at Wellesley College), especially as it constrains our understanding of female development, new areas of interest are emerging. Rather than a study of development as movement away from and out of relationship, this approach posits growth through and toward relationship. Delineation of different kinds of relationships becomes important as a way of understanding what people are seeking in relationships and why certain relationships are a source of joy and meaning, while others become deadening and destructive. People often speak of the search for mutuality in relationship as a goal in their lives, particularly in dyadic love relationships. Its absence is a frequent complaint bringing people to therapy. Relational mutuality can provide purpose and meaning in people's lives, while lack of mutuality can adversely affect self-esteem. The traditional therapy model of looking at intrapsychic factors, the "I," the one-person system provides important insights, but acknowledging the importance of the relationship, context, the quality of interaction and the deeply intersubjective nature of human lives greatly expands our understanding of the people with whom we work.

MUTUAL INTERSUBJECTIVITY

What does a mutual relationship mean? Dictionary definitions indicate that mutuality involves being "possessed, entertained, or performed by each toward or with regard to the other; reciprocal" (Oxford English Dictionary, 1971) or "having the same feelings one for the other; characterized by intimacy" (Webster's Ninth New Collegiate Dictionary, 1984). In a mutual exchange one is both affecting the other and being affected by the other; one extends oneself out to the other and is also receptive to the impact of the other. There is openness to influence, emotional availability, and a constantly changing pattern of responding to and affecting the other's state. There is both receptivity and active initiative toward the other.

Crucial to a mature sense of mutuality is an appreciation of the wholeness of the other person, with a special awareness of the other's subjective experience. Thus the other person is not there merely to take care of one's needs, to become a vessel for one's projections or transferences, or to be the object of discharge of instinctual impulses. Through empathy, and an active interest in the other as a different, complex person, one develops the capacity at first to allow the other's differentness and ultimately to value and encourage those qualities that make that person different and unique.

When empathy and concern flow both ways, there is an intense affirmation of the self and, paradoxically, a transcendence of the self, a sense of the self as part of a larger relational unit. The interaction allows for a relaxation of the sense of separateness; the other's well-being becomes as important as one's own. This does not imply merging, which suggests a blurring or a loss of distinctness of self.

In the broadest sense, this topic might be called mutual intersubjectivity; by that I mean an interest in, attunement to, and responsiveness to the subjective, inner experience of the other at both a cognitive and affective level. The primary channel for this kind of mutuality is empathic attunement, the capacity to share in and comprehend the momentary psychological state of another person (Schafer, 1959). It is a process during which one's self-boundaries undergo momentary alteration, which in itself allows the possibility for change in the self. Empathy in this sense, then, always contains the opportunity for mutual growth and impact.

While relying on mutual empathy (Surrey, Chapter 3, this volume) in the sense that one finds knowledge of the inner state of the other through empathy, mutual intersubjectivity also encompasses other aspects of relationship. Empathy is the affective-cognitive experience of understanding another person. Intersubjectivity carries with it some notion of motivation to understand another's meaning system from his or her frame of reference and ongoing and sustained interest in the inner world of the other. Intersubjectivity could be thought of as a relational frame of reference within which empathy is most likely to occur. It is a "holding" of the other's subjectivity as central to the interaction with that individual. Surrey (Chapter 3) has pointed to the centrality of mutual empathy in psychological development and of intersubjectivity in relationship. The concept of intersubjectivity stresses understanding the other from her or his subjective frame of reference. What is developed here is the notion of the importance of an "intersubjective attitude" on the part of each member of the relationship (hence "mutual intersubjectivity").

A model of mutual intersubjectivity, then, suggests the following for each person in a relationship: (1) an interest in and cognitive-emotional awareness of and responsiveness to the subjectivity of the other person through empathy (Surrey, Chapter 3; Atwood & Stolorow, 1984); (2) a willingness and ability to reveal one's own inner states to the other person, to make one's needs known, to share one's thoughts and feelings, giving the other access to one's subjective world (self-disclosure, "opening" to the other); (3) the capacity to acknowledge one's needs without consciously or unconsciously manipulating the other to gain gratification while overlooking the other's experience; (4) valuing the process of knowing, respecting, and enhancing the growth of the other; (5) establishing an interacting pattern in which both people are open to change in the interaction. It is not merely a balancing, an "I'll scratch your back if you scratch mine," but a kind of matching of intensity of involvement and interest, an investment in the exchange that is for both the self and the other. The process of relating is seen as having intrinsic value.

EXISTING THEORY

Few psychological theories have explicitly addressed mutuality, likely in part because there has been a bias toward viewing development as a progression away from initial dependence toward greater autonomy. Emphasis on innate instinctual forces, increasing internal structure, separation and individuation have characterized most Western psychological theory. Mutuality suggests an ongoing interdependence that many theorists disregard or sometimes even view as pathological. Classical Freudian theory sees relationships as secondary to or deriving from the satisfaction of primary drives (such as hunger or sex); thus the initially unrelated, narcissistically bound infant develops a cathexis (attachment) toward the mother who satisfies its primary drives (Freud, 1959).

Sullivan moved away from the instinct/drive model and explicitly noted, "A personality can never be isolated from the complex of interpersonal relations in which the person lives and has his being" (1953, p. 10). He nevertheless tended to perpetuate a picture of unidirectional influence, conceiving of the self as made up of "reflected appraisals" (1953, p. 22), but not considering the other side, that is, what the self contributes to others.

The object relations theorists of Britain greatly enlarged our appreciation of the importance of relationships in psychological development, but continued the Freudian-inspired model that made the other an "object" of the drive; hence, the very language used to describe this theory honors the biologically determined and one-directional model which it sought to modify. Melanie Klein, whose work predated the object relations theorists, contended that "object relations are at the center of the emotional life" (1952, p. 3). Her notion of reparation to the loved one suggests at least the beginning of a kind of mutuality, as she notes that "the attempt to save the love object, to repair and restore it, attempts which in the state of depression are coupled with despair, since the ego doubts its capacity to achieve this restoration, are determining factors for all sublimations, and the whole of ego development" (1934, p. 290). She stated that "feelings of love and gratitude arise directly and spontaneously in the baby in response to the love and care of his mother" (1953, p. 65). And there is Winnicott's now much-quoted statement: "The infant and the maternal care together form a unit; there is no such thing as an infant" (1965, p. 39).

Winnicott's paper, "The Development of the Capacity for Concern," traces the infant's path from viewing the mother as a "part-object," there to satisfy needs, to seeing this part as fused with the "environment mother," or affection-giving mother: "It was the opportunity to contribute that enabled concern to be within the child's capacity" (1963, p. 171). This description indicates the importance of an active, concerned attitude on the part of the infant-child rather than only the neediness of the baby for the mother and the one-directional flow of caring. But both Klein's and Winnicott's theories are still anchored in an aggressive-libidinal impulse model, in which guilt over destructiveness and aggression, or pleasure from need satisfaction, form the basis of relationship.

Fairbairn presents development entirely as relational growth. He states: "It is impossible to gain any adequate conception of the nature of an individual organism if it is considered apart from its relationships to its natural objects, for it is only in its relationships to these objects that its true nature is displayed" (1946, p. 39). He notes that we move not from dependence to independence, but from "infantile dependence" to "mature dependence." "In mature dependence the emphasis shifts from taking to giving and exchange"; it is characterized "by a capacity on the part of the differentiated individual for cooperative relationships with differentiated objects" (1946, p. 145). Guntrip most explicitly acknowledges mutuality. He writes: "But personal object relations are essentially two-sided, mutual by reason of being personal, and not a matter of mutual adaptation merely, but of mutual appreciation, communication, sharing and of each being for the other" (1973, p. 111).

Recently Kohut (1984), in his recognition of the importance of empathy and of the ongoing need for selfobjects, has pointed to the lifelong centrality of relationships. But the selfobject relationship is hardly characterized by mutuality, at least as presented so far; it serves the narcissistic needs of the individual and is presumably under the fantasied control of the self. The selfobject operates in lieu of structure of the self to regulate self-esteem and to ensure cohesion of the self. While this formulation marks an important departure from traditional psychoanalytic thinking in that it does not emphasize independence and autonomy from objects as the primary endpoint of development, it remains one-directional; the selfobject is used by the self for self-maintaining functions.

Interest in the other as a separate, subjective being is not a part of this model. Kohut does not consider the possibility of intersubjective relating of two or more people; nor does he address the experience of being a selfobject for another. In selfobject relations, both members are affecting and being affected by the interaction; by limiting our understanding only to the "self" who is receiving selfobject functions from another, a great deal of the process is lost. Perhaps Kohut's retention of the term *selfobject* for this lifelong turning to another for empathic resonance also does the theory a disservice. It is possible that what Kohut acknowledges in the ongoing need for selfobjects is the more general need for empathic relationships throughout life. This need should be differentiated from the need for archaic selfobjects. The latter derives from more serious failures of early empathic figures.

Daniel Stern specifically rejects the energetic assumptions in the term *object*. In his studies of the early mother–infant relationship he creatively delineates several modes of "being with the other." They are (1) "self–other complementarity," in which "each member's actions are the complement of the partner's; one person performs the action, another receives it" (e.g., mother–infant cuddling, babbling and alternate listening; 1983, p. 73); (2) "mental state sharing and tuning," in which "there is some sense of commonality of experience or sharing of similar external or internal experience" (vocalizing together, simultaneous imitative events, affect contagion, empathy); (3) "state transforming" events, which are "the experiences that originally and traditionally preoccupied psychoanalysis, namely gratifying the hungry infant and causing the shift in state from hunger to sleep" (1983, p. 78).

Recent infant research suggests that patterns of differentiation of self and other exist almost from birth; the notion of primitive merging may not provide an accurate description of this early phase. There are also early forms of relatedness and ways in which the infant actively participates in mutual regulation with the mother, for instance, initiating and terminating contact through gaze aversion. Sander's research (1964) notes both the mother's and the infant's participation in "regulation of reciprocal exchange" by the age of 3 to 6 months. Self with other, according to Stern (1986), is also "an active mental act of construction not a passive failure of differentiation."

Precursors to empathy, necessary to the development of mutual intersubjectivity, have been studied in infants as young as 3 days, and there are numerous studies of empathy in children. While noting that the infant is probably quite unable to appreciate fully the subjective experience of the other, Kagan suggests that children as young as 2 years are "capable of inferring a psychological state in another person based on their prior experience" (1981, p. 132). The self, however, is not spoken of as a subject until the third year; an appreciation of the other's subjectivity as a totality is unlikely before then.

THE RELATIONAL SELF

Internalization of the caretaker's (typically the mother's) empathic attitude and development of mutual empathic responsiveness with the mother contributes to the capacity for later relational mutuality. An evolving theory of self in women, tentatively called self-in-relation, and developed by Miller (see Chapter 1, this volume), Surrey (Chapter 3), Jordan (Chapter 4), Stiver (Chapter 8), and Kaplan (Chapter 12) at the Stone Center at Wellesley College, suggests that for women the experience of self is intimately bound to relationship. Development proceeds through relational differentiation (Surrey, Chapter 3, this volume) and elaboration rather than through disengagement and separation. Emergence from and integration in a relational context form an ongoing dialectic in women's lives. A nurturing figure of the same gender strengthens the young girl's sense of relatedness and connection; the nature of the mother–daughter identification and the formation of flexible self-boundaries enhance empathic sensitivity in females (Jordan, Surrey, & Kaplan, Chapter 2; Jordan, Chapter 4; Surrey, Chapter 3). While there appear to be clear sex differences, with women demonstrating more investment in connection and "we-ness," more empathic attunement and identity anchored in relationship, it is likely that the emphasis on relationship and interaction in this theory will be useful for understanding male development as well. Lack of cultural investment in relationship as a primary value, however, has led to the neglect of study of this line of development in both males and females. This is part of the highly individualistic, agentic ethic of American culture, typified by the Lone Ranger legend.

The needs to receive, to be given to, to depend on, and to be loved are well covered in the psychological literature. Much relational exchange and growth, however, is overlooked in this one-sided model. Because the model of the needy infant is so compelling in our most prominent theories, the less mutual relationship, the relationship based on need gratification, has been the keystone in developmental theory. The model of genital primacy, with orgasm as its goal, rests on a similar bias of "state transforming" need fulfillment as the bottom line in relationships.

Trevarthen (1979) has suggested that there is a "primary intersubjectivity" that is innate and unfolding. I would like to suggest that in addition there is intrinsic pleasure in mutuality in relationships. This pleasure may grow from the early spontaneity and joy that exists in the mother–child interactions characterized by cuddling, hugging, babbling, smiling, "oohs" and "aahs." Both participants in these early exchanges often seek to extend these engagements, and there is true pleasure and growth for both people in the back-and-forth interplay. While there is clear asymmetry in the mother–infant pair, particularly with regard to regulation, there are almost from birth, episodes of mutual regulation (e.g., in gaze aversion or sucking). In the early days one sees the empathic attunement flowing largely from mother to infant, but, as Sullivan (1953) notes, there is early empathic responsiveness of the infant to the mother. I remember vividly when I was doing mother–child observational research an incident that convinced me of early empathy. A mother inadvertently jammed her hand in the door of the playroom and was in obvious pain. Her 18-month-old daughter immediately picked up a soft, cuddly toy with which she had been comforting herself earlier and took it to the mother, standing close to her, looking worried and rubbing it against her mother's cheek. When the mother smiled and said she was all right, the child's face lit up.

Even in a relationship that is mutual overall, every interaction will not be mutual. But there will need to be sufficient mutuality in important areas so that all members feel that their need for mutuality is met. Something we might call mutual relational responsibility (Surrey, Chapter 3, this volume, refers to taking "care of the relationship") is crucial to the maintenance of such a relationship; both (or all) partners must put attention and energy into caring for the relationship as well as the individuals in it.

FEMALE–MALE DIFFERENCES IN MUTUALITY

A central aspect of mutuality is having an impact on the other, seeing that our actions, feelings, or thoughts affect the other, and opening to the influence of others on us. Emotional reaction is one clear way that this impact is conveyed. We feel moved. Change in behavior or thought is another way impact occurs. It may be that, in general, males and females tend to differ in the cues they attend to regarding these changes. Women may be more attuned to shifts in feelings, while men may be more alert to behavior or ideational changes in the other. This difference often becomes a source of conflict in female–male relationships. An example occurs in the differing ways of dealing with painful affect. Women often want the man's presence and acknowledgment, the witnessing of their feelings, while the man often seems propelled into action to change or remove the "offending feelings." (I'm reminded here of Haim Ginott's advice to parents of adolescents: "Don't just do something, stand there").

For men there may be more attentiveness to actual physical outward movement or change in positions vis-a-vis ideas, while women may be focused more on inner action, if you will, a change in feelings conveyed either subtly or through verbalization. Zella Luria's (1981) research on play behavior of latency-age children supports this point. Little boys engage in active, structured, often competitive games with rules and goals. Little girls, on the other hand, form groups, "simply talk," attend to each other's feelings. In organized sports, boys are literally trained over and over again to move something from one place to another, usually a ball or a person. When this goal is achieved, often in a competitive, aggressive context, they experience pleasure; they believe something has been attained. One can see how coming together in mutual exchange can become quite problematic for many men and women, as they actually meet using different channels of communication or meaning. Women are often attuned to and want sensitivity to feeling, while men tend to focus more on action. Goals for couples might then include articulating, expanding, and differentiating ways of "being with the other." Too often when these differences are not recognized they become part of a power or control struggle. People become locked into feeling misunderstood or feeling that their particular needs are devalued or overlooked. Because male–female relationships are so laden with stereotyped expectations, particularly around dominance and submission, it is often difficult to establish mutuality even though both partners deeply long for it. Often mutuality comes more easily for women in woman-to-woman relationships, which can provide wonderfully sustaining mutual empathy and care.

Mutual empathy occurs when two people relate to each other in a context of interest in the other, emotional availability and responsiveness, cognitive appreciation of the wholeness of the other; the intent is to understand. While some mutual empathy involves an acknowledgment of sameness in the other, an appreciation of the differentness of the other's experience is also vital. The movement toward the other's differentness is actually central to growth in relationships and also can provide a powerful sense of validation for both self and other. Growth occurs because as I stretch to match or understand your experience, something new is acknowledged or grows in me. In Piaget's terms, I accommodate to your experience and therefore am changed by our interaction. I am *touched* by your experience. The validation occurs because the person being empathized with feels her differentness or uniqueness can be accepted. It is not simply a static mirroring process but an expansive growth process for both. In the excitement of exploration, getting to know one another—who are you? who am I? who are we?—there is the opportunity for new self-definition; new aspects of self are expressed and each provides that opportunity for the other. This is growth through relationship.

In sexuality the significance as well as the failure of mutuality can be experienced keenly. To see sexuality as a process of discharge, a pressure of impulse toward gratification, is to take an extraordinarily limited view. If this were the primary motive for sexuality, surely masturbation would be the preferred modality. But in fact it is the intersubjective, mutual quality of sexual involvement that gives it its intensity, depth, richness, and human meaning. In the interplay of bodies and heightened feelings, in finding interest in the response of the other, in coming to know the impact of one's own action on the other and opening to the other's affecting us, there is opportunity for such intensity, pleasure, and growth. When sexuality becomes mechanical meeting directed toward orgasmic discharge only, a performance of the ego or narcissistic exercise of the self, a conquest of one by another, it becomes one of the most profoundly lonely and limiting experiences. Part of the awful aloneness in such a case occurs because in sexual engagement there is such a rich potential for expression of exquisite attunement and the possibility to give one's attention in equibalance to self and other. There can be mutual surrender to a shared reality. It is the interaction, the exchange, the sensitivity to the other's inner experience, the wish to please and to be pleased, the showing of one's pleasure and the vulnerability that that implies which distinguish the mature, full sexual interaction from the simple release of sexual tension.

A patient who by all superficial standards enjoys an active sexuality (that is, she and her husband have frequent, orgasmic sex) reports a powerful sense of alienation in the relationship. She sees her husband as mechanically "a skilled lover." She says he pays attention only to her physical arousal, and she feels he is interested in her orgasm as proof of his sexual prowess. While she appreciates the fact that he does not attend only to his own pleasure, she does not experience a sense of his interest in her inner state, in her full experience of their exchanges. She feels like an object to him. She also feels he treats himself like an object and feels both of them are thereby diminished. It makes her sad. Thus, despite physiological excitement and discharge for both, she feels a core longing for intersubjective attunement and mutuality for a better sense of wholeness in the interaction.

IMBALANCES IN MUTUALITY

Imbalances in mutuality stem from many different sources and, if they occur in primary relationships, create significant pain. Boundary rigidity (discomfort with self-disclosure and difficulty allowing another to have an emotional impact) is a major impediment to relational mutuality. In this case, one member of a dyad may be "walled off," inaccessible, or disconnected. In couples this is a frequent complaint of the woman; the man does not feel emotionally present or available to her, does not talk about his deepest hopes and fears, does not reveal that about which he feels most vulnerable, and expresses little interest in his inner world as well as hers. At the core the man often feels deep fear of strong feelings and great anxiety about being in what he may define as a more passive or exposed position vis-a-vis his own feelings and the other person. This position is not at all passive in a model of mutuality.

The narcissistic individual who uses others to shore up his self-esteem also fails to engage in mutual relationships. The other does not exist as a whole person about whom he feels concern and caring. The goal of this kind of narcissistic relating is, in fact, ultimately to be free of the need of the other, to achieve a grandiose state of self-sufficiency and encapsulation. Developmentally, one would expect that this individual suffered early injuries not only to self-esteem but also in the formation of mutual relationships, thus failing to acknowledge the deeply interdependent nature of peoples' lives. (The Don Juan who compulsively uses others to reassure himself about his sexual and masculine adequacy is such a person).

Depression also impairs the capacity for mutuality. Withdrawal into the self to repair and heal, as well as frequent feelings of helplessness, lead to a regressive wish for nurturance and ministration from others. While all relationships must develop the means for tolerating increased needs at times, such intensified needs interfere with an ongoing mutuality. Depressed people suffer from a diminished interest in the inner world of the other and little ability to attend to, let alone minister to, the needs of the others. In many angry depressions there is also difficulty receiving from others.

For the person who becomes depressed there is often deep pain in seeing oneself as incapable of transcending self-interest. Self-blame for "selfish preoccupation" augments the depressive feelings. Very often the old advice of "you need to get out of yourself and think of someone else" actually has some validity. However, to someone paralyzed with depression, this admonition often sounds like condemnation, one more obligation he or she cannot fulfill. Often becoming interested in another, giving of oneself, moving toward another does help lessen the depressed feelings—not when it follows from a moral imperative but when it derives from (and ultimately strengthens) a tentative sense that one has something of worth to offer another. Development of a time perspective in which the person can see that this period of depressive self-preoccupation can lead eventually to reengagement in a more mutual relationship can be of great help. This help can work to ameliorate the fear of remaining stuck in a relationship of infantile dependency and helplessness in which one does not feel capable of giving to others.

Mutuality will also suffer from imbalances of a different sort.

These occur when one individual in a couple begins to do most of the accommodating and giving, expecting less and less in return. While it takes two to create this pattern, societal pressures foster these tendencies. One individual might be characterized as self-sacrificing and the other as self-preoccupied. The inevitable consequences of a self-sacrificing position are a devaluing of the self and resentment of the other, who comes to be seen as powerful and more worthy.

A clinical example offers some sense of this problem. A young artist came to treatment because of depression, a sense of discomfort with people because she had "nothing to say," and increasing difficulty leaving her home to go to work. She commented in the first session that the only thing she did not need to examine in therapy was her marriage, which was "terrific." As she described her relationship with her husband, however, it became clear that there were imbalances that were quite destructive for her. She expended large efforts taking care of his every need, often sensitively anticipating them. She completely adjusted her work schedule to match her husband's, and gave up an important evening course because it prevented preparing his dinner every night. In social situations she stood quietly by his side, feeling invisible and finding ways to draw him out about his successes so that he would appear in a favorable light to others. When alone with him, she spent much time helping him sort out his inner world. At the same time, she felt he rarely expressed interest in her feelings, tended not to notice her presence in social situations, and sexually rarely stopped to find out whether or not she was interested in making love, acting on his own arousal only. The level of mutuality in this relationship was clearly low, and this woman's self-esteem was linked to the ways in which she did not feel attended to, empathized with, or acknowledged. She did not feel respected by her husband. She felt increasingly worthless; before her marriage she had considered herself a rather competent and assertive individual. In the course of therapy, as she began to notice her own longings for mutuality, she began to challenge the existing patterns. She and her husband went to couples treatment to see if they could move out of what finally felt to her to be an intolerable lack of mutuality, a state in which she felt cut off and unseen.

Another client, a warm and expressive woman in her 50s, said of a love relationship that was ending: "It seems like I was always trying to tune in to what he wanted, how much intimacy he could tolerate, whether I was crowding him emotionally and physically. It never occurred to him to pay attention to my needs that way. Then when I'd try to tell him what I wanted, he seemed bothered. If I persisted or said it louder, he'd say I was harping and bitching. I don't regret all the tuning in and giving I did. I want to do that. It feels good. But when it doesn't flow back, it starts to gnaw at you. I started to feel less valuable, like I needed him too much. He seemed more important. . .very powerful to me."

Often women accept an imbalance of this sort and move into a one-sided nurturing that can lead to a sense of being used and devalued. Too often clinicians viewing this pattern diagnose it as "masochism" in women, a diagnosis which most dramatically points to the limitations of a psychology that does not attend to relational context. Clearly both partners contribute to this problem. This woman did not enjoy the pain she experienced in this relationship, but she felt herself to be the "keeper of the relationship." As such, she felt she had to make more of an effort to sustain the sense of connection. Her husband felt no such need. As a result, she made many accommodations, often at the expense of her own self-esteem. Only in the process of therapy could she begin to acknowledge that she could expect more interest in her inner world from a partner.

Power dynamics, where there is an investment in personal ascendancy or dominance of one person over another, clearly interfere with mutuality. In fact, a motivation for personal power and ascendancy directly contradicts the notion of mutuality presented here. If one is primarily concerned with the establishment of a position of dominance vis-a-vis another, that motive eliminates the possibility of a real interest in the subjective experience of the other. Rather, one's own interests are felt as uppermost. Manipulation of others to achieve ends that are unilaterally defined becomes the focus of the interaction. Whenever an individual's own needs become so primary that they obscure the perception of another's needs, mutual concern and empathy cannot exist. Furthermore, when the emphasis is on instrumentality or striving to maintain power, often through competition, self-disclosure decreases. Disconnection and inequality are basic to a power model, along with a prevailing sense of competing subjectivities. Models of mutuality depend on interaction, a capacity for empathy, and reciprocally enhancing subjectivities. The two ways of approaching relationship really stand at odds with one another.

PROBLEMS IN THE WORKPLACE

For women in the workplace, particularly at high levels in business or professions, relating with others on the basis of roles for instrumental ends can bring significant stress. A lawyer in treatment commented that a colleague told her she could be a terrific lawyer if only she did not get so involved with her clients' problems. She accepted his criticism, feeling perhaps she "cared too much" for the people with whom she worked. Her colleague further advised her that the client "needed her" and that meant she did not need to "put herself out" so much. If she did, the client might even lose respect for her. Expressing a concern for the subjective well-being of the client, engaging in a relationship with some mutuality, was seen as threatening an important power base. He added gratuitously that the problem with women lawyers was that they did not understand how to use power and were not politically savvy enough. Instead of feeling validated for the particular way she was practicing law, which included caring and mutuality, she was left feeling as if she had to keep those more "female" characteristics out of the office.

Another client, a businesswoman who is also warm and caring, placed a high value on relationships with others in her department. These daily personal contacts gave her pleasure. She felt confused when a senior colleague suggested she was "squandering" her resources and should think long and hard about who would be "of use" to her in climbing the corporate ladder and should expend her energy in that direction. These examples represent small indications of the kind of invalidation that occurs almost daily when one expects relational values to prevail in the workplace; the very notion of mutuality or interdependence is seen as threatening to "the job at hand." Often women feel quite betrayed when they discover that relationships they thought were of intrinsic value are part of another's Machiavellian plans for power and success.

At present, most work settings are not structured to attend to, let alone foster, mutuality or relational bonding. Rather, there is a strong emphasis on productivity, and in our society that is seen as enhanced by competition and highly developed individualism. In such a system, hierarchy and lines of individual power and dominance are developed as incentives to individual achievement, but the inevitable interdependence that underlies any institutional power structure is devalued.

THE THERAPY RELATIONSHIP

The therapy relationship is a complex dialogue that superficially seems to have clear roles and boundaries between participants. In conceptualizing the science/art of therapy we have used natural science models (no longer applicable even in the natural sciences) that posit discrete, separate selves and others, honoring the Cartesian distinctions of observer and observed and the old notion from physics of separate, static entities causing objectively measurable changes in other bodies. But if we really look closely at the therapy relationship we begin to ask important questions. In therapy there are two (in some forms, more than two) active members who are both (all) open to change through their interaction. The relationship is central to the process, whether we talk about transference, corrective emotional experience, or empathic attunement. As Fairbairn (and others) note, "the relationship existing between patient and analyst is more important than details of technique" (1957, p. 59). In his last book, *How Does Analysis Cure?*, Kohut states that the aim and result of cure is "the establishment of empathic in-tuneness between self and selfobject on mature adult levels" (1984, p. 66).

Rather than independence from others, therapy leads to an enhanced ability to engage in relationships. Similarly, Kohut sees analysis as helping the patient realize that "the sustaining echo of empathic resonance is indeed available in the world" (1984, p. 78). The relationship with the therapist engenders and sustains this change. Further, in good therapy I think both people are affected. Both client and therapist grow and in that sense are involved in a relationship of mutuality. This is a dialogue. But in several ways it is not a fully mutual relationship, and awareness of both of these dimensions is useful. In therapy, one individual discloses more, comes expressly to be helped by the other, to be listened to and understood. The client's self-disclosure and expression of disavowed or split off experiences, in a context of nonjudgmental listening and understanding, forms a powerful part of the process. In order to facilitate this process there is a contract that puts the client's subjective experience at the center, and there is an agreement to attend to the therapist's subjective experience only insofar as it may be helpful to the client. The therapist offers her-or himself to be used for the healing. But within this context there can occur real caring that goes both ways. There is an important feeling of mutuality, with mutual respect, emotional availability, and openness to change on both sides. And the experience of relationship, of mutuality often grows with the therapy.

In summary, while some theorists have questioned the line of development from helpless infant to autonomous, self-reliant, independent adult, this goal has remained a psychological ideal, certainly in Western culture. As we learn more about early development, we see that the infant begins life with many capacities for relatedness, that there is far more organization and differentiation suggestive of an early "sense of self" despite the absence of language and formal representation. Infants also demonstrate early recognition of organized patterns in the environment, especially in the human environment, indicating early appreciation of and relatedness to others. These data alter our old notion of the merged, undifferentiated, disorganized infant. At the adult end of the developmental line we are beginning to appreciate the healthy adaptiveness of ongoing connection, identity within relationship, a sense of "I" that is rarely separate from some sense of "we," and a need for mutuality. Views of identity are changing toward concepts of a process involving interaction and interpenetration of self and other, rather than a static structure with fixed boundaries. The development lines of relatedness and mutuality clearly need further study. In the meantime, clinicians can pay particular attention to the quality of interaction and to clients' desires for mutuality. (Unfortunately, the language used to describe this relational model at times becomes cumbersome and inexact; we are working toward finding words that better capture this process.)

Mutual relationships in which one feels heard, seen, understood, and known, as well as listening, seeing, understanding, and emotionally available, are vitally important to most people's psychological well-being. In many ways we know ourselves through relationship. While we have the capacity to stand back and observe ourselves to some extent (the observing ego, if you will), our deepest sense of our inner reality often occurs in relationship. In intersubjective mutuality, then, we not only find the opportunity of extending our understanding of the other, we also enhance awareness of ourselves. We provide for the other, and we also receive the gift of what Kohut calls "the accepting, confirming and understanding human echo" (1978, p. 705).

This paper was presented at a Stone Center Colloquium in December 1985.

6

Beyond the Oedipus Complex: Mothers and Daughters

IRENE P. STIVER

Serious questions about the female Oedipus complex have been raised for a long time, but the theory is still dominant in clinical circles. Moreover, the current renewed interest in psychoanalysis has led some modern feminists to accept many of its basic premises. I will examine the theory in the light of recent theoretical research and clinical evidence, and then suggest alternative formulations based on clinical experience with women.

It is probably not too surprising that it has been primarily (but not only) women who have been able to raise serious questions about feminine development in Freudian theory. It is also of interest that these women have not been adequately acknowledged by the psychoanalytic community. In an interesting paper, Fliegel (1973) traces a historical reconstruction of ideas of feminine psychosexual development. She notes that some of the important early contributions by Horney were largely ignored by Freud and other analysts. While Ernest Jones joined her in some of her observations, subsequent literature has tended to credit the ideas developed by Horney to Jones and sometimes did not credit either of them.

Even more relevant, however, is the absence of acknowledgment of the significant contributions of Chodorow, Gilligan, and Miller in contemporary discussions of early female development in psychoanalytic theory. Chodorow (1978), in particular, examines in considerable detail the extent to which gender difference significantly affects the asymmetrical developmental paths of males and females in the "pre-Oedipal" stage and in the resolution of Oedipal conflicts; Gilligan's (1982) work on moral development empirically addresses and challenges the earlier psychoanalytic notion that the superegos of females are less developed than those of males. Miller (1976), of course, has offered us a path toward a new psychology of women but also has brought together in a separate volume (1973) some of the classic papers that critically examine female development in psychoanalytic theory. Yet it is a rare paper in the current psychoanalytic literature on female development that mentions any of these in its list of references.

There has been some decline of psychoanalytic interest in the Oedipal conflict in some quarters. For example, the Kohutians have moved it from the center of classical theory to more peripheral positions, but many other psychoanalysts have long given more attention to "pre-Oedipal" development. Recently there has been an emphasis on the infant–mother dyad around issues of separation and individuation. Still, I believe it would be safe to say that psychoanalysts and other clinicians remain wedded to the centrality of the Oedipus complex for maturation and sexual development. Schafer (1974) notes that the use of the terms "pre-Oedipal" and "pregenital" to name early phases betrays a bias that "anchors the roots of personality to Oedipal issues." More telling, however, is that when voices have been raised seriously questioning the central components of the female Oedipus complex and other aspects of psychosexual development, one still sees "the need to salvage Freud's formulations even at the expense of their internal logic" (Fliegel, 1982, p. 24).

But my purpose is not to demonstrate that since I am a woman, I have less castration anxiety than do men and thus can brave the authorities by challenging something as central to the theory as the Oedipus complex. This would be foolhardy, I have learned, as the following vignette illustrates. Recently, while having lunch with colleagues, I brought up this sensitive subject mainly to check out my sense about the current standing of the female Oedipus complex. A heated discussion followed, and I left after lunch. One of these colleagues is reputed to have said afterwards to the other, "Well, if they don't get it on the couch, they certainly won't get it over lunch." So I do know the dangers of exposing myself to such unsolicited analyses.

What I hope to accomplish here is to demonstrate how the inflexible application to female development of a concept derived from male development, without sufficient attention to the quality and nature of women's experiences, leads to a significant misunderstanding of women. While this would be bad enough, it also blinds us to seeing the unique nature of female development in the areas of sexuality, affect, and cognition.

FORMULATION OF THE OEDIPUS COMPLEX

As a step toward this goal, I would like first to examine the formulations for the male and next the female Oedipus complex. In particular I will be reviewing the theoretical analyses of the female Oedipus complex and the empirical data available in order to illustrate how weak are its underpinnings. I will then offer some alternative ideas to help us think about those features that do seem relevant at some level to female experience. Finally, the implications of these observations for psychotherapy with women will be considered.

The Male Oedipus Complex

The original formulation of the Oedipus complex described a crucial stage of development for boys (Freud, 1924). Around 3 to 4 years of age, a little boy's attachment to his mother becomes genitally centered, and he soon sees his father as a rival for his mother's love. In the service of his wish to replace his father, he has fantasies of taking his father's penis, wishing him dead, and murdering him. He also fears retaliation in the form of castration by his father, a notion so terrifying that he gives up his loving attachment to his mother, represses his sexual feelings toward her, and identifies with the aggressor, his father, with the hope that in this way he will ultimately possess the mother exclusively. The parental, that is, father-aggressor, prohibition against his sexual wishes toward his mother is incorporated internally to form his superego. The boy then moves forward in his development as a male through identification with his father—which also means moving away from his mother and into latency, with further repression of his sexual wishes.

This model stresses the competitive and aggressive qualities of male-to-male relationships and also seems consistent with clinical observations of men's tendencies to distance from their mothers, as well as of the powerful influence of castration anxiety on the experiences of young boys and adult males.

The Female Oedipus Complex

Freud's original efforts to apply this paradigm directly to females involved the assumption that little girls, before the Oedipal stage, were undifferentiated from little boys, were, in fact, "masculine" in orientation (1931). Little girls were presumably aware only of the clitoris, which was experienced as phallic: "We are now obliged to realize that the little girl is a little man" (1933, p. 118). Thus, Freud saw a complete identity of the pre-Oedipal phase in boys and girls. Lampl-de Groot (1927), a woman analyst, supported this view with her notion of the negative Oedipus complex in girls; again, little girls were seen as exactly like little boys, since they were erotically aroused by their mothers, believed they could actively, phallically penetrate them with the clitoris, and were rivalrous with their fathers for their mother's attention.

What I believe Lampl-de Groot was observing was the intense connections of both little boys and little girls with their mothers. It is rather amazing that the little girl's passionate attachment to her mother could be tolerated and acknowledged only in the guise of a "negative" or "phallic" attachment to her. Ironically, Lampl-de Groot's contribution did draw Freud's attention to the fact that girls remained attached to their mothers longer than he had originally believed. This led him to say that girls had a longer pre-Oedipal period than did boys, entering the Oedipal stage later, at 4 years of age or older. This was the beginning of recognition of some crucial differences between girls' and boys' sexual development.

Indeed, Freud seriously grappled with the problems he encountered in trying to understand how girls differed from boys in modes of entry and modes of resolution of the Oedipus complex. The resulting struggle to force-fit a male paradigm to females led to rather complicated theoretical acrobatics on Freud's part as well as in other psychoanalytic literature. It is striking that there is so much written on the subject, with so many psychoanalysts trying somehow to account for, or hold on to, the various components of the female Oedipus complex even when it does not seem to fit together. Nothing similar occurs in the examination of the male Oedipus complex. As Miller (Chapter 1, this volume) states, the difficulties analysts keep encountering trying to find the female Oedipus complex may be due to the fact that it does not exist.

Let us outline now the specifics of Freud's last version of the female Oedipus complex, as formulated in 1931. He noted that while the male child begins to resolve the Oedipus complex because of terror of castration, it is the belief that she has already been castrated that ushers little girls into the Oedipal stage. That is, when the little girl becomes aware of the anatomical differences between her and the little boy, she discovers that she does not have a penis. This leaves the little girl feeling that she had one and lost it. Since she now realizes that her mother is also without a penis, she blames the mother for depriving her of that valued member. The little girl becomes so deeply disappointed in the mother because she is penisless, and so deeply enraged because of what her mother has done to her, that she then turns to father who has the penis. It is the belief in her castration and her envy of the penis, then, that accounts for the little girl's rejection of her first love object, her mother, and her turning instead to her father.

The little girl feels competitive and rivalrous with the mother and has murderous wishes toward her. She longs for her father to give her the penis she has lost; since that seems unlikely, she then yearns for a baby from her father as a substitute for the penis. She ultimately gives up this wish because it soon becomes clear that her father will reject her and will not give her a baby. Only if she identifies with her mother will she some day possess her father and get a baby— that is, a penis—from her father. The threat of retaliation by castration is, however, not an issue for girls. Since they have already been castrated, Freud believed there was not as strong an impetus to leave this stage as was the case for boys, and therefore the dissolution of the Oedipal stage takes longer for girls.

Thus, girls enter latency more gradually but cease all masturbation and repress their sexuality, although they continue to be attached to their fathers. As a consequence, girls' superego is less well developed than that of boys, since they are not subject to the powerful prohibitions and fear of punishment that boys experience in their competitive struggles with their fathers. One other important point is that Freud believed that true femininity does not develop for girls until adolescence, when the shift from the clitoris to the vagina needs to occur. Despite the identification with the mother as the mode of resolution of the Oedipus complex for girls, the dominance of the clitoris in the girl's sexual experience precludes true feminine gender identity. For years women have been taught that true adult femininity required the capacity for vaginal rather than clitoral orgasm, and it was assumed that only neurotic women were unable to make the shift. The components, then, for the female Oedipus complex include the following: (1) Girls are undifferentiated from boys until the Oedipus complex is resolved; (2) castration anxiety is a central experience for little girls and ushers in the Oedipus complex; (3) penis envy plays a powerful role in female development—for Freud it was the "bedrock of a girl's neurotic problems"; (4) the mother is seen as defective by the daughter because she has no penis and punitive because she is presumed responsible for the daughter's castration; (5) the girl turns away from her mother, and is erotically drawn to her father, wanting him to give her a baby, which serves as a substitute for the penis; (6) there is a more gradual resolution of the Oedipus complex, continued attachment to father, and the development of a weaker superego than the boy's; (7) latency follows as a period in which female masturbation ceases because it is a reminder of castration and penis envy, and it is the stage at which repression of prohibited sexual aims occurs; and (8) a shift from clitoral to vaginal sexuality is necessary to attain mature feminine identity.

COMPONENTS OF THE FEMALE OEDIPUS COMPLEX EXAMINED

While Freud himself and other psychoanalytic writers have scrutinized and questioned each of the above components to some extent over the years, they have had the greatest difficulties accounting for exactly how or why the girl makes the shift from her mother to her father? For little boys there was no need to explain a moving away from mother since no change of love "object" was involved. But does the girl really turn away from her mother and what really draws her to her father? Freud's major explanation rested on the concepts of castration and penis envy. Other kinds of explanations have been offered. Horney (1926), who questioned the function of penis envy in the construction of the Oedipus complex, believed that there was a biological drive of heterosexuality that led the girl to turn naturally to her father as the object of her erotic feelings. Later analysts, interested in the issues of separation and individuation, believed that the turning to the father represented the little girl's efforts to ward off engulfment by the mother, with whom boundaries were so fluid (Abelin, 1971; Loewald, 1979). Thus, the need to differentiate from the mother through the attachment with someone so different, the father, the one with the penis, presumably accounted also for the girl's turning away from mother to father.

A somewhat different version is offered by Chassequet-Smirgel (1970), who presumes that the little girl longs for a penis and the father defensively, to counter her sense of helplessness with the mother, who seems to be omnipotent and powerful. It is notable that, despite all the attempts to account for the reasons little girls turn from their mothers to their fathers in the Oedipal stage, it is noted repeatedly in the literature that the relationship between mother and daughter neverthe-less remains powerful, enduring, and continuous through it all.

This phenomenon is often misunderstood since the psychoanalytic literature has emphasized the potential pathological implications, while the more positive aspects of the continuity in mother–daughter relationships still need an explanation.

However, before addressing the mother–daughter relationship, I would like to examine the different components of the female Oedipus complex and demonstrate how tenuous they are in the face of more recent empirical data. The data are of several types: more systematic clinical observations of children; research data on sexuality and gender formation; and the writings of women clinicians. Data from all of these sources have raised central questions about the internal consistency, validity, and usefulness of the concept of a female Oedipus complex. Yet I could find very few instances in the standard literature in which the concept itself is seriously questioned.

Gender Identity

The first point, that girls begin life undifferentiated from boys and do not experience themselves as female until they resolve the Oedipus complex, now appears completely untenable. Stoller (1968) has shown unequivocally that by the age of 18 months both girls and boys have developed what he called a "core gender identity," largely a function of cognitive development, parental attitudes, and gender labeling of the child; this occurs, then, before girls are presumably aware of the anatomical differences between themselves and boys. Other studies (Kleeman, 1977; Kohlberg, 1966) have also reported that boys, although strongly attached to their mothers, experienced themselves as boys; and girls as early as 1 year of age showed pleasure and pride in being a girl.

Castration Anxiety

The next point is that castration anxiety is a central experience of little girls and ushers in the Oedipus complex. The data here are either absent or confusing. In an intriguing paper, Roiphe and Galenson (1972) report finding castration anxiety in girls as early as during the second year of life. While recognizing that this is much earlier than Freud's observation, they conclude that there must therefore be two stages of castration anxiety: one very early, reflecting fear of object and anal loss, and a later stage connected with the Oedipal constellation.

While there has been much criticism of their research on the differences between boys and girls concerning the time of onset and the quality of early genital play, the criteria they report for castration anxiety include: increased negativism, increased dependency on the mother, nightmares, fear of being bitten by animals, and questions asked by little girls about why they do not have a penis. In addition, the authors note that their sample was, in fact, limited to children who had

had early experiences that tended to produce unstable body images. Apparently later a new level of castration anxiety resurfaces, ushering in the Oedipus phase for girls.

Still, it is puzzling how to make sense of such early putative signs of castration. The theory states that castration anxiety arises at the time that anatomical differences between the sexes are noted by the little girl, thus propelling her into the Oedipal phase, with fixation on the father, and so forth. But, if girls move into the Oedipal stage later than boys, after 4 years of age, and castration anxiety is already evident by 16 to 17 months, how can we then account for the girl's ultimate need to turn from her mother to her father. Why does she not enter the Oedipal phase much earlier? It is another example of holding onto a concept even when the internal logic of the theory cannot be sustained.

Another study (Parens et al., 1977) reported such observations as little girls' distress with broken crackers and broken toys as an index of castration anxiety. In the enthusiasm for the concepts upholding the theory, the authors omit alternative considerations, such as the possibility that young children of both sexes might feel some tenuousness of their body integrity and become anxious in the face of any symbolic or actual bodily threat. Horney (1926) very early noted that "castration is a male, not a female, fantasy." I believe that is absolutely correct. In my clinical experience with women, issues around castration are neither as central nor as pervasive as they are with men, for whom concerns about castration are often a powerful and repetitive theme.

Penis Envy

Now let me address the role that penis envy is presumed to play in the female Oedipus complex. This concept has been the most hotly challenged of all the ideas about female sexuality. Horney and Thompson early took issue with both Freud's formulation of the concept itself and his notion that it was "the bedrock of neurotic problems." Horney (1924) attempted to distinguish primary penis envy, which she saw as early narcissistic mortification of girls possessing less than the boy, and secondary penis envy, which she saw as a complex and defensive formation against the girls' hostility to men. Horney (1926) also made a strong case for male envy of motherhood, pregnancy, childbirth, the breast, and so forth, which she felt was more enduring into adulthood than penis envy was for females. Thompson (1943) also challenged the concept of penis envy and introduced a broader cultural orientation. For example, she noted the general competitive tendencies in our culture, which stimulate envy, and the tendency to place an inferior evaluation on women. Ruth Moulton (1973), a more contemporary critic of penis envy, believed that it simply reflects one aspect of universal childhood curiosity and interest in anything new; penis envy, then, she saw as quite transitory if the girl is encouraged and valued. She believed that the notion of penis envy ought not to be taken literally and instead needed to be understood in the context of how little girls experience the ways their mothers are treated by their fathers, how much they feel valued as females, and the like.

Irene Fast (1978) offered a somewhat different understanding of behaviors previously identified as penis envy. She noted that both boys and girls begin with the assumption that they have the characteristics of both sexes and both feel a sense of loss as they discover certain attributes that they must give up as not belonging to them. As an example, she quotes Little Hans' assertion that boys could have babies and other clinical data which show that male children insist that their fathers have the capacity to bear children. Bettleheim (1954) also reported on boys obsessed with the wish to possess both male and female genitalia, with corresponding wishes to become a girl. Greenson, in a paper entitled, "Disidentifying from Mother: Its Special Importance for the Boy" (1968), talks about males' intense envy of women and makes the point that transvestism is a male disease, an extreme statement of men's not infrequent dissatisfaction with maleness and wish to be female.

Equation of Penis with Baby

We can now explore the notion that the girl looks to the father to give her a baby as a substitute for the valued penis. Again, the data are skimpy at best. Internal logic of the theory would dictate that the wish for the baby from the father should follow the discovery of differences between boys and girls and turning away from the mother out of disappointment in her defectiveness. Yet the clinical data suggest that the girl's wish for a baby precedes awareness that the boy has a penis, and seems to be primarily a function of identification with the mother (Parens et al., 1977). As early as 1940, Brunswick wrote, "Contrary to our earlier ideas, the penis wish is not exchanged for the baby wish which has indeed long preceded it" (p. 311). In fact, it is reported that both boys and girls as young as 1 year of age express interest in having babies (Parens et al., 1977). It is again quite remarkable to note that such complicated explanations are necessary to understand little girls' wishes "to mother" and to have a child.

Superego Development

The next component, which we can address briefly, is the notion about how the superego develops differently for girls and boys. Freud believed that girls' superego was weaker because there was a less abrupt ending of the Oedipal conflict than occurs for boys. Yet observations of latency-age girls show no lack of superego development (Blum, 1977); they are, in fact, less aggressive than boys, more socially conforming, and demonstrate more self-control. Even more far-reaching in its implications, however, is the work of Gilligan (1982), which finally laid to rest the often repeated observation of women's weaker superegos. For Gilligan, the psychology of women is distinctive in its greater orientation toward relationships and interdependence, which implies a more contextual mode of judgment and a different, rather than lesser, moral understanding than men.

Latency and Sexuality

It is worth making some comments about latency here, too, since part of the theory does suggest that as girls emerge from the Oedipal phase, and move into latency, their masturbation essentially ceases and their sexuality is repressed. Again the data are not supportive. Clower (1977), a child analyst, makes some telling comments, such as "all analysts today realize that girls in latency age do masturbate" (p.109) and later, "it is interesting to speculate whether repression, formally thought of as normal, was as common as believed" (p. 111). In fact, in another paper, Fraiberg (1972) speculates that adult women who experience frigidity are those who did more completely repress their sexuality in latency and were very afraid about being unable to contain the excitement of genital stimulation. So the notion that little girls, as they emerge from the Oedipal stage, continue to feel castrated, and cannot tolerate to touch themselves, and repress their sexuality remains unsubstantiated. In a classic paper by Scherfey (1973) some of the myths of female sexuality have been finally dismissed. Based on the empirical work of Masters and Johnson, she rightly concludes that there is no such thing as "a psychological clitoral fixation" and that the vaginal orgasm as distinct from the clitoral orgasm does not exist.

Turning Away from Mother

We now come to the most central feature of the Oedipus complex—which maintains that for a girl to develop normally she must reach a point where she moves away from her mother, erotically fixates on her father, then gives up sexual wishes for him, longs for a baby from him, and returns to identify with her mother.

The core of the complex assumes that somehow or other the girl turns away from her mother and turns to her father. The dynamics of the castration complex and penis envy, which require that the little girl see her mother as defective and inferior, were offered to account for this phenomenon. However, as Lester (1976) notes, quite the opposite has been reported in normally developing girls, who show continuous identification with their mother; only when the mother has been grossly inadequate does the father become the main love object for the girl, around the ages of 3 to 5 years.

In reviewing the literature I could not find any systematic studies supporting the notion that little girls turn away from their mothers and instead become intensely attached to their fathers at this stage of development. As more interest in fathers has emerged, however, new studies observing young infants and children have raised some new questions about how children relate to both parents. For example, in one study Schaffer and Emerson (1964) found that infants with a strong tie to their mothers were likely to be responsive to other specific people as well; and by 18 months most infants of both sexes were attached to both father and mother. Girls were noted to attach very early and positively to their fathers.

In a paper entitled "The Development of Self," Stechler and Kaplan (1980) note that the young infant learns to relate to more than one person right from the beginning. In one case in which the father actively participated, the little girl showed a clear capacity to discriminate between, and to attach to, both mother and father, but she developed different modes of relating to each. In particular they note that the child developed a series of dyadic relationships with each person, and each offered a different kind of stimulation. Chodorow (1978) stressed the continued importance of the girl's external and internal relationships to her mother and the way her relationship to her father is added on to this. Thus it is not a turning away from mother so much as a new relationship added on to the existing one.

As it becomes more apparent that fathers are important figures to little girls much earlier than the Oedipal stage, a different level of observation about little girls' sexual development emerges in the analytic literature. For example, they are described as being seductive very early indeed (Abelin, 1971). In one paper (Galenson & Roiphe, 1982) a little girl of 6 months was described as coy and flirtatious, and she was presumed to look out with lowered eyelids; this look, we are told, was experienced as attractive and appealing to her father and to various other men. A 15-month old girl was described as flirtatious with male staff.

This brings us to another possible hypothesis to explain the girl's turning erotically to her father; that is, the father's seductiveness toward the little girl, and his projection of sexual wishes onto her, may stir up the little girl's sexuality and direct it to him. While there has been some recognition of the seductiveness of the father in the literature on counter-Oedipal attitudes (Benedek, 1959; Leonard, 1966; Moulton, 1973), it is quite limited. This discrepancy is striking when compared to the frequency with which it is assumed that it is the little girl who is sexual and flirtatious toward the father because he is not defective and, therefore, more desirable than her mother.

Summary of Analyses of the Female Oedipus Complex

Let us now review quickly this lengthy analysis. I have raised serious questions about the viability of the Oedipus complex in women, since it seems as if each of the components represents rather forced and unsubstantiated attempts to fit a male model to female experience. The development of gender identity seems more related to parental attitudes and cognitive development; castration anxiety and penis envy may describe something about some little girls' experience, but these ideas hardly seem central to female development and adult experience; girls do not appear to turn away from their mothers; and girls become attached to their fathers in different ways starting very early indeed; Gilligan (1982) and others (Blum, 1977) have described the nature of women's different but not weaker superegos, compared to men's; latency continues to be a period of some passionate feelings for many little girls; and vaginal sexuality is not consistent with our current knowledge of female sexuality.

When all is said, I believe two pieces of observation—not Oedipal theory—need our attention. To address them in a way which has any value, however, requires that they be taken out of their previous context of the female Oedipus complex and examined freshly. I am talking about two important observations about women—first, that their relationships with their mothers, although intense, are often quite conflictual; and second, that there is frequently an intense, and sometimes passionate, attachment to their fathers, which may continue well into adulthood. To reduce these observations to castration anxiety and the search for the penis reflects a model in which fear and envy are the propelling forces underlying normal growth and development.

The self-in-relation conceptualization offers another perspective in which forces enabling growth are considered in terms of relational models, with mutual empathy and mutual empowerment playing central roles (Miller, 1986; Jordan, Chapter 4, this volume; Surrey, Chapter 3, this volume). That is the concept I would like to use to explore daughters' relationships with their mothers and fathers, beginning at the age in life when cognitive development and maturation allow for movement from more limited to more complicated relational connections.

ALTERNATIVE VIEWS TO OEDIPAL EXPLANATION

One of the most common observations in the process of psychotherapy is that while men may express the wish to be like their fathers, women more often express the wish to be the opposite of their mothers. There are women in other social and cultural settings who may not share these attitudes, yet the women I know in my practice and among friends and colleagues are often quite critical of their mothers, focus on those qualities in their mothers they most dislike, and struggle against showing any sign of such qualities in themselves. Even those women who have identified themselves with feminist causes are often quite unforgiving of what they see as their mothers' offenses against them, and they resist modification of such attitudes in therapy. Paradoxically, as noted above, it is also evident that strong bonds are often established between mothers and daughters, bonds which continue throughout life. I believe these observations can be examined more fruitfully by exploring the specific features in women's progression from more limited to more complex interrelationships in the family.

As the recent developmental research has demonstrated, infants are highly responsive to environmental stimuli from birth and are very much attuned to their fathers and siblings, as well as to their mothers, at an earlier age than had been previously considered (Lamb, 1981; Abelin, 1971). We know that rapid growth in all areas occurs during the early years. For example, the significant cognitive changes identified at 18 months contribute to the young child's greater capacity to imagine significant people even when they are not present and, thus, to tolerate better interruptions in relational contact. In the same way, the maturation of perceptual and motor skills and of language stimulates the child's curiosity to look out into the world and thus helps children make more sense out of what they see and experience. Changes in bodily sensations and awareness of sexual excitement contribute further to the complexity of the child's relational experiences. The most rapid changes in both mental and physical development seem to occur in the first five years of life. Indeed, one sees considerable awareness in very young children of rather complicated interactions among family members.

Freud, as everyone knows, and as reviewed above, believed that the little girl as early as 3 years of age was profoundly shocked when she became aware that she did not have a penis—and, furthermore, was devastated to learn that her mother did not have one either. I would suggest that both little girls and little boys experience shock and devastation when they confront indications that their beloved and highly valued mothers are devalued and are often treated with contempt and harshness, and sometimes with cruelty.

A woman in therapy reported a powerful memory which she felt had haunted her all her life. The memory is of herself around 3 years of age, walking hand in hand with her adored father while they were on vacation, exploring the hotel at which they were staying. This was an unusual treat, since her father was rarely around and was perceived as quite wonderful and powerful. During their exploration, her father opened a door leading into a room in which a rehearsal was going on for that evening's entertainment. The irascible director was very annoyed by the interruption, and in an angry and insulting way told her father to, in effect, "get the hell out." The little girl was very shocked that anyone would talk to her father like that. She even recalls the look on her father's face, which she knew somehow reflected this embarrassment and great discomfort, although she did not label it as such at the time. But she remembers his "taking it," smiling back at that awful man, and even apologizing as they sheepishly left and closed the door. She felt she could never look up to her father in the same way again, and she reported this with great sadness. This was a particularly interesting memory, because in her family her mother was very much devalued by her father. She realized in our work together that she probably had seen or heard her mother insulted by her father many times. But that had become so much part of her experience, repeated so often, that she could not as keenly identify the moment of disillusionment as she had with her father.

Mother–Daughter Relationships

Lewis and Herman (1986) believe that the major source of anger in the mother–daughter relationship is the mother's "fall from grace" in the family. They feel the girl suffers a double blow; that is, "the denigration of the person to whom she had been so deeply attached, and the awareness that becoming an adult like her has no future reward or superior power" (p. 150). The daughter feels outrage and fury as a consequence and accuses her mother: "Why didn't you fight harder?"

That is indeed a frequent lament of my women patients. While reporting with some feeling the ways in which their fathers demeaned their mothers, they express anger at their mothers, saying, "Why did she take it? Why didn't she leave him? It's her own fault."

We need to wonder about the absence of compassion for the mother while reporting such observations, as well as the resistance to truly perceiving the mother in context. Here it is necessary to begin to explore the relationship of the daughter to the father, since I believe she has very much identified with and taken on some of the father's perceptions and attitudes toward the mother. As a consequence, the daughter is very much caught between the strong emotional-relational connections with each parent as well as between parents.

The Role of the Father

As noted earlier, we now recognize that fathers become very important to both male and female infants very early. Abelin (1971) reports that the recognition of the father with happy smiles occurs before the age of 6 months and that by the age of 9 months most of the infants observed were strongly attached to their fathers. Interestingly, girls attached themselves earlier and more intensely to their fathers than did boys; yet fathers are said to prefer their sons and to be more responsive earlier to their male children. (Margolin & Patterson, 1975). This observation may account in part for the little girls' yearning and struggles to capture the interest and attention of their fathers in order to feel loved by them.

It is important to note how these new data about early response to the father are assimilated into psychoanalytic theory. While previously fathers did not enter significantly into developmental interpretations before the Oedipal phase, now they are seen as absolutely essential to protect the child from the "engulfing mother": "The infant seems to be ready for the relationship with the nonmaternal parent long before the phallic Oedipal phase" (Abelin, 1971, p. 229). Mahler and Gosliner (1955) write, for example, "the father is a powerful and perhaps necessary support against the threat of engulfment of the ego into the whirlpool of the primary undifferentiated symbiotic stage" (p. 209). The father is seen as "an uncontaminated mother substitute" (Abelin, 1971).

The Engulfing Mother

This is a very common theme in the literature that stresses separation-individuation as the major goal of mature development. The need for both male and female children to move out of the relationship with their mothers, who are said to be experienced as overwhelming and powerful, is emphasized repeatedly. Even Chodorow (1978) talks of the need for the girl to defend against potential engulfment by the mother. On the one hand she recognizes that there may be more permeable boundaries between mothers and daughters, which in turn contribute to girls developing more relational selves; and on the other hand she concludes that mothers cannot adequately differentiate themselves from their daughters and that daughters as a result cannot readily differentiate themselves from their mothers. The father, then, is presumed to play a significant role in helping the daughter to differentiate from her mother by attaching to him as someone who is different and "the other."

There are a number of problems inherent in these views. They suggest that in normal development mothers are naturally engulfing and cannot differentiate themselves from their children, especially their female children. It assumes that the normal mother must somehow be so primitive that she cannot have more permeable self-boundaries and know the differences between herself and her daughter. Jordan's paper on empathy (see Chapter 4, this volume) nicely demonstrates how empathic a mother or therapist can be without losing her experience of self in the process. We are well aware that boundary confusion can occur with our more disturbed patients, and that they are often caught in very intense and destructive relationships with one or the other or both parents. However, this clearly does not represent the norm.

How do we understand why this point of view is so prevalent in the current literature? It is, of course, not too different from a long history in our field of blaming the mother for all developmental failures. She is seen as both powerful in this respect and yet so unimportant compared to the father in every other respect.

Let me suggest that this attitude has at least two sources. First, if men need "to disidentify" (Greenson, 1968) from their mothers in order to gain acceptance, value, and prestige in the eyes of men— namely their fathers—this may lead to attributing excess power to their mothers. Defensively, we know, this may lead to the need to devalue women in order to deny their power. Second, women do sometimes hold onto their relationships with their children in order to feel connected with someone when other adult relationships fail them. This theme is particularly developed by Miller (1972), who indicates that mothers may become overinvolved with their male children because they cannot fully engage with a male adult.

If the analytic community displays such a bias against the mother who is seen in normal development as engulfing, it is not surprising that fathers may communicate to their daughters their perception of their wives in a similar way. Daughters then may adopt their fathers' views as their own.

Fathers and Daughters

There are other observations about fathers and daughters that can help us understand both the intensity of their relationships and the nature of the conflicts between mothers and daughters. In a paper exploring father–daughter relationships, Contratto (1986) notes that the daughter's observations of the father–mother interaction contribute significantly to the daughter's psychological development. In particular, early recognition in many families that men have more power and authority than do women may lead daughters to overvalue and idealize their fathers from a young age.

Contratto reports also that many of her women patients' earliest memories of their fathers were that they were fun, clever, and more exciting than their mothers, who were seen instead as familiar, reliably present, and less interesting. These women patients also saw their fathers as controlling and often belittling their mothers, which led them to try to earn their fathers' respect by being different from their mothers. Contratto believes, too, that since the mother is more familiar and more present, there is less need and less motivation for the daughter to figure out the relationship to the mother; the father, on the other hand, because he is unfamiliar, becomes a more intriguing figure of excitement and delight. Surrey (see Chapter 3, this volume) has noted that girls' needs to understand as well as to be understood are apparent very early. Thus, in fact, they do inquire about the mothers' feeling states, and so forth. Mothers are more likely, however, to respond and become, therefore, far less mysterious figures than fathers.

In the literature on the role of the father in early childhood development, there are additional observations that may help us understand further the father–daughter relationship (Lamb, 1981; Machlinger, 1981). We now know that fathers become important figures very early for both boys and girls.

Still, in most families mothers spend much more time with their children than do fathers. When fathers do interact, they have significantly different styles from mothers. While mothers engage in more conventional play and assume primary responsibility for caretaking, fathers engage in more physical and often more stimulating interactions (Lamb, 1981). They are quite action oriented with their

daughters, though less rough and tumble than they are with their sons
(Biller & Meredith, 1974). Very early, then, fathers become associated
with play and adventure.

Other data suggest that fathers also put more pressure on their
children to conform to sex role stereotypes (Biller, 1981). For example,
fathers focus on achievement and dominance in their expectations for
their sons, while for daughters their stress is on submissiveness and
pleasing others (Aberle & Naegele, 1952). Thus, little girls may face a
dilemma in attempting to gain the respect of their fathers who are so
valued in the family. To be like their brothers would perhaps gain more
of their fathers' attention, but, as girls, they learn early that they are
expected to be "feminine" to please them.

SEXUAL COMPONENT OF THE FATHER–DAUGHTER RELATIONSHIP

This brings us to the sexual component of the father–daughter
relationship. As noted earlier, there has been some awareness that the
father's seductiveness and projection of his sexual wishes onto his
daughter contribute significantly to the girl's passionate attachment to
him. Still, this observation has not been given central importance in
current theory. Recent data on father–daughter incest are, however,
impressive and disturbing (Herman, 1981); for example, over 5% of all
girls are incestuously involved with their fathers or stepfathers, and
women who have become sufficiently disturbed to require hospitalization show an alarming history of sexual abuse (54%) (Bryer, Nelson,
Miller, & Krol, 1987), more often than not occurring in the family.

However, let us consider much more subtle expressions of the
father's seductiveness, or the mode of interaction between fathers and
their daughters, which may help us understand the ways little girls
establish relationships with both parents.

In talking to fathers, it becomes apparent that they often get great
pleasure from what they see as their daughters' adoration of them and
presumed "flirtatiousness." Recently, one male psychiatrist remarked
that he believed girls who felt they could titillate their fathers grew up
to feel good about their femininity, while another psychiatrist added,
"How else do little girls learn how to be flirtatious with men when they
grow up?" Both of these comments were given with a kind of pleasure
and pride in contemplating the early father–daughter relationship in
this way. A woman colleague recalled that when she was 15 her father,
a highly respected figure in the community, took her to lunch at a
glamorous restaurant and introduced her to the maitre d' as "my

mistress," which warranted a big laugh all around. Yet if mothers should talk with such apparent pleasure about their son's sexuality or so-called flirtatiousness with them, I suspect a horrified reaction would follow. These more subtle expressions of the father's sexualization of the relationship with his daughters are quite prevalent. Yet it is notable that they are addressed only minimally in the literature. It is a kind of "given" for men, and the implications for the growing girl are not taken seriously. Instead, as we have seen, little girls are labeled repeatedly as being sexy and seductive.

How do we understand this propensity of many fathers to see so readily expressions of their daughters' excitement, glee, and love as seductive, and what are the implications for their daughters' experience? We know that fathers' play with their daughters is often physical and can be quite stimulating. During the early years of such rapid growth, the little girl's intense physical sensations will often accompany her interactions with both her father and mother—although those with the latter are not as regularly "noted." Tessman (1982), in describing father–daughter interactions, reports, too, that there are often rapid shifts from peaks of involvement to valleys of minimal attention, which may be quite confusing and disturbing to the little girl.

I believe that men have difficulty learning how to relate to their daughters, who behave differently from their sons in important ways. From an early age, little girls reflect more relational qualities than do little boys. They are certainly less aggressive, are noted to smile earlier and, to show more sensitivity to the affective states of other children, and are generally seen as more affiliative and sociable than little boys (Oetzel, 1966; Moss, 1974). The identification with mother as "mother" contributes to their developing more nurturant, empathic capacities (Chodorow, 1978; Surrey, Chapter 3, this volume). Both Miller (1976; Chapter 1, this volume) and Surrey (Chapter 3, this volume) have addressed the ways little girls very early show the need to take care of the important relationships in their lives—which involves an attentiveness to the feeling states in both parents. It has also been suggested that little girls take care of their mothers by helping them feel better—less sad, depressed, or angry—and take care of their fathers by helping them feel more important, adored.

The tendency to misinterpret these relational behaviors as seductive and flirtatious represents a significant misunderstanding of what little girls may be looking for when they try to engage with their father. Tessman (1982) sees in the daughter's relationship with her father an excitement that includes the wish to adapt to a new kind of mutuality with him; and she notes, too, how much the daughter's need to give love actively has been underestimated—and, I would add, misunderstood when observed.

Fathers more typically interact with their sons in task-oriented, aggressive activities and may feel at a loss about how to connect with their daughters' more personal, relational styles. A man I saw in therapy returned to see me after his daughter was born; he had a 3-year-old son. While he had great pleasure and pride about both children, he reported that only recently had he been able to start to relate to his son—now that he was old enough "to do things with"; with his daughter he felt uneasy, saw her as too fragile, and was afraid he would not know how to be with her.

This uneasiness in fathers becomes even more marked in adolescence, when their daughters' sexuality does begin to develop more clearly. We know some fathers become overly involved with their daughters at this stage, either by being openly sexual or overly possessive and restrictive, stating the need to protect them from the sexual dangers in the world. Another common response is for fathers to withdraw and distance themselves from their daughters to ward off their own sexual impulses.

A 15-year-old girl who was admitted to the hospital after a suicide attempt reported that she had become increasingly depressed because she felt completely ignored by her father, who attended instead to her two brothers. Her mother was chronically depressed, and she felt very protective of her. The family history revealed that the father had had a series of affairs, was very much involved in body building in an open, exhibitionistic way at home, and had persuaded his wife to engage in some unusual sexual activities. At the same time, this father seemed to care sincerely about his daughter and wanted to be involved in her treatment. It became clear that as his daughter moved into adolescence, he was quite threatened by his sexual feelings toward her and, thus, needed to ignore her and focus his attention elsewhere. At the same time the daughter was very aware of his sexual activities and did often sexualize her relationship with him, for example, by staying up late to "catch him" after he was out with another woman. She was alternatively enraged with him and despairing about ever gaining his love and attention.

Not only do fathers need to see little girls' behaviors as flirtatious, sexy, and coy; mothers also may encourage their daughters in such interactions by labeling their behaviors in such a way. This, I might add, is in sharp contrast to the propensity of fathers to be deeply resentful and jealous of their sons' strong connections with their wives. The mother's encouragement of her daughter's development of "feminine wiles" with her father may also reflect the mother's efforts to help her daughter get on in the world and to learn how "to get a man" who will ultimately presumably take care of her, and so forth. Even more to the point is that this behavior probably also speaks to the mother's yearnings for a father's attention and love, which she can play out through the relationship between her daughter and her husband.

At the same time, if she feels devalued and abandoned by her husband, she will also be deeply resentful of her daughter; and she may express these feelings in critical and hostile attitudes. Daughters, of course, in such instances, recognize that their mothers seem to value men more than women, through their perceptions of how their mothers relate to husbands and sons, and in the ways they encourage the daughters' relationships with their fathers. Lewis and Herman (1986) observe that the daughters can experience their mothers' apparent preference for their husbands, sons, and other males as a deep betrayal of their close connections, which contributes to the underlying anger in mother–daughter relationships.

Competence and Mastery

Another facet of the father–daughter relationship that requires attention is what Tessman (1982) calls "endeavor excitement." This term refers to the ways in which fathers can help daughters achieve a sense of competence and mastery in the world. This can occur, she believes, only if the father can both acknowledge his daughter's wish to bestow her love freely and seriously on him and also integrate her growing competencies into his view of femininity. Fathers have more traditionally represented links to the outside world, and an important piece of their relationships with their daughters is to help them master tasks and feel competent and effective. We might expect that over time, as women move out of the home into the work arena, mothers will also become associated with the development of competency and achievement. In those many families where the mother is still devalued, however, the daughter's sense of accomplishment may lead to significant inhibitions in the work arena in later years (Stiver, Chapter 12, this volume). Instead, if positive relational connections between parents are apparent to the child, learning to become competent occurs within a relational context and contributes to further growth and development.

Let me share an example of watching my nephew help his 3-year-old daughter learn to cut her food with a knife. This father and daughter are deeply connected, and since a sister was recently born they are together even more than previously. He was sitting with her while she was eating and apparently decided in the middle of this process to show her how to cut her own food. She was intensely interested and completely focused on the task as he guided her hand with the knife several times until she finally did it herself. It was a rather glorious experience to see the marvelous enthusiasm they both expressed at this event, both smiling from ear to ear, and then rushing in together to the other room to share this great accomplishment with the mother who, though nursing her baby, had full opportunity to show and share her delight and great pleasure.

Birth of a Sibling

I would like to address now the enormous significance of the birth of a sibling to a little girl's development and her relationships within the family. While it is probably the first new relational challenge for a young child, it has not been given much attention compared to the centrality of the Oedipus complex. In fact, some of the powerful, highly varied feelings children do have toward their siblings are often dismissed by interpreting them simply as displacements from their parents in the Oedipal drama. Yet the entry of a new person into the household significantly alters the family equilibrium and changes the exclusive experience a child has with her parents, particularly the mother, as the primary caretaker. While this can be painful for the child, it also offers an opportunity to enlarge her relational capacities and a may help her move forward into more complicated interactions.

Obviously, the age of the child when a sibling is born, the family constellation at the time, and other features offer many variations, which cannot be addressed now. Still it is important to note that the little girl is often torn among many feelings: her own identification with her mother in the mothering of the new baby, rage at being displaced, enthusiasm about the opportunity to spend more time with her beloved father, which sometimes occurs, and empathic interactions with a mother who often feels quite burdened and torn herself.

A woman I was seeing in therapy who had a 3-year-old daughter was pregnant and struggling with what it would be like for her daughter to have a sibling. This struggle replayed in part some significant events between her and her brother, but it was also a reflection of how deeply tied she felt to her daughter, how much she felt what she imagined would be her daughter's pain, and how much she also resented her daughter for interfering with her simultaneous wish to bond with her new baby. All of these issues I believe contribute to the power of the mother–daughter connection and the underlying conflict that is also present.

In the above discussion I have tried to address the ways in which conflict-ridden relationships between mothers and daughters do not seem to arise out of penis envy, castration anxiety, and rivalry between them, but from other sources. The mothers "fall from grace" when she is seen as less valued than the father, the sense of betrayal by the mother for her apparent preference for men, and the fury at being replaced by her mother's relationships with others are some of the relevant factors.

Also, the passionate attachment to the father is seen as having its source in part in the style of the father–daughter interactions, which are often physical and stimulating. At a stage of rapid growth and development of the little girl, such intense physical sensations may inform experiences of love with intense excitement, joy, and other feelings. Also, it seems likely that fathers, being men, project their own sexual interests onto their daughters and need to see them as adoring and flirtatious as a way of understanding their own loving feelings (since men often interpret any loving and close feelings as sexual [Stiver, Chapter 12, this volume]). Fathers, as more mysterious figures who are not as present as mothers, are perceived to be more in the world and more valued than the mother; this perception, in turn, leads to an overidealization of the father in contrast to the mother, who is seen as more familiar and real and whose flaws are more visible in day-to-day interactions.

I would like to add, too, that this lack of full, day-to-day interchange accounts in part for the continuation of the idealization of the father into adulthood; that is, since the father is often not very present with his daughter in her growing-up years, she does not have the opportunity to resolve, and come to terms with, a real relationship with him. This tendency is exacerbated by the father's difficulties in knowing how to relate to his daughter in a nonsexual way. In an analogous fashion, sons may have a difficult time resolving their relationships with their mothers when the culture puts such pressure on boys to move away from their mothers in early development, thus depriving them of more opportunity to truly work through this relationship over time—even though their mothers are physically present in this case. Unhappily, boys, like girls, have little opportunity to work out their relationships with their fathers, who are relatively absent to boys as well. This prevalent situation often leaves the boy quite alone, and with much unfinished business. It is important to note that while girls do have major conflicts with their mothers, they are also able to work out much more positive relationships over the years.

Of course, in adolescence, many of these issues come to the forefront again, and with more power. This period has been addressed elsewhere, along with the suggestion that mother–daughter relationships may become more intense and problematic at this stage for many reasons (Lewis & Herman, 1986). However, despite such intensification, the data are still impressive that mothers and daughters continue to maintain close, if complex, ties. Gleason (Chapter 7, this volume), in a survey of Wellesley College students, reported that the majority identified with their mothers as the most important person in their lives.

All of these issues need to be addressed in our therapeutic work with women, but we lose sight of them easily if we allow a theoretical formulation to guide our observations. It can blind us to what is truly going on in the lives of women. I hope I have shown how the components of the female Oedipus complex do not hold up when empirical data and clinical work with women are considered, nor does this formulation help us understand women's development.

The conceptualization of the self-in-relation as a model of female development helps us in a more powerful way to understand the meanings of the different relational connections that evolve over time. Surrey (Chapter 3, this volume), in discussing women's capacity and pleasure in relatedness, notes that these involve the ability to identify with the other, the sense of connectedness through feeling states and empowerment based on the complex awareness of the needs and realities of another person.

A CASE EXAMPLE

Let me close with a clinical example that illustrates these qualities in lieu of an explanation based on the dynamics of the female Oedipus complex. A young woman was referred for treatment after developing a hypomanic reaction of psychotic proportions. This reaction was apparently triggered by her stepfather's close brush with death after a stroke. During his recuperation, this woman became increasingly excited, domineering, and bossy; she called herself Scarlett O'Hara, predicted the date of her father's death, and repeatedly talked of wanting to sleep with her father. By the time I saw her, she was no longer acutely psychotic, although she was rather overactive and talked with glee and pleasure about wanting to be Scarlett O'Hara.

As I pursued her history, I learned of several significant events. Her biological father had died when she was only 1-1/2 years old. She had no memory of him, but she did remember that a year later, when her mother remarried, her stepfather was very kind to her, brought her a Bugs Bunny doll, and so forth; but then he "disappeared." What that meant was that he was a very successful businessman who traveled all over the world and was at home less and less. She saw her mother as quite inadequate, and her mother was often called "stupid" by the stepfather. When I asked what was so terrific about Scarlett O'Hara, she said that Scarlett was a strong woman who knew what she wanted. She then talked about how weak she saw her mother to be and how upsetting this was to her. Still she remained high, often rather giddy and grandiose.

When she spoke again about wanting to sleep with her father, I asked her what that meant—and as she answered, her demeanor began to change. In a much more subdued fashion she explained that this powerful stepfather became quite terrified after his stroke. He believed he was going to die. He was afraid of the night and thought if he closed his eyes and slept he would die. She was quite shocked and upset to see such vulnerability in someone who had had such contempt for any sign of weakness in others, but she could not bear his pain. "I thought," she said, "if I slept with him, if I put my arms around him, comforted him, he would be less afraid, that he would sleep, and he would stay alive." As she told me this, tears were streaming down her face and she was truly able to feel deep sadness about losing this beloved stepfather— and her real father many years before.

This paper was presented at a Stone Center Colloquium in May 1986.

7

Women's Self Development in Late Adolescence

ALEXANDRA G. KAPLAN
NANCY GLEASON
RONA KLEIN

The Relational Self in Late Adolescent Women

ALEXANDRA G. KAPLAN
RONA KLEIN

Prevailing theoretical views portray late adolescence as part of a broader developmental framework—one that equates psychological maturation with increasing levels of autonomy, separation, and independence and that stresses competitive achievement as an important basis for self-evaluation. Yet observations and clinical experience at the Stone Center and elsewhere reveal that neither this general developmental pattern nor this description of late adolescence fits women's actual mode of growth (Miller, 1976; Jordan, Surrey, & Kaplan, Chapter 2, this volume; Josselson, 1980; Gilligan, 1982).

In this paper we will suggest some reinterpretations of the late adolescent developmental paradigms based on the model of the

Rona Klein, M.D., is Instructor in Psychiatry at Harvard Medical School, and Division Director in Community Residential and Treatment Programs at McLean Hospital.

"self-in-relation" that is being developed at the Stone Center (Miller, Chapter 1, this volume; Surrey, Chapter 3, this volume). Within this model, women's core self-structure emerges out of experience of a relational process. Beginning with the earliest mother–daughter interactions, this relational sense of self develops out of women's involvement in progressively complex relationships, characterized by mutual identifications, attention to the interplay between each other's emotions, and caring about the process and activity of relationship. Note that in speaking of relationships, we are referring not only to actual relationships but also to important inner constructions of the relational process.

The dynamic of the early mother–child relationship initiates the development of the core relational self. This dynamic is characterized by a finely tuned affective sensitivity and responsiveness of the mother to the child and vice versa. The child identifies not with a static image of the mother but with an image of the mother as an active caretaker. From this, the earliest mental images of the self are of a self whose emotional core is responded to by the other and who responds back to the emotions of the other. Miller (Chapter 1, this volume) has noted that this "interacting sense of self" is probably present initially in all infants but is then discouraged from full evolution in boys, at least in this culture. In girls, however, it becomes the kernel around which additional dynamic images of the self are organized. As a result, for women the sense of self is refined, enhanced, and strengthened not through a series of separations but through the inner experiences of relationships marked by mutuality and affective connection. Being in relationship, empathically sharing with another, and maintaining the well-being of relationships function as important motivations for action, and sources for self-esteem and self-affirmation.

As we turn to describing the development of the core relational self in late adolescence, we will focus on how the relational nature of the self shapes women's experiences of the situations facing them at this time. Although we will be drawing on experience with college women in this paper, we postulate that these formulations will hold up as well or better for other women of this age. We will be taking a somewhat arbitrary slice out of what we see as an ongoing, expanding, and fluctuating process that ebbs and flows in response to life conditions. Development of the core relational self, as we see it, cannot be described within the confines of standard epigenetic theories. Such theories paint a picture of development as a discrete series of stages, each of which represents a developmental advance over previous stages (Freud, 1905; Erikson, 1950; Sullivan, 1953; Alexander, 1963). Evidence of continuing patterns from an earlier stage is often considered a sign of regression or retarded development. By contrast, we are describing a much more fluid and interconnected process in which early modes of being become the base for a continuation and expansion of the relational self.

THEMES IN THE LITERATURE ON ADOLESCENCE

In the literature on adolescence, the most prominent current models of growth pose a dichotomy between self-differentiation and interpersonal connection. It is as if these were mutually exclusive human processes (Benedek, 1979; Slaff, 1979; Gilligan, 1979, 1982). This view of development is buttressed by several broad themes embedded in the literature. One theme, stemming from early Freudian tenets, holds that a primary task of late adolescence is the consolidation of an autonomous identity via a process of increasing disconnection from internal and external primary love objects (Freud, 1905; Deutsch, 1944, 1967; Blos, 1962, 1979; Galenson, 1976; Ritvo, 1976; Erikson, 1968). Deutsch and Blos are prominent among those who describe adolescence in terms of a "loosening of affectionate ties," "emotional disengagement," and "severing" of family bonds. And when talking about late adolescent girls in particular, they stress a maturational demand to turn away from the early mother–daughter relationship.

A second theme is that of the "firmly-bounded" self. Blos was the first to posit a "second individuation" process, at the close of which the adolescent should have attained a distinctly separated self, with firm demarcations between self and others. Following from this, theorists have typically described as regressive and pathogenic the very same continuity of mother–daughter closeness and mutual identification that we believe enhances a daughter's maturation (Jones, 1935; Lample de Groot, 1960; Deutsch, 1967; Blos, 1962; Easser, 1976; Ritvo, 1976; Ticho, 1976). From Deutsch on, theorists have focused on a threat to feminine development inherent—as they see it—in the "regressive pull" of the internalized pre-oedipal mother. Further, they emphasize the role of this pull in the pathogenesis of such problems as promiscuity, infantilism, or sexual inhibition.

These formulations about the firmness of self-boundaries and the repudiation of early maternal ties are now being questioned in relation to female adolescent development. Blos, for example, has acknowledged recently that "the adolescent girl tolerates ... a far greater fluidity between the infantile attachments to both parents and her adult personality consolidation" (Blos, 1980, p. 16). The girl, he states, "has never abandoned her preoedipal attachment to the mother as fully as the boy has. When blending these earliest attachments with oedipal passions, the girl's range of empathy broadens and her fluid potential for identification unfolds, going far beyond anything available to the male" (Blos, 1980, p. 19).

Although he now sees that sustained early mother–daughter attachments do play a role in the unfolding of positive capabilities, Blos, nevertheless, continues to locate these attachments in the pre-oedipal phase of development and to stress the part they play in the dynamics of female adolescent symptomatology. Basically, he does not see the mother–daughter relationship as a base for a *positive* relational mode of development, which also has evolved over time and is no longer to be characterized as "pre-oedipal." Thus this relationship's contribution is, on the whole, minimized, devalued, and not well described.

Finally, in the standard adolescent literature, conflict emerges as the key dynamic by which the "necessary" tasks of separation take place. To quote Blos: "... personality growth and psychological differentiation come about only through the elaboration of conflict and its transformation into adult personality structures" (Blos, 1980; p. 21). By contrast, we see conflict as one way of elaborating the continuity of connection to significant others. We would argue that the ability to engage in conflict, without losing touch with the more basic affirming aspects of these connections, is an important part of healthy development. The experience of conflict, then, must be understood as but one aspect of personality, which gains its meaning to the adolescent girl in terms of her inner relational self.

CONFLICT, CONNECTION, AND RELATIONAL GROWTH

In this sense, we see conflict as one mode of intense and abiding engagement, not as the leading edge of separation and disconnection. Conflict is a necessary part of relationships, essential for the changes that must be made so that the relationship and each person in it can change and grow (Miller, 1976). The intense affective quality with which conflict is expressed can represent a means by which young women work out differences within relationship, moving into a relationship to confront differences, not away from it. Disconnection, or separation, would more accurately be characterized by indifference, withdrawal, diffidence, or "false compliance." Further, the capacity to engage parents in conflict without disrupting the underlying qualities of care and commitment is an important step toward expressing this same stance within later adult relationships.

In our work, college women often demonstrate their wishes to keep conflict from distorting basic relational ties and to work out conflict within key relationships. One student, for example, had struggled throughout adolescence to be understood by her critical and anxious mother and to act so as to please her. This student was now considering a study trip abroad, a trip that she knew her mother would oppose. Her concern was with how she could go on this trip without damaging to her already fragile relationship with her mother. The issue was not how to manage the trip without her mother's consent, because she did have the means to do that. What was important was that the decision be resolved within relationship. She knew that if she chose to take the trip against her mother's wishes, her feelings of self-blame for upsetting her mother would far outweigh any personal gains that the trip might otherwise have offered. Thus, while this trip would have enhanced the student's vocational skills and her growing capacity to act in the world, the more basic gains in self-esteem and competence were linked to her ability to take care of the relational aspects of the endeavor.

It is important to perceive and to give proper weight to the desire to "take care" of relationships—as a valuable motivation—and not to leap to the conclusion that this was a "regressive pull." In addition, it is important to stress, again, that a large part of the young woman's sense of self-worth is based in her ability to take care of relationships— a basically very valuable mode of living that has to be weighed along with other factors such as the gains in experience afforded by a trip abroad.

We have found in our clinical work that conflict between late adolescent daughters and their mothers is typically encapsulated around specific issues that can coexist with the feeling that "my mother is my best friend," a feeling reported by a number of women students. For example, in structured interviews done with students at Wellesley College as part of a project exploring women's development, the majority of women identified their mothers as the most important person in their lives.

At times, conflict serves as a test of these relationships. The adolescent daughter wonders: Can I remain emotionally connected to my parents as my own views and values grow to differ from theirs and as I expand my own capabilities and relational involvements? In part, the adolescent is testing whether her parents can evolve in their relationships with her in keeping with her mode and tempo of growth. This suggests, though it is seldom explored in the literature, that successful resolution of adolescent–parent conflict requires flexibility in the parent as well as in the child (Fulmer et al., 1982). It may be that much of the conflict that emerges during this time results from the fact that the parents are fixed on earlier, more controlling modes of relationship, which contrast with the daughter's age-appropriate expansion of spheres of ability and competence.

The student described above, engaged in resolving conflict so as to minimize further damage to her relationship with her mother, had a number of close women friends and a steady boyfriend of several years' standing. From our clinical and educational experience with college women, we have found that there is generally a correlation between a daughter's fundamental core of connection with her parents, even in the face of conflict, and a healthy capacity for relationships with her peers. The consistent dynamic remains that of being in affective connection with the other and establishing a basic mutuality of concern, even if that concern is expressed in conflicting ways.

This pattern represents a contrast to those women students who are disengaged and affectively separated from their parents. This disengagement often has its beginnings early in life, highlighted by the daughter's increasing sense of estrangement from her family, and resulting in a growing emotional distance between them. Rather than conflict, there is a paucity of emotional connection, with the daughter taking pains to minimize contact with her parents. These women who "have nothing to say" to their parents are, by and large, the most inhibited and constricted in their movement toward evolving new and intimate relationships with their peers, and they are most uncertain of their own capacities as relational beings. As one of these students put it, "I have no idea how to go about making friends here." For this student, emotional separation from the family occurred in the context of an *absence* of conflict, and resulted in a significant lowering of self-esteem and general well-being. In clinical work with women who are disengaged in this way, it is still important to see how much the lack of a growth-promoting relational context has hurt them and to help them work toward developing such a context—rather than seeking only more separation (Miller, Chapter 1, this volume).

For healthy development of college-age women, then, a basic sense of affective connection with one's parents remains the core out of which a positive sense of relational self-esteem emerges. Students able to become affectively connected to others remain in internal dialogue with their parents' beliefs and values, regardless of their ultimate degree of acceptance of them. Mother at times serves as a model of caring and concern, or as the base for a form of "practicing" (Mahler, 1972) involving differentiation of self within a basically connected context. The relational *process* between parents and daughter becomes a formative model in the daughter's evolving relational self.

THE COLLEGE SETTING

In a residential college setting late adolescence can be seen as a time of rapid evolution of a student's relational matrix, with a sudden and developmentally arbitrary break in daily contact with parents and home. The adolescent is confronted with a dual relational task: maintaining a continuity of relationship with family under conditions of distance and less commonality of experience, and evolving ways of finding people in the new network (students, faculty, staff) to supplant some of the relational roles previously filled by parents and longtime friends.

The context in which these dual tasks occur is significant. College is defined as a time for academic pursuits, almost always seen as competitive success as measured against one's peers (Sassen, 1980). And yet the college years are also times of rapid consolidation of female friendship and intensification of sexual relationships. Within self-in-relation theory the task for the college woman is to build on parental and peer relationships so as to enhance her sense of self as a competent and able being, thus becoming empowered toward the fullest utilization of her abilities.

While empowerment emerging out of relationships is also a developmental aim during the high school years, the situation then is quite different. The high school girl remains in proximity with her parents and close friends of many years' standing. These relational ties can be strengthened by, as well as supportive of, her achievements. In other words, actions and strivings during the high school years can serve to enhance rather than threaten most relationships. Further, parental approval of her accomplishments can leave a daughter with the sense of giving to her parents and of being in a situation of mutual affirmation that is a central component of her self-image. (There are other, countervailing forces during adolescence, but they will not be discussed now because the main focus here is on the change in conditions with the move to college (Miller, Chapter 1, this volume; Gilligan, 1982).

However, much of this is altered when the daughter goes to college. Parents often intensify their concerns about their daughter's level of achievement and choice of a major, applying increased pressure on her to do well and provide for her own economic future. A number of students in recent years have sought counseling out of concern, in part, with the conflicts between following a course of study consistent with their own wishes or pursuing a course that is more in keeping with parental pressure. Inevitably, their question is not "what to major in" but how to fulfill their own aspirations without damaging their ties with their families. Distance from parents and the absence of the mutuality of daily experience often intensify this dilemma and its subsequent burden on the student.

The academic setting may create conditions that lessen the student's capacity to grow intellectually through mutually supportive and validating relational connections. To the extent that schools emphasize grades and competitive endeavors, students come to feel that learning is a private matter, that sharing of ideas may lessen their competitive stance vis-a-vis others, and even that sharing their academic status with friends may disrupt feelings of trust and support. This can have several results. For one, it increases students' isolation from others, curtailing their opportunities for relational enhancement, especially relational enhancement as it is intertwined with intellectual growth and empowerment. For another, the college environment tends to segment student's experiences into the "personal" topics of interest and of real meaning to them versus the "academic" topics that are the focus of their classroom studies. This division can result in a narrow approach to learning, cut off from students' broadest realms of curiosity and inquiry, which are in fact the wellsprings from which the deepest learning occurs. This explains why many women students feel invalidated even in the face of academic success and diminished in self-esteem to the extent that their successes have cut them off from avenues of relational growth. For example, Locksley and Douvan (1979) have documented that adolescent girls with high grade point averages (GPAs) show more depression and more psychosomatic symptoms than do a similar group of boys, or girls with lower GPAs. We think the basic contradiction between the heavy pressure for individual, competitive achievement and women's motivations for action within a relational context may underlie these kinds of findings.

Relationships with faculty members can also contribute to this process. Faculty members can be a source of personal validation for students in their work, such that academic studies become an integral part of human connections. This does occur, but unfortunately it is too often limited only to a few very successful students. For others, steps they may take to reach out for connection to faculty members can be seen by teachers as signs of the students' dependency or neediness rather than as the legitimate seeking of connection. Thus students feel that their own academic work neither brings them closer to the adults in their college setting nor contributes in any mutual way to the intellectual development of individual faculty members.

SOME PRACTICAL APPLICATIONS

Self-in-relation theory suggests some of the pathways by which the college environment may contribute to the relatively high incidence of depression and bulimia currently found in college-age women in this country (Weissman & Klerman, 1979; Stangler & Printz, 1980; Wechsler et al., 1981; Halmi et al., 1981; Halmi, 1983; Pope et al., 1984). In particular, college can exacerbate certain dynamics that have been identified as key aspects of clinical depression in women, including low self-esteem, vulnerability to loss and inhibition of assertive action and of anger (see Kaplan, Chapter 2, this volume). Women students tend to be cut off from key relational sources of self-esteem, while they identify with a college ethic that often devalues these sources. Instead, as they struggle toward the more valued goals of independent endeavor and competitive achievement, they believe that they are doing what they "should be doing," but somehow they find themselves feeling worse and worse.

The experience of one young woman, Ann, offers an example. Ann was a 19-year-old junior on leave from a small, previously all male, elite college. Throughout her childhood, her parents had shared her view of herself as "self-confident" and "self-motivated." As a result, they refrained from offering her what they saw as unnecessary and unwanted support, guidance, and encouragement. Ann had felt alienated and misunderstood because of their lack of involvement, but during her high school years she had close friends to whom she could turn for the validation and support that was missing at home.

Her situation changed dramatically in college. Ann lost the sense of mutual understanding with her old friends, while the norms of her college impeded her ability to seek new relationships as a source of self-affirmation. She felt she "had to focus on work . . . I couldn't have feelings or need people. . . . It was easier to be distant from people than feel the pain of what I needed but didn't think I could get." In this context, Ann developed feelings of shame and confusion. She then blamed herself for these feelings, leading to further loss of self-esteem and culminating in the depression that precipitated her year's leave and brought her to therapy.

Contrary to the traditional emphasis in psychotherapy with adolescents on separation from the family, the major task here was to allow a new parent–daughter dynamic of closeness to develop, involving open sharing of each other's needs and fears as well as open acknowledgment of differences. On the basis of feeling her relational needs validated in the therapy, Ann was able, in a family meeting, to express to her parents that her wish for "continued guidance" from them represented a need for recognition, not a "dependent need for them to give her the answers." Ann's mother responded by sharing her feeling that Ann was the family member by whom she always had felt most understood. Ann, deeply moved, smiled through her tears and expressed her sense of affirmation at hearing this. This exchange was a turning point for Ann's establishing mutually rewarding affective connections with her family and subsequently with new friends. Concomitant with her seeking new ways of being with others, Ann began to experience a renewed sense of self-worth and self-confidence.

This student's experience is a good illustration of how emotional difficulties can develop when young women's basic relational needs are not given recognition and avenues for development or are misinterpreted as dependent behaviors. We can see that the college setting can include conditions that undermine women's optimal mode of growth and that promote pathology. Ameliorating these conditions would require a fundamental examination of the assumptions upon which all educational institutions are based—assumptions that devalue relational paths to learning and growth. Such an examination could, in turn, lead to new programs designed to promote a relational path of self-development.

Late adolescence is an important period in the development of women's core relational self-structure. Charting the course of development during this phase involves identifying and describing the paths by which the young woman's relational self grows in complexity, flexibility, sensitivity, and adaptability. The many planes along which this growth occurs include (1) an increased potential for entering into mutually empathic relationships characterized by being able to share one's own affective states and to respond to the affect of others; (2) relational flexibility, or the capacity to permit relationships to change and evolve; (3) an ability and willingness to work through relational conflict while continuing to value the core of emotional connection; and (4) the capacity to feel more empowered as a result of one's inner sense of relational connection to others, particularly to mothers. As illustrated further in the following paper, the relationship between a late adolescent daughter and her mother is often characterized not by disengagement but by qualities of mutual empathy, understanding, acceptance, and forgiveness. This ongoing, albeit changing, engagement between mother and daughter is a crucial aspect of women's self-development during late adolescence.

Thus, the late adolescent woman does not develop "out of" the relational stage, but rather adds on lines of development that enlarge her inner sense as a relational being. This process occurs within a desire for continuity of core emotional connection to family members.

Daughters and Mothers: College Women Look at Their Relationships

NANCY A. GLEASON

Kaplan and Klein have provided a framework for a relational model of the psychological development of women in late adolescence, specifically in the college years. My paper offers an example of this model as it describes a specific project designed to explore and elucidate the relationships college-age women have and aspire to with their mothers.

In the fall of 1983, the Stone Center offered Wellesley students the opportunity to join a Search-Research Group (which I will describe shortly) entitled simply "Daughters and Mothers." The preliminary sign-up yielded 30 students—demonstrating far more interest than any other topic for these groups before or since. Because of the numbers, we divided into two groups. I will report on the work of one of these groups.

After defining the Search-Research Group, I will describe the three phases of the work of this particular group—first the exploration by the members of their own relationships with their mothers, then the expansions of that inquiry through a survey of other students, and finally the compilation and analysis of the results of the survey.

SEARCH-RESEARCH GROUPS

The Search-Research Group is a unique concept originated by the Stone Center (and especially Janet Surrey) in 1981 to "foster conditions whereby women's experiences and learning styles can be validated and translated into active learning projects." At least three such groups have been offered each year, covering such topics as eating patterns, the experience of minority women, procrastination, relating to men, women and sports, and living with alcohol. Meeting weekly in a group, students explore and learn about the subject as they learn about themselves. Each member becomes her own expert. The group itself lends support to this process of exploration, sharing affectively and

Nancy Gleason, M.S.W., is a Senior Social Worker at the Stone Center Counseling Service, and Director of Project WAIT (Wellsley Alcohol Informational Theater).

cognitively in the relational setting. The "leader" essentially sustains the process and is a learner with the others.

Following the "search" phase, those interested students continue with a "research" or action phase of their choosing. The personal interest becomes an academic pursuit and a bridge is formed between subjective, experiential learning and objective, academic discipline. Thus, for example, the first "Eating Patterns and Weight Control" group did a survey of student attitudes and behavior, while the second developed and negotiated with the college a healthy eating program (which continues to this day).

THE SEARCH

In the "Daughters and Mothers" Search-Research Group the themes that emerged included th. qualities the students valued in the relationship, such as closeness, friendship, trust, and the wish for approval. Daughters perceived their mothers' pain in "letting go." They wondered if patterns were repeated from generation to generation, and some talked with their mothers about their mothers' own experiences as daughters. Fighting and arguments were mentioned infrequently, as were extended rifts. Changes in the relationship over time were noted in the past and anticipated for the future, but these changes reflected different needs mother and daughter might have for each other rather than disruptions. Some members discussed their awareness that their mothers needed them, and three students came together in their discovery of the supportive role each maintained with her mother around the need to care for another member of the family who was ill. They were concerned with the effect of stress on communication in the family but were aware, too, of a healing process that not only brought people back together but seemed to strengthen the bond.

At the end of most meetings, we stopped for 5 minutes to write. These writings constitute an informal journal of the group. In one meeting, for example, people talked about an underlying understanding with their mothers—they called it "reading between the lines"— that seemed to help them know how to act within the relationship without threatening it. One student wrote of that session: "I had never realized before how little my mother and I actually fought. Stress usually found an outlet in some other way; we often would sit down with a cup of tea and talk about it."

The most frequently repeated theme in these writings was the expectation that the relationship would continue and, in all likelihood, would grow. Roles might change, as might the quality of their "friendship." Issues creating strain between parent and child might differ, but the basic affiliation would be expected to continue. One daughter wrote: "In the next five or ten years I am quite sure that I will be depending on her for advice and support as I define my goals in life and begin to establish myself either in a career or possibly in a marriage. I want to stay close to her, as I always have been, but I know that I have to develop a certain distance from her as a mother. Of course she will always be my mother, but if our relationship grows to incorporate two adults instead of one child and one adult, I will be satisfied. A fine balance exists between a concerned mother, who can be resented by a child/adult (me) for interfering, and a concerned friend who lets that person know that she is there if needed. I don't want to lose the strong emotional bond with my mom, but I do want us to be close as friends—and I think she knows this."

Members expressed the wish, in different ways, that their mothers would forgive their actions when necessary in their love, acceptance, and approval of the daughter. "There is a real need still, and I can't rationalize it away, to tell my parents. I don't usually want their advice but I need to know that they still like or accept me." Another wrote: "The issue of testing the unconditional love that a mother and father give seems to be very important to me right now. I want them to know that I can handle this (difficult situation) on my own, yet somehow I still need them to approve. I feel as if I have violated their trust in not sharing this large part of my life—and I guess what I am afraid of is that they will feel betrayed. Their acceptance of my ability to deal with my own problems means even more to me than their acceptance of (my actions)." Another expressed concern about her mother, "knowing that she will always love me, but will she like me?" Still another reported that, for her, "approval is important—I like that reassuring feeling I get when I say something, and they say, 'Darling, we trust you.'" Students wrote that they often feel apologetic or embarrassed for wanting approval. If autonomy is the goal, searching for approval would appear regressive. There was no suggestion here, however, that regression was occurring.

The daughter may be aware of ways in which her mother adapts to her growth, usually without discussion. "As I've grown up and become more mature, I've found that my mother has been surprisingly accepting, so much so that I haven't realized until later that I've changed, that she's noticed and that she misses me." These daughters do not feel smothered or trapped by their mothers—struggling to get free and go their own ways.

We must now ask whether the students who chose to participate in this group had unusually strong attachments to their mothers. Was their commitment to the relationship atypical? Did the culture of the group encourage positive statements contrary to actual feelings? As one student wrote, "One of the things that I most enjoy about this Search-Research Group is that I always seem to leave feeling very good about my family." Might it have been otherwise? The results of the research should shed some light on these questions.

THE RESEARCH

Three students chose to continue on to the research phase, making a commitment to creating a survey, disseminating it, and tabulating the results—a major undertaking in one semester while carrying a full academic course load. In designing the survey, the students decided to focus on whether the mother–daughter relationship changed during the daughter's college years. We wondered whether entering students would experience intensification of early adolescent issues, leading to a need for some distance, that would abate into more comfortable relationships as the students aged or, conversely, that leaving home more recently would intensify the wish for closeness. With this in mind, we chose to survey 100 freshmen and 100 juniors selected by random sample.

In order to measure closeness in the relationship as it currently exists, we asked about frequency and duration of telephone contact and about subject matter discussed. We asked whether mother and daughter missed each other when separated. We asked about unspoken sensing of each other's moods. Then we asked respondents to look ahead 5 years after college and portray their idealized relationship with their mothers in terms of identification, closeness, roles, and values. Finally, we asked respondents to answer two open-ended questions—"What is especially important to you in your relationship with your mother?" and "How would you like to change the relationship you have with your mother?"

Ninety-seven of the 200 surveys, or nearly 50%, were returned by 52 juniors and 45 freshmen. This constituted a statistically representative sample of these two classes and slightly less than 5% of the total student body. To our surprise, no statistically significant differences were found between freshmen and juniors. Juniors call home as often, discuss the same subjects, and seem to be as close to their mothers as the freshmen.

The typical student talks with her mother once a week for between 15 and 30 minutes. Calls are initiated equally by mother and daughter.

The daughter talks about daily happenings (her own and her mother's), about family members, and about academics. In these phone conversations, she rarely talks about disagreements, intimate relationships, sex, or, surprisingly, money. She tells her mother more about her life than her mother reveals of hers. She feels closer to her mother than to her father, her siblings, or to anyone but her best friend. (But the relationship with her mother does not appear to interfere with that with her best friend.) When at Wellesley, she misses her mother at least occasionally and worries about her as well. She is also likely to be glad to be away. However, as she describes it, her mother misses her considerably more, is rarely glad to have her away, and is more likely to worry about her than the reverse. We really do not know whether this is an accurate perception on the daughter's part or the expression of her sense of her mother's involvement with her as she has moved away from home.

Response to the question about sensing moods without being told was striking. Sixty-five students, more than two-thirds of the respondents, report that they often sense their mothers' moods. Only one student never does. Fifty-seven, or slightly less than two-thirds, believe that their mothers often sense their daughters' unspoken moods, as opposed to three who never do. It is not clear if this is merely the familiarity of spending years together or a particular alliance in this dyad.

Looking ahead 5 years after graduation, few students anticipate asking their mothers to help them raise their children, while most anticipate caring for their mothers if needed. Most expect to understand their mothers better when they, too, are mothering. They do not, however, expect to discuss the personal concerns with her any more or less than they do now, to be more honest with her, or to fight more openly with her than they do now. In sum, these relationships are ongoing, changing perhaps, but not ending or even diminishing.

THE COMMENTS

The two open-ended questions—"What is especially important to you in your relationship with your mother?" and "How would you like to change the relationship you have with your mother?"—repeatedly elicited the themes we have noted already.

Of the 80 who described what was especially important to them, 69 used strongly positive terms, with relational words such as "closeness," "trust," "acceptance," "caring," "love," "openness," "confiding," "sharing," "enjoyment," "support," and "friend"; as well as such phrases as "we can talk about anything," "there when I need her," and "we respect each other." Responses ranged from effusive—"She is very understanding and extremely special. We enjoy each other's company. We share great times, wonderful memories. . . we communicate"—to more cautious—"The fact that she cares so much about me. Although it's hard for me to open up to her, I know she's always ready to listen to me and help me if I ask her to. She is extremely respectful of me as an individual. She doesn't try to manage my life. She's not at all detached from me."

Only one student described no caring for her mother—"I don't really have a relationship with my mother. I haven't lived with her since I was 15. . . ." The remaining ten reported less comfort, more distance, or more tension with their mothers. "I feel that we both attempt to understand one another even though we totally disagree with each other. We also try to refrain from putting too many expectations on the other." Another wrote: "I wish I could understand her better (and she, me) but she is from such a different background and we are so different. I wish I could accept her more for what she is because I know she loves me and is not perfect." One said that what was important to her was "confidence—brutal honesty at times; harsh; ultimate forgiveness after extended periods of torture. Stability, someone who knows me. No explanations necessary. She knows me."

To the second question—"How would you like to change the relationship?"—13 chose not to answer and 18 stated that there was nothing they wished to change. They liked the relationship as it was. The responses of two suggested serious difficulties that created problems in the relationship.

Thirty-eight, nearly two-thirds of the remaining, stated in one way or another that they would like more closeness, greater openness, trust, or friendship. The direction of their interest is in more relationship, not less. "I wish I could talk a bit more freely and openly with her, although we do get along very well." "I would like to be able to discuss more personal types of things with her, such as my sexual relationship."

In contrast, only six explicitly desired less involvement with their mothers. "She sometimes leans too heavily on me. She forgets that I get upset about family problems and that it makes me feel even worse now that I am away." (This student also liked the fact that her mother "treats me as an equal, respects my opinion and asks my advice.") "I have been very close with my mother—to an extent that it has affected my personal growth. I/we have to become more autonomous." Another would like her mother to back off. "I wish that my mother would become more independent and have more of "a life of her own."

She is bright and creative but has put her own interests aside to raise her children. I feel that as soon as she reestablishes her independence, she'll be able to accept mine." Finally, "I would like to be completely independent of her so that I can make my own mistakes and then ask her about stuff, rather than having her try to prevent me always. I appreciate it sometimes afterwards, but the times I do not tend to seem more prominent in my mind."

Most describe the changes they would like as a responsibility shared by mother and daughter. "Not having my little quirks bother her so much" expresses one student's wish that her mother would be more accepting. Another would like to "be somewhat more open about my innermost feelings, emotional, sexual, etc." More students place the burden of change on their mothers' attitudes but a number are ready to risk being more open as a route to greater closeness.

Kaplan and Klein see conflict between mothers and daughters as compatible with the closeness described above and suggest that dealing with conflict serves to maintain the engagement between the two. While we did not explore this issue specifically, our results suggest that the daughters want to resolve conflict and will work to achieve resolution, but that expressing anger or arguing does not feel like a means to that end. Those few who specifically refer to open expression of conflict see it as a threat to the relationship. Five state they are grateful that it is *not* a problem. "I enjoy her company and we hardly ever fight." "We rarely fight and that's important to me."

Eight who complain about anger or fighting would like to argue less. "Less fighting and more mutual comprehension," is what one student wishes for. Another gives more insight into the process: "I wish we could have a greater tolerance for each other's fallibilities and weaknesses. We can make each other very angry at times for not fulfilling our internal standards for each other. Because of this, we are reluctant to confide our problems at times and to trust each other." These daughters are not backing away from their mothers but are seeking other ways to resolve conflicts. Resolution, then, is sought within the context of the relationship.

SUMMARY

We have heard the voices of college women not in pain—voices that we who are therapists do not often hear. These women may have concerns they wish to negotiate with their mothers, but at the same time their energies are directed toward growth within the relationships with their mothers. In this study this pattern does not change between freshman and junior years, nor do the daughters anticipate any lessening of the ties. Changes are sought in the quality of the relationship as the daughter matures and sees herself as adult. She looks to mutual adjustment between them as her mother accepts her maturity; maturity alters the balance but not the closeness. No suggestion was made by any student that her relationship with her mother interfered with her forming other relationships. As she sees herself maturing and her relational network expanding, the daughter feels her interest pulling her toward her mother.

At the same time, these daughters want to be loved, approved of, trusted, and supported. They want to talk more, not less, and about intimate topics, including sex. And they want their mothers to do likewise.

We asked earlier in the paper, after reporting on the statements of the group members in the search phase, if these statements were atypical, representing a self-selected group with unusually positive feeling about their mothers or reflecting a culture in the group that encouraged positive statements. The answer seems clear, at least for a significant segment of young college women. The results of the survey are strikingly consistent with and confirming of the statements of the members of the group. We still cannot know, however, whether those who did not return the survey have a different outlook.

While not addressing the above question, another way to examine these results would be to repeat the study with women in coed colleges and women not in college. We do not know whether women who choose Wellesley College are more closely identified with their mothers, or at least more comfortable with their womanhood. We might ask whether Wellesley women, because they have achieved academic success, have less need to compete with or deny the attachment to their mothers. Within the scope of this group and this study, we have strong evidence of a model of development in which the closeness of the mother is enriching and empowering, where mutuality enhances the relationship, and where striving for "independence" is strikingly absent.

The following quotation, written by one of the students in the group, describes the evolutionary process of growth and change in the relationship through adolescence:

"Perhaps the best way to summarize my feelings about my mother is to use an analogy a religion professor told me about religion. He said that true faith in a religion is to listen to the tenets, and agree with them. Then, gradually you realize that you doubt some of the tenets, so you come to disagree with the tenets. Somehow, after a period of questioning, you come to believe the tenets in a new way. Then a new level of belief is reached. This growing process occurs throughout your life. So, too, I can feel this with my mother. When I was young, I never questioned what she said to me. Perhaps when I began college I began to doubt what she said and then the arguments began. Gradually, I answered the questions about values and thought processes I had raised and came to believe in her in a new way. It's not that I don't believe in my mother anymore; it's just that she doesn't always know how I feel about everything and I don't always agree with her philosophy. Deep down, there is a lot of trust in one another."

These papers were presented at a Stone Center Colloquium in February 1985.

II

APPLICATIONS

8

The Meanings of "Dependency" in Female–Male Relationships

IRENE P. STIVER

In this paper I will be examining the role of dependency in relationships between women and men. As the title indicates, this will involve exploring the meaning of the word *dependency*, a relational term. I hope to demonstrate how unclear is its meaning and how differently it has been used in different contexts. In particular, I would like to make the point that it is a term that has acquired such pejorative connotations precisely because it has been considered for so long to be a feminine characteristic. I will then attempt to speculate about why women and men have trouble depending on each other and the modes they have taken to be gratified and to defend against the gratification of their needs. My focus will be on women and men in heterosexual relationships, although I believe many of the observations can be applied to women and men in their lives in general.

In considering women's and men's struggles around dependency, we see how each sex adapts differently and each fares better or worse in some settings than in others. The capabilities for working and loving, as Freud said, are the hallmark of mature adulthood. Yet women and men are both limited in different ways in the development of these capabilities. While men may have been said to manage better at work and women seem more expert about love, we shall see that conflicts around dependency interfere with the optimal functioning of both women and men in *both* work and love.

THE DIFFERENCES IN WOMEN'S AND MEN'S EXPERIENCE

For women, their sense of femaleness seems jeopardized by the expectations of how they ought to behave at work; for men, their sense of their maleness seems jeopardized by what is required to establish close interpersonal relationships. Women in work situations experience considerable dissonance between the expression of such interpersonal qualities as nurturance, emotionality, and empathy and what they see as the qualities expected of them to succeed at work—namely drive, ambition, and competitiveness.

The conceptualization presented in recent writings on female development—that a woman's sense of self is a relational one and that her need to feel related to others is a crucial aspect of her identity (Miller, 1976; Gilligan, 1982; Surrey, Chapters 2 and 3, this volume) —allows us to understand why women are so threatened when there is the danger of alienation from both men and women, something they often experience in the work arena. At "home" and in other interpersonal settings, a woman's relational self seems to serve her better. To be attentive to the needs of others, to want to connect with others, to be expressive of feelings—all these presumably allow her to feel more comfortable with herself. We shall see, however, that it is not quite this simple.

Men at work usually experience the demands to be competitive, to suppress emotions, and to maintain an impersonal attitude as syntonic with their sense of themselves as men. One needs to question how adaptive these qualities are, even in the working arena, since it is an interpersonal context; still the more successful a man is at work, the more manly he feels. The pressures to demonstrate self-sufficiency and independence as signs of adulthood allow men to tolerate possible alienation from others in the course of competitive work situations. Paradoxically, men are more accepted, more admired, and less apt to become alienated, the more they succeed at work (see Stiver, Chapter 13, this volume).

At "home," however, men's capacity to develop, express, and own qualities that facilitate close relationships and intimacy appears to conflict with their sense of themselves as "masculine," self-sufficient, and independent. To acknowledge a need for others, to be open about one's feelings, and to be sensitive and empathic with women are all apparently quite threatening to the sense of manliness for many men.

In a study of the images of violence that appear in stories written by college students to pictures on the Thematic Apperception Test, Pollack and Gilligan (1982) found statistically significant sex differences. Men see dangers more often in close personal affiliations than in achievement, and they construe danger to arise from intimacy. Women, on the other hand, perceive danger in impersonal, achievement situations and construe danger to derive from competitive success.

The danger men describe in their stories on intimacy is a danger of entrapment or betrayal—being caught in a smothering relationship or humiliated by rejection and deceit. The danger women portray in tales of achievement is danger in isolation—fear that in standing out or being set apart by success, they will be left alone. As people draw closer in pictures, the images of violence in men's stories increase; as people move further apart, violence in women's stories increases. The authors conclude that men and women experience attachment and separation in different ways and that each sex perceives a danger that the other does not see: men in connection, women in separation.

In the book *Couples in Collusion*, Willi (1982) describes the different ways in which women and men present themselves as they enter couples therapy. The "prototypic" woman is usually one who initiates the therapy, since she feels so dissatisfied, then takes on the role of the plaintiff, accusing her husband of indifference, lack of understanding, and oppression. She complains about raising the children alone and presents a range of physical symptoms, moodiness, and suicidal ideation. She seems clearly quite emotionally upset and expresses disillusionment in her search for intimacy and togetherness.

Willi acknowledges that in current psychiatric circles she could easily be labeled as "hysterical." Her complaints would be considered excessive, devoid of objectivity, and often as evidence of regressive and infantile behavior. She might then be called immature and dependent.

The "prototypic" male is described as resistant to therapy, because he feels marital conflict should not be open to a third party. Also, the man typically believes that voicing disputes in therapy only makes matters worse. He reacts defensively to the woman's complaints, controls his reactions, trivializes reproaches, and reduces points of argument to objective practical problems. Despite the woman's clear dissatisfaction, he is apparently content with the marriage and does not wish to make any changes.

Willi notes that the man's style of presenting himself in couples therapy does not seem as amenable to psychiatric diagnosis as does the woman's. There is no ready label of psychopathology in the man's presentation. Yet men have shorter life expectancy, they have higher incidences of serious psychosomatic difficulties and alcoholism, and they make more successful suicide attempts (Willi, 1982; Pleck, 1981). One could, of course, interpret the woman's behaviors as indications of strengths rather than of pathology. That is, she can be seen as putting more effort into the relationship by initiating couples therapy. She can ask for help, reveal weakness, and show more emotional openness. Finally, her reaction may reflect "feelings of desperation in the face of the emotional imperviousness of the man" (Willi, 1982).

Thus whether at "home" or abroad, women's "reality" or perception of the world based on a relational self-identity is frequently considered as pathological, or, at best, immature, and it is demeaned and often misunderstood. The importance of relationships to women and their need to be engaged with others are often seen as indicators of "dependency." Men's "reality," or perception of the world based on a model of independence and autonomy, is considered to be more normative and mature. It is rarely devalued, although it is as often misunderstood by both women and men. I believe it is this difference in perspective—in the cognitive and affective modes of entering relationships—that makes the notion of "dependency" so problematic.

DEFINING DEPENDENCY

One of the most difficult problems I had in writing this paper was to find a useful definition or some consensus about the meaning of the term *dependency*. Our own study group spent at least two long evening sessions struggling with this problem. We finally felt we were up against something both very elusive and highly value laden. A review of the literature is most confounding and more often infuriating than helpful. The most benign definition can be found in *Webster's New Collegiate Dictionary* (1971): The adjective *dependent* is defined as "relying on or subject to something else for support"; the noun *dependent* is defined as "one who is sustained by another or relies on another for support." So far not very value laden, but not especially helpful.

In the most recent *Psychiatric Glossary* (American Psychiatric Association, 1980a), dependency needs are defined as "vital needs for mothering, love, affection, shelter, protection, security, food and warmth; may be a manifestation of regression when they appear openly in adults." This is quite an array of needs to begin with, but note also the implication that to need *anything* in adulthood is "regressive." In the psychoanalytic model, dependency needs have their origin in the oral stage, the stage of the earliest attachment to the mother. Dependency needs in that context are synonymous with oral needs. The oral personality is, in fact, considered to be a dependent personality who has a fixation at this early stage and who consequently cannot move toward maturity. In clinical settings, patients who appear to be "dependent" on others (parents, spouses, therapists, etc.) are often described as "infantile," "helpless," and *feeling* too needy." Again, the message is that such feelings belong to childhood. In the *Glossary of Psychoanalytic Terms and Concepts* (American Psychiatric Association, 1980a), dependency is not defined at all. I then looked up *orality* and found that "oral conflicts . . . manifest themselves in specific character traits and abnormalities," of which dependency is listed along with "demandingness" as well as "restlessness, impatience, and curiosity." Other characteristics used to describe the oral personality are passive, helpless, and needy—terms used frequently to describe the more normative female in our culture.

I could not find a clear or consistent differentiation between pathological dependency and normal dependency except for some "quantitative" criteria, (e.g., "too dependent" or "too needy") to describe more disturbed states. Essentially, the prevailing belief seems to be that dependency needs belong in childhood, and if these needs, whatever they are, are not satisfied in childhood, they continue to exert influences in a negative fashion, either in the form of counterdependent personalities (Post, 1982) or more directly in the form of clinging, demanding, helpless personalities. I am not addressing here more disturbed indications of personal relationships seen in those men and women who experience boundary confusion and who are terrified of loss of self in these relationships. These are less expressions of "dependency," I believe, than of wishes in those who lack a cohesive self to fuse and merge with the other.

I submit that the pathological expressions of dependency are more a function of the underlying rage about unmet needs than of the "dependency" itself. Those who are called "too dependent" are often those who ask for help in a way that makes it very difficult to respond because of the communication of underlying rage at both self and others. When one is able to give a person the help he or she asks for, one usually experiences a sense of gratification and pleasure. When one feels, however, that no matter what one does, the other's discomfort is not allayed, one is apt to become angry and quickly label that person as "too dependent." To ask for help with underlying hostility, or with the conviction that one does not deserve anything, or with fear of refusal typically will result in failure to get one's needs fulfilled. There are others who ask for help in various guises but are unable to take or accept the support and help offered to them—a dynamic that also results in significant frustration and anger for both the person asking for help and the one attempting to respond. It is not the request for help, the turning to the other person, that is so problematic, but the ease and comfort with which one is able to identify what one wants and then ask for help. I believe both women and men have trouble with this.

Considering all the above, one notes that the term *dependent* has been used to describe a need state (longing, oral needs), an affective state (feelings of helplessness, neediness), a personality trait (dependent, demanding), and even a personality type (passive-dependent, oral). Other literature (Seligman, 1974) refers to "dependent" behavior as "learned helplessness" and/or as a strategy to engage others to do things for one or to please others who presumably expect childlike, dependent behavior. Sometimes it refers to behavior that involves counting on or relying on more than one person in order to get a job done.

An overview of these definitions indicates a lack of understanding of dependency and considerable influence of value-laden judgments. The prevailing assumption, despite inadequate definitions and data, is that women are more dependent than men. If men behave in a self-sufficient and independent fashion, it is because they *are* independent. If women behave similarly, they must be covering up a basic dependency—that is, they must be counterdependent. As an aside, let me say that I know that both men and women clinicians are aware of those men who are so defended against any expression of their passive longings that they develop psychosomatic ailments and/or manifest exaggerated expressions of independence and hypermasculinity. Yet the term *counterdependent* is not typically used in describing such men. For women, then, to be dependent and adult is usually understood as being immature, childish, and, at best, neurotic. In my clinical experience, I have not found women to be basically more dependent than men. Some women, however, have an investment in presenting themselves as "dependent." While there are many reasons for such behavior, primarily it allows them to become engaged with others and is the established mode of relating to men in the expectable direction. Men, we know, have their own investment in seeing women as being more dependent than they are. In a paper on female dependency, Lerner (1983) discusses how women's display of passive dependency often has a protective and systems monitoring function. That is, in the family system, the underfunctioning of one spouse can allow for the overfunctioning of the other. Thus the helpless, dependent stance of one partner has an adaptive, ego-bolstering effect on the other. For the woman to move out of this position is often perceived by others, and consequently by herself, as aggressive and hurtful. She may then hold on to or stay in the position of relative weakness in order for this most significant relationship to survive.

Men also need to be attached to others, to engage with others, and to have their needs met, but they have considerable difficulty acknowledging their needs openly. Men are, in fact, often very threatened by their own needs for connection and attachment; while disowning them, they also project them as undesirable qualities onto women.

MOTHERS AND SONS

That men have more difficulties in acknowledging their vulnerability, their needs for others, and feelings of helplessness has captured the attention of several theorists. Dinnerstein, in her interesting book *The Mermaid and the Minotaur* (1976), takes the position that because the first important figure in every child's life is a woman, special problems emerge for men and women. The man especially, however, in his efforts to achieve a different sexual identity, needs to repudiate powerful early experiences that encompass both exquisite joy in the early physical contact with mother and terror and rage associated with her imperfections and his inevitable disappointments at not having all his needs met. The child then needs to disown his powerful yearnings to recapture the early moments of ecstasy with his mother by seeing his mother and other women as outside of him and very different from him; he then projects onto them his terrors and rage associated with the earliest experiences of deprivation. As a consequence, women take on for him, unconsciously, powerful images of magical omnipotence and are seen as the source of ultimate gratification as well as of frustration and denial. According to Dinnerstein, the man struggles throughout his life to defend against temptation to give way to "voracious dependence" and to recover feelings of competence, autonomy, and dignity. As a consequence, his relationships with women embrace "both worshipful and derogatory feelings, grateful and greedy, affectionate and hostile feelings." Since the man attributes such great power to his mother, he must render all women powerless by keeping them in a dependent position, and he defends against acknowledging his longings to recapture early experience.

Rochlin presents a somewhat different model, more consistent with psychoanalytic theory. In his book *The Masculine Dilemma* (1980) his central thesis is that male development involves an energetic resistance to identification with the mother in the early years and that, throughout a man's life, his masculinity is "precariously held and endlessly tested." Because of the close interactions between little boys and their mothers, a feminine identification develops. But soon little boys discover their mothers do not have a penis and, therefore, are devalued; boys must struggle against such dangerous identification. Instead they must identify with the man, the father (also seen as the aggressor), as a means of asserting their masculinity and establishing pride in their manliness. He states that the boy's incentive to establish his masculinity is at odds with a compelling identification with his mother; the unconscious solution the boy reaches is to defend against the identification with his mother by repression. Given this precarious masculine identification, men must not allow any expression of what might be associated with femininity—for example, nurturance, sensitivity, or open statements of needs.

Both Dinnerstein's and Rochlin's theories suffer from oversimplification and reductionism. While each differs in what aspects of the early mother–son experiences are deemed so significant, they both assume a rather fixed and irreversible effect of these experiences on subsequent development, and both place the ultimate responsibility for the son's development on the mother. Neither acknowledges the process of change nor the ongoing dynamics of the mother–son and father–son interactions.

DIFFERENT DEVELOPMENTAL PATTERNS OF WOMEN AND MEN

The "self-in-relation theory" of female development (Miller, 1976; Gilligan, 1982; Surrey, Chapters 2 and 3, this volume) considers the mother's interactions with her children as part of a process of connectedness and differentiation. The theory states that female identity formation takes place in the context of an ongoing relationship, since mothers tend to experience their daughters as more like and continuous with themselves. This is the beginning of a particular bonding between mothers and daughters with expectations of mutual caretaking and mutual empathic interactions and interdependency. Daughters can then experience more continuity with their past relationships, such as early dependency on their mothers and on others, without seeing it as a threat to their "growth" or "maturity." In Chapter 3, a paper on the development of self in women, Surrey talks about the identification with mother as "mother," which contributes further to women's playing a more nurturant role than men in most relationships and becoming highly sensitive and vigilant to the nuances in interpersonal interactions. The daughter then develops early the capacity to flow back and forth between being the receiver of supplies, with an acknowledgment of an attachment and connection with the mother, and being the mother herself in her interactions as caretaker with her mother and others. This serves as a precursor to women's fluidity, moving back and forth as needed, between the roles of givers and receivers of support. At the same time, women often enough experience their mothers as devalued to contribute to their struggles to defend against their identification with them and their dependency on them. Despite this struggle, however, women typically continue to experience, consciously and unconsciously, strong connections with their mothers.

The dynamic of the mother–son relationship follows another developmental path. Mothers experience their sons as different from them and are under both inner and outer pressures to affirm this difference. The cultural expectations of how boys should be are internalized by many mothers; they believe that, in order to help their sons develop a strong masculine identification, they need to encourage aggressive behaviors and separate strivings. Thus sons have fewer opportunities than daughters to learn how to move back and forth in the giving and receiving dynamic of healthy interpersonal connections. However, a mother's sense that she must help her son achieve individuation and independence through pushing him away from her often conflicts with her natural inclination to maintain the attachment while affirming the differences between them. While the mother consequently feels very torn, the pressures to conform to social expectations are usually strongly supported by the father. I believe it is extremely important for fathers that their sons conform very early to a stereotypic notion of masculinity. Any signs of strong attachments to mother, of fearfulness, of not being aggressive or active enough, and so forth, usually evoke in the father fear that his son is a "sissy" (see Miller, Chapter 10, this volume). He typically reacts by treating his son with ridicule and contempt and becomes angry at the mother for presumably encouraging such unmanly behavior. Fathers' attitudes and behavior toward their sons then reinforce the pressures on the mother to push the little boy toward separation, and on the little boy to negate *his* wishes to maintain more open and continuous contact with his mother.

ADULT DEVELOPMENT

In reviewing the studies that have explored the process of becoming an adult, it is interesting that the major efforts to date have been about male development—for example, investigations by Levinson (1978) and Vaillant (1978). While both of these authors, in different ways, talk about the importance of interpersonal relationships for men and discuss their effect on overall growth, their studies are organized largely around the career development of men in their samples. For Levinson, the relationships with women are often seen as subordinate to the man's occupational growth:

> [for the man] in entering the adult world . . . occupation and marriage and the family are the components most likely to be given central importance. One task is to choose and follow an occupational direction that permits him to define important parts of himself. A related task is to form a marital relationship with a wife who supports his aspirations and is ready and able to join him on his journey. (p. 83)

Later he talks about how a man's energy is directed toward forming a dream and gratifying this dream. The "dream" is largely organized around achievement and acclaim in the eyes of the world. Finally, in the later state of "settling down," which Levinson refers to as "becoming one's own man," the man's effort is to be more independent and self-sufficient and less subject to the control of others; he notes that these goals are to be found at all stages of adulthood but represent the culmination of the "settling down" phase. Vaillant (1978) studied the lives of a sample of men over a 30-year period after they graduated from a highly competitive liberal arts college. He reviewed the lives of these men from the point of view of exploring ego defenses, or modes of adaptation, and established a hierarchy of defenses to help define adult mental health. Vaillant does recognize that close, loving relationships as children affect the capacity to love as adults, but his emphasis is again mainly on the career development of these men and the importance of gaining recognition by society. While concern with others is of interest, it often takes the form of more abstract societal concerns than that of intimate interpersonal relationships. It is important to note that there is not yet a well known long-term follow up study of women's journey into and through adulthood. Carol Gilligan's work on moral development in women, however, demonstrates how powerfully "the relational self" shapes the development of moral judgments for women (Gilligan, 1982).

In my own clinical experience, I am impressed over and over again with the differences between women's and men's experiences of work and love. Women with careers do not keep their lives at work and interpersonal connections outside of work very separate. When they talk about their work, it is typically in the context of personal relationships, past and present. Men, when talking about their work, seem more apt to split off thoughts, feelings, and concerns associated with their personal relationships outside of work, both past and present. In reading Theodore Reik's (1960) book *Sex in Man and Woman*, I came across this curious paragraph:

> A woman who cooks and cleans and brings up children, shops, dresses and undresses is rarely, in her thoughts and her emotional life, separated from her husband and lover. Almost everything she does or wants to do has some reference to him. A man in his laboratory or office rarely thinks of his wife while he works; she is psychologically as distant from his thoughts as if she lived on a far away island to which he sometimes transmitted his thoughts and feelings in moments of lessening attention during his work. He feels consciously or unconsciously as if this were the wrong thing to do, as if he had gone astray when he thinks of his wife or mistress while he works. What woman would have a guilt feeling when she, during her occupation as typist, secretary, nurse, etc., would sometimes think of her beloved man? And what man would not have sometimes a guilt feeling in the analogous situation? (p. 56)

While I think Reik was onto something, I do not think he appreciated the implications of his observations. That is, women do keep connected with the important people in their lives by more continuity of thoughts, and men, as a rule, are able to split off and shut out more effectively their personal connections with people outside of work. Again this illustrates the degree to which women function in the context of relationships—much more than most men. Reik's depreciation of women's emphasis on relationships reflects a general point of view in our culture—which values single-mindedness, "objectivity," task-orientation, and so forth without considering the importance of meaning and context. There is, then, a significant asymmetry in the developmental process that women and men follow as they move from their earliest relationships to their mothers and fathers, through adolescence, into adulthood. Men try to move from attachment to separation, to individuation and autonomy, with the goal of independence as the traditional sign of maturity and mental health. Women move from attachment to continued connection, always developing in the context of relationships; they experience the goal of "independence" as lonely and isolating.

SEX DIFFERENCES IN STYLES OF RELATING

Given these different lines of development, how can we understand the ways in which women and men attempt to establish relationships with each other? What strategies do they use to try to get their needs gratified? How do both sexes sabotage their efforts at gratification through significant disavowals of important aspects of themselves?

I would like to begin this part of the discussion with an examination of the common assumptions that (1) women are more dependent than men and (2) women experience these dependency needs as more syntonic than do men. If one reviews female—male relationships, it is apparent that men are usually better taken care of than women. Wives, as caretakers and nurturers, readily respond to their husband's physical and emotional needs. They cook their meals, clean their homes, do their laundry, and attend to their emotional needs by listening to them at the end of the day. This is so much within the realm of the traditional wife's "job description" that the man does not usually need *to ask* for these things; rather he has learned to expect them. He, in turn, is supposed to provide or take care of the woman's need for economic security and sometimes other more "physical" aspects of household maintenance. The fact that men are bigger and often stronger than many women contributes to the view of them also as protectors against dangers from the outside world.

This has been the traditional view. We all know there are many variations on this theme, and we have been seeing significant changes in this pattern over the past decade. We also know that women are not necessarily protected but sometimes are at great risk in their own homes (Carmen, Russo, & Miller, 1981; Herman, 1984). Still, in many marriages, it is the woman who plays the caretaking and nurturant role more than does the man—especially around the gratification of emotional needs. There are some data about depression in women and men as a function of their marital state which support the hypotheses that, in marriage, men are better taken care of than women and that women experience considerable underlying anger and despair as a consequence. Studies on depression consistently show that women become depressed more frequently than men (Radloff, 1975; Weissman & Klerman, 1977). However, among the single and widowed, men are more likely than women to become depressed (Briscoe & Smith, 1973). Women are more likely than men to become depressed during their marriage. Men are more likely than women to become depressed during marital separation (Radloff, 1975).

I believe that women and men both deny their needs to be taken care of, but for different reasons. On the one hand, men experience the acknowledgment of neediness as threatening to their sense of manliness; to need others is experienced as endangering their autonomy and independence. On the other hand, women experience their needs as expressions of selfishness; they feel they have to take care of others before attending to their own needs. A lifetime of training to put others ahead of themselves and to be sensitive to others' emotional states has not helped women to identify their inner need states nor to feel entitled to pursue their own gratification.

Responding to the needs of others does allow women some vicarious gratification. Through identifying with those whom they care for, they can experience indirectly some sense of gratification and fulfillment. There are, however, significant and unfortunate consequences of this strategy. Vicarious satisfaction is never a substitute for direct gratification, so that deep feelings of deprivation must emerge; in addition, it often involves the woman's projecting her needs onto others, which interferes with her ability to differentiate appropriately her needs from those of others. To be attentive to the needs of others without feeling the right to ask also that others respond to her would inevitably lead to feelings of envy and deep resentment. Considering how difficult it is for women to own and express their anger (see Miller, Chapter 10, this volume), a typical consequence is a sense of powerlessness and despair about their ability to have any impact on others. But even more important is the effect on a woman's self-esteem if she feels less entitled than everyone else to ask that others respond to her and if she feels that her anger is both unfeminine and dangerous. In a paper on intimacy, Miller (1981) presents an analysis of one family to illustrate how the wife/mother's depression was a consequence of her feeling second-rate and unworthy after years of suppressing both the examination and expression of her feelings and needs. A growing awareness of her dissatisfaction with her marriage only made her feel "selfish and horrible." These feelings served to maintain her in a more helpless and, therefore, dependent position, even though she was, in fact, responding effectively to others' needs more than her own.

"Dependency" as a Female Style of Relating

Earlier I mentioned the tendency for some women to present themselves as helpless and dependent as a way of engaging with others; but these are also expressions of how they feel about themselves. Women's low self-esteem comes from many sources: To put others first carries the message that one is less worthy. In addition, women do not usually have the opportunity or training to develop many of the skills needed to deal with the world, including more assertive modes of negotiation with others outside of the home. These "worldly skills" are valued in our culture much above the many skills involved in household management, childrearing, and other areas requiring empathic, sensitive interactions. Thus many women feel inadequate and lack confidence in their being able to cope without a man to help manage their lives. Often it is striking to note the incongruity between the profound lack of self-confidence expressed by some women and the objective signs of their effectiveness and competence.

One woman I see in therapy has returned to school since her children have grown; she is studying engineering and getting high grades. She also received a brown belt in karate, which she took up after she had been raped. She is personally very attractive, charming, and sociable, and she has a wide network of friends. As she struggles about deciding whether to divorce her husband, from whom she is separated, she worries about whether she will be able to manage. Her husband, she says, always said "I'll take care of it" to a notice about insurance, a legal issue, trouble with the car. She is afraid she could not manage these things herself. This same husband whom she feels will "take care of everything" also was physically abusive to her.

While women hold to this image of themselves as helpless and dependent, they are also deeply ashamed of it. They often feel there is something wrong with their being unable to manage alone, and they are guilty about burdening their husbands. Yet if one looks at the dynamics of many marital relationships in which the wife experiences herself as "too dependent" on her husband, one often sees that the husband is very much in collusion, supporting that dependency at the same time he grumbles about it.

The case of Diane is illustrative. She said in one therapy session that she was quite upset because her fear of driving her car alone for long distances was confronting her again. It was another sign of her inadequacy. Some years ago her husband had registered her car in another state, where they have a summer home. This arrangement required that the car be taken there periodically for inspection. The time had come again and, in this instance, he could not go and told her she had to do it herself. She was very reluctant and fearful, but too ashamed to admit it. After discussing it in therapy, she realized that she did not want her car registered out of state and instead wanted to take care of her own car and assume responsibility for it herself. She went home and told her husband just that. He said, "Great! It's been a nuisance for me! You take care of your own car now, but if anything goes wrong with your car," he admonished, "it's all your concern now." In other words, all or nothing. Nevertheless, she agreed. The following morning he got up very early and, without consulting her, left to reregister her car in the other state. While in the past she would have seen this as his making a sacrifice again to take care of her and put up with her neurotic symptoms, she had to recognize this time that he needed to keep her in a dependent position.

This last example points to the miscommunications between women and men when each sex has trouble examining, identifying, and expressing her and his needs. Women's skills at listening and empathizing allow them to respond readily to other's emotional needs. Men, since they have less experience in close personal relationships, are not apt to be sensitive to women's need states, whether spoken or unspoken. Thus the frequent lament: "What do women *want?*" or "Why can't a woman be more like a man?" Typically, men try to be helpful through adopting the more active mode—to *do* rather than to listen. It is easier for men to give material things and sometimes physical care that requires specific and concrete activity. Indeed, men can be very caretaking in these physical and material ways. Men also feel very threatened by the woman's expression of painful feelings, since they need to ward them off in themselves; thus the man often reacts with impatience and anger—which communicates again to the woman that her needs are not legitimate and that she is not worthy. Women, in turn, feel deeply frustrated when they know they are not getting what they need—that is, to be listened to, understood, affirmed—yet feel guilty because they are not at all clear that it is reasonable to want something different from what they are getting. Certainly when women feel deprived in all quarters, they are more apt to focus on their needs for physical and material signs of caring.

I believe that often the "demanding woman" who puts such emphasis on wanting more and more material goods may be "settling" for these when she is not even aware of how much her emotional needs are unrecognized and unattended. The underlying rage at unmet needs contributes to her pathological dependency on "things" over more personal concerns.

Rubin (1976) reports that working-class women, in response to what they value most in their husbands, will say, "He's a steady worker, he doesn't drink, he doesn't hit me," while middle-class women focus on issues of intimacy, caring, and communication. Yet one finds that one of the major factors contributing to depression in working class women is the *absence* of an intimate and confiding relationship with a husband or boyfriend (Brown & Harris, 1978).

Men's Self-Esteem Threatened by "Dependency"

Let us now examine some of the strategies men use to gain gratification of their needs and the frustration they encounter in the process. While men also deny their needs, we know that, as a rule, they are better taken care of than women. As long as the man experiences the caretaking as a "given," he has to acknowledge neither his own neediness nor the extent of his dependence on his wife. When events occur that disrupt these expectations, such as the arrival of children, then the man is confronted with changes in the care and attention previously experienced. It is not uncommon to hear of a husband's jealousy of the attention his wife directs toward a new baby, although again it is rarely acknowledged as such by the man. The more typical reaction is for the husband to become angry and either withdraw and detach from the family and/or to become more aggressively demanding, usually around issues displaced from the original needs.

An interesting study found that upper-middle-class fathers often were critical of their sons, devalued and ridiculed them, called them names like "little dumbo" and "peanut head," despite consciously expressed loving feelings toward them (Gleason, 1975). I believe that these fathers were very envious and resentful of their sons, who as children can openly show their needs for their mothers. One might speculate that these fathers find their own needs to be cared for as so alien to their sense of manliness that they hate that part of themselves and must disown it—so much so that when their sons express such needs, they are treated with contempt.

While women's denial of their needs has its source in a fear that they are too selfish or not worthy, for men the denial of their needs has its source in maintaining their self-esteem as based on a manly image in the eyes of the world—namely, other men. Thus it is extremely important for men to hide any sign of their neediness or vulnerability from others. The difference between the ways women and men respond to the breakup of a relationship is significant. The more typical response for women is to become sad and to isolate themselves as an expression of how alone and abandoned they feel; at the same time they also reach out very often to other women for support, revealing their pain to them. While men also experience such painful feelings at the end of an intimate relationship, they are rarely as apparent. Instead, they quickly move into brief sexual liaisons with different women in order to make the statement to the world that they are not feeling rejected or humiliated about the breakup. A male client reported after a recent breakup, "I no longer have to run around showing all my friends that I do not give a damn." As a consequence of therapy, he was able to acknowledge his sadness and to recognize that he had no emotional energy at that moment to connect with anyone else.

This brings us to the sexual arena, one in which men express their needs more openly. Our culture does allow men to be more explicit about their sexual needs since, again, they appear as "rights" divorced from emotional neediness. As long as men can experience their sexual needs simply as needs for physical release, they can feel entitled to expect women to be there for them sexually and not feel that this betrays any weakness in them. In listening to male clients talk about their sexual needs, one is often struck by how much their search for intimacy is primarily through the sexual experience. For many men, one of the few settings in which they can give expression to their needs to be given to and cared for and can experience deep feelings, and still feel manly, is in the bedroom. There the man can be at his macho and phallic best, while also allowing himself to be entitled to gratification of his needs for closeness and connection. We know that for some men the regressive pull is so enticing and so frightening that they need to split off entirely their tender and loving feelings. Men do report in therapy their yearnings to recapture the ecstatic experience of being enveloped by a woman, while at the same time feeling sexual and powerful.

A more complicated picture emerges when one examines how the woman reacts to any indications, explicit or implicit, of the man's need for her. As long as the woman feels her needs are not being met, she will, unconsciously at least, be resentful and hostile toward any expression of the man's neediness. I believe that is part of the reason why women sometimes resist responding to the man's needs in the sexual arena; it is because at some level they recognize the underlying meanings of his yearnings for nurturance and resent them. But as long as women experience their own neediness as shameful, they will have difficulty tolerating signs of dependency in men. The wish for the man to give them the strength they feel they lack is part of the woman's propensity to idealize the man, attribute great power to him, and feel disappointment when he deviates from the ideal. Interestingly, I have also found that women who realize that their needs to see men as so strong and powerful are unreasonable also are apt to accept more open signs of the man's vulnerability. They feel contemptuous, however, of the man who covers up his vulnerability with transparent bravado, as, for example, in the sexual arena.

Yet both women and men want to be needed by the people they care about. A woman experiences the need to be needed as part of her identity. Her self-esteem is enhanced when she experiences herself as a "giving" wife and mother. A man also wants very much to experience himself as a good husband and father and feels frustrated when the efforts he makes at trying to please are not appreciated.

In the final analysis, of course, in heterosexual relationships both women and men need each other; each sex suffers from shutting off and denying the needs and longings to be cared about. Each sex experiences anger and disappointment when these needs are not met. Women sacrifice the identification of their needs and acting on them because they do not want to be selfish. Men sacrifice the identification of their needs and acting on them because they depend so much on gaining the respect of other men and defend themselves against humiliation and rejection. Each is cheated as a consequence.

A NEW VIEW OF DEPENDENCY

In concluding, I will attempt a different definition of dependency from the ones we have heard—a definition which takes into account that "to depend" involves an interpersonal dynamic. I would like to define dependency as: A *process of counting on other people to provide help in coping physically and emotionally with the experiences and tasks encountered in the world when one has not sufficient skill, confidence, energy, and/or time.* I have defined it as a process to stress that it is not static but changes with opportunities, circumstances, and inner struggles. While the meaning of "physical" help may be more apparent—for example, actual physical support, economic support, feeding, caretaking of an ill or otherwise helpless person, and so forth—the meaning of "emotional" help needs further elaboration. I believe that what each of us requires emotionally from others is to feel affirmed and validated in our feelings and perceptions. This notion of dependency would allow for experiencing one's self *as being enhanced and empowered through the very process of counting on others for help.* In these terms, dependency would be seen as normal and growth promoting.

When, however, turning to others for help maintains one in a more static place, or worse, pulls one back to a position in which one feels awful about oneself and/or desperate about getting anything from the other, then pathological expressions of dependency emerge. Typically, such expressions of dependency are a function of a number of conditions—for example, an interpersonal dynamic in which one person needs to keep the other in a subordinate position, or relationships that mirror or reactivate early histories of severe deprivation and abuse.

One can see "healthy" dependency, then, as offering a context for growth and development. The more one feels one can count on others and be heard, understood, and validated, the more one feels worthy and the more solid is one's sense of self. Women have long played the role of listening and affirming with men, their children, and their friends. However, as long as they do not feel they have the right to want this for themselves, and as long as they feel their needs are not reciprocated, they will unconsciously sabotage their efforts to support those they love and resent demands made on them. Men, in turn, need more opportunities for emotional experiences in relationships so that they can become more empathic and begin to acknowledge their vulnerabilities and not feel ashamed of them.

In my therapeutic work with women, my focus is to help them not only to attend to and identify what is important to them, but also, even more crucially, to value their needs and inner feelings—what Jordan, in Chapter 4, refers to as "self-empathy."

When women can feel more free to express and communicate what they need from others, they will be less likely to become depressed and more able to respond in a less ambivalent fashion to men's expressions of dependency on them.

In my clinical experience with men, they show considerable relief when they realize that I recognize and appreciate their manliness because, and not despite, their growing capacity to reveal and express their fears, their sadness, and their loving feelings. Another intervention that can be very helpful for men is a couples group. In that setting a man can learn about himself in a relational context. He can feel validated by the other men in the group while at the same time learn from the women something about their inner feelings and their capacity to relate to others. In this larger group context, the man does not have to deal with the dangers he often experiences in the dyad of husband–wife interactions—in which issues of power and control often preclude the possibilities of being able to hear what the other person is saying or respond to the feelings expressed. Only if women and men can learn to accept and value their dependency on each other and assimilate it with positive self images will they be able to reach higher levels of adaptation and maturity.

This paper was presented at a Stone Center Colloquium in May 1983.

9

Relationship and Empowerment

JANET L. SURREY

Often when I speak about the relational self in women, people ask, "What about action, work, and creativity? A person has to be able to act, to work, to stand, and to move *on her own.*" Even among clinicians, our typical models of action tend to evoke the image of a single actor, agentic for her or his own interests, autonomously achieving, self-expressing, and self-maintaining. Relationships are something you *have* when you are not working or living your life, at night or on weekends. The idea of "doing" or "acting" or "working" appears to be separated from "relating" and, at best, relationships are seen as meeting needs for support, affection, and contact, and not as opportunities for action or growth. Further, we too easily fall into the trap of equating "relationship" with our "primary relationships" (this term also needs further exploration) and often with our sexual relationships. For most of us, however, much of our life activity occurs in a larger relational context—both formal and informal.

The notion that action occurs in a relational mode seems to challenge our usual perspectives or paradigms. Bakan (1966) described the two basic human modes of "agency" and "community," and I think this is still a widely held dichotomy. In Chapter 1, Jean Baker Miller wrote about "agency in community," and in our Colloquium Series she described the empowerment to act as a part of healthy interaction (Miller, 1986). Here I want to continue the examination of relationship and empowerment and to explore how women's early self-experience as connected *with* others ("self-and-other" or "self-with-other" experiences) can form the basis for shaping new visions of relational action, power, and movement: new visions that acknowledge the power inherent in "being together," "moving together," and "acting together."

In this paper, I will focus on the *motivational* and *action* components of our evolving self-in-relation model and on the concept of psychological empowerment as it relates to these aspects of women's development. Three questions will be explored:

1. What is *empowerment* and *empowering* in relationships?

2. What constitutes an *empowering relationship* or relational context? This allows me to talk about more than a two-person dyad.

3. How can we help to *create* and *support* relational contexts that facilitate women's empowerment? As a step toward this, I will give an example of a workshop designed to empower women to work for nuclear disarmament.

EMPOWERMENT IN RELATIONSHIP

Women and Empowerment

Why has the concept of empowerment become so popular, and why have we been using it increasingly over the past few years to describe this essential aspect of women's development? First, the use of this concept has encouraged a redefinition of traditional power models. In our first colloquium, Jean Baker Miller (see Chapter 11, this volume) proposed a use of the word *power* as "the capacity to move or to produce change," to replace the notion of power as dominion, control, or mastery, implying "power over." She suggested that women would have difficulty embracing a power model that involves competition or winning over others. "Empowerment" does not have such a connotation.

An alternate concept of personal power as inner strength and self-determination has appeared throughout the psychological literature (e.g., Rogers, 1975; Maslow, 1954), but this concept still evokes the image of the highly individuated self-actualizer. We have needed a different concept to suggest power with others, that is, power in connection or relational power. Thus we have talked about mutual empowerment (each person is empowered) through relational empowerment (the relationship is empowered).

Recently the concept of group empowerment has begun to appear in the community psychology literature (Rappaport, 1984) and in writing on methodologies for oppressed groups to gain political and social power (Freire, 1970). These writings describe widely diverse ends and means of empowerment. Rappaport (1984) has contributed a thoroughgoing review of the definitions and uses of the word and has suggested that empowerment is an evocative but not yet totally definable idea that varies among groups, settings, times, and purposes. For the present, I define psychological empowerment as: the motivation, freedom, and capacity to act purposefully, with the mobilization of the energies, resources, strengths, or powers of each person through a mutual, relational process. Personal empowerment can be viewed only through the larger lens of power through connection, that is, through the establishment of mutually empathic and mutually empowering relationships. Thus personal empowerment and the relational context through which this emerges must always be considered simultaneously.

The literature on group empowerment suggests that this process varies for any particular population according to the strengths to be mobilized and the means appropriate to that group. In this Colloquium Series we have explored one of women's particular sources of strength—the power to empower others, that is, to participate in interaction in such a way that one simultaneously enhances the power of the other *and* one's own power (Miller, Chapter 11, this volume, 1986; Surrey, Chapter 3, this volume). While this basic model (often referred to as "nurturing") is inherent in healthy parent–child development, it can be applied to all growth-producing relationships. "Nurturing," however, sounds more like feeding or gardening and describes a more one-directional growth process. Mutual "empowerment" better connotes the true potency inherent in a growth-promoting, life-enhancing, interactive process (Surrey, Chapter 3, this volume). As Jean Baker Miller has written (1976; Chapter 1, this volume), this process, perhaps because it has been in women's domain, has been underestimated, trivialized, and misunderstood. For example, a common misinterpretation of the relational process of "nurturing" or empathic interaction between mother and child is that the mother "takes herself out of the picture" to focus on the child's needs or that the mother becomes "identified with" or "mirrors" the child. This misinterpretation overlooks entirely the highly complex and creative interactive process of empowering. In an earlier paper (see Chapter 3, this volume), I used the words "taking care of the relationship" as a way of describing relational activity. Again, this process can be more accurately described as "empowering the relationship," that is, acting to create, sustain, and deepen the connections that empower. (I might note parenthetically that I have experienced enormous difficulty in trying to find language to describe these interactive processes; as Jean Baker Miller has said, our current language feels inadequate to this task.)

Alternative Models of Power and Action

The concept of empowerment is inextricably linked with ideas about action. For example, traditional thinking usually connects the two dichotomies of "powerful–powerless" and "active–passive." In the "power over" or "power for oneself only" model, there is an assumption of an active agent exerting control through the actual or threatened use of power, strength, or expertise. Women often feel unable to act when considering action in the "power over" or "power for oneself only" model. They anticipate that their action will not take others into account or may lead away from connection. If power or activity is viewed in this model, women will often choose to focus on the needs of the other person in order to allow the other to feel powerful. Therefore, when viewed from this dichotomous model, women's behavior often looks "passive" or "inactive" or "depressed." The alternative model of interaction that we are proposing might be termed a "power *with*" or "power *together*" or "power emerging from *interaction*" model. It overrides the active/passive dichotomy by suggesting that all participants in the relationship interact in ways that build connection and enhance everyone's personal power.

The "power with" or "mutual power" model grows out of a synergistic and nonhierarchical model of growth through the development of mutually empowering relationships. We have described the dynamics of the early mother–daughter relationship as laying a foundation for such a model (Surrey, Chapter 3, this volume). By contrast, the more traditional vertical or hierarchical "power over" model views power as a scarce resource. Competition for power pits people against each other in zero-sum power contests. Freud's construct of "healthy" Oedipal resolution of the father–son relationship provides a classic developmental model of power in an authoritarian power-over framework. Put too simply, the boy (who is small) wants the resources (mother), but father (who is stronger and bigger) has them. Since he is frightened of the father's power to castrate, the boy surrenders his wishes, chooses to "identify" with father, and begins to internalize control through the development of a strong, mature superego. The boy is willing to enter into a hierarchical system of power because he will eventually grow up and gain the power and resources, or at least feel entitled to them. This vertical definition of power and authority as a zero-sum commodity is fundamental to a hierarchically ordered developmental model in which little self/big other has the possibility of becoming big self/little other, where power is defined by size, strength, and power of dominion. Our alternative model assumes that power or the ability to act does not have to be a scarce resource, nor based on zero-sum assumptions—certainly not in interactions between human beings.

The problems of women's disempowerment have received considerable attention in both psychological and social writing, in part because of the prevalence of this deficiency model in explaining women's psychological problems. Concepts such as "fear of owning one's power," "identification with the victim," "fear of success," and the "Cinderella syndrome" describe women as they deviate from the more traditional models of power and action. These concepts have shaped the questions we ask about ourselves and our women clients: Is she being *too passive*? Can she learn to be *more active* on her own behalf? Perhaps the questions we need to ask are: Is she being responsibly "interactive"? Has she established a relational context where mutual power is encouraged and facilitated?

Disempowerment, then, is difficulty in creating or sustaining a healthy relational context. Kaplan (1984) suggests that the constellation of factors that can lead to depression includes inhibition of action, which follows from the loss or distortion of a relational context. Steiner-Adair (1986) and Surrey (Chapter 14, this volume) have viewed eating disorders as a reflection of the disempowerment experienced when women become alienated from their own relational needs. Jordan (Chapter 5, this volume) has described the psychological difficulties arising from nonmutual relationships, especially for women in heterosexual couples. Stiver's papers (see Chapters 8 and 15, this volume) discuss the terrible personal and clinical misunderstandings that ensue when women's relational motivations are viewed as "dependency" needs and are not validated and fulfilled.

Empowerment through Interaction

It is often easier to describe the problematic or pathological aspects of relationships than the positive, growth-enhancing dynamics. However, some theorists have discussed empowerment more positively within a relational framework. The British object relations theorists (e.g., Fairbairn, 1950; Winnicott, 1965; Guntrip, 1973) have written beautifully about the primary importance of the relational context in psychological development. In America, Kohut (1971) and Rogers (1975) have emphasized the fundamental significance of empathy in the development of the person within both developmental and therapeutic frameworks. But these formulations do not focus on the two-directional relational process. In our work we are focusing on the characteristic aspects of mutually empathic relationships that facilitate psychological growth and empowerment. This formulation recognizes that for women, the motivation to understand and foster development of the relationship (which includes the other) is equally as important as the need for empathy or "self–objects" (Kohut, 1971). It further recognizes that empathy does not just exist mysteriously. For the persons to become empathic, the development of the capacity *for* empathy must grow in the context of mutually empathic and empowering relationships.

In an earlier paper (Surrey, Chapter 3, this volume), I suggested the basic "process" of women's development as a relational self and described this development in the context of the early mother–daughter relationship. Girls learn to grow in relationship through healthy interaction with their mothers and other significant people. The fundamental processes of mutual relationship are mutual *engagement* (attention and interest), mutual *empathy*, and mutual *empowerment*. Both mothers and daughters are empowered as relational beings through their capacity to "see" and "respond to" the other and to engage in interaction that leaves both people feeling more aware of self and other and, therefore, more energized to act. This capacity "to act in relationship" has been described as response/ability. Further, this ability leads to the capacity to "hold" the psychological reality of the other as part of an ongoing, continuous awareness beyond the momentary experience and to "take the other into account" in all one's activities. This awareness we have called cognitive and emotional intersubjectivity (Surrey, Chapter 3, this volume; Jordan, Chapter 5, this volume). Response/ability, then, is not limited to the momentary process of interaction but implies an ongoing capacity "to act in relationship," to consider one's actions in light of other people's needs, feelings, and perceptions.

Miller (1986) has described in further detail the nature of an empowering interactive process resulting in increased zest, empowerment, knowledge, self-worth, and desire for more connection for all participants. The capacity to engage in an open, mutually empathic relational process rests on the maintenance of fluid "ego boundaries" (Jordan, Chapter 4, this volume) and the capacity to be responsive and "moved" by the thoughts, perceptions, and feeling states of the other person. In such empowering interaction, both people feel able to *have an impact* on each other and on the movement or "flow" of the interaction. Each feels "heard" and "responded to" and able to "hear," "validate," and "respond to" the other. Each feels empowered through creating and sustaining a context that leads to increased awareness and understanding. Further, through this process, each participant feels enlarged, able to "see" more clearly, and energized to move into action. The capacity to be "moved," to respond, and to "move" the other represents the fundamental core of relational empowerment.

This process creates a relational context in which there is increasing awareness and knowledge of self and other through sustained affective connection and a kind of unencumbered movement of interaction. This is truly a creative process, since each person is changed through the interaction. The movement of relationship creates an energy, momentum, or power that is experienced as beyond the individual, yet available to the individual. Both participants gain new energy and new awareness since each has risked change and growth through the encounter. Neither person is in control; instead, each is enlarged and feels empowered, energized, and more real. Empowerment is based on the capacity to turn toward and trust in the relationship to provide the ongoing context for such interaction. This action or movement of relationship, then, transfers to action in other realms as the person has become increasingly response/able and empowered to act.

We have postulated that the early and continuing emphasis on building connection is necessary for the growth of the capacity for mutual empathy. For boys, however, emotional and physical separation and the ability to disconnect—to separate from the emotional context—are seen as fundamental to the development of the independent, self-reliant, and courageous soldier, explorer, thinker, achiever, or worker. Boys are encouraged to make this early disconnection from *both* parents. The hallmark of male identity formation has been seen as the willingness to "identify" (*not* connect) with the father's way of being powerful. Boys, it is said, are taught to renounce the pleasures, safety, and growth within emotional and physical connectedness to mother (the representative of the "weaker" sex) as well as the open expression of vulnerable feelings (Miller, 1976; Bernardez, 1982; Jordan, Surrey, & Kaplan, Chapter 2, this volume; Stiver, Chapter 8, this volume). Thus men do not have as many opportunities for developing their relational capacities and do not learn to develop trust in their capacity to engage in mutually empathic, mutually empowering interaction. They can come to view connection as if it were associated with loss of identity, control, power, and the capacity to act on one's perceptions and interests.

Girls, in contrast, are encouraged to act and work in connection. Girls do not tend to see relationship and activity as mutually exclusive. Boys tend to believe they must feel themselves more clearly defined as emotionally distinct and separate and to believe that their action comes from each self alone. Thus adult men are more likely to attribute their

successes to their own efforts, while women more frequently acknowledge the impact of the whole context (Miller, 1986).

I am suggesting that early connectedness for women can lead to a
"moving with" others, what Jean Baker Miller (1986) calls "movement
in relationship." Unfortunately, this is not a model of action or
achievement that is fully encouraged or developed in families or in
academic and social institutions, for either girls or boys.

Relational competence can be defined as the interest and capacity
to "stay emotionally present with," to enlarge or deepen the relational
context to create enough "space" for both or all people to express
themselves and to allow for possible conflict, tension, and creative
resolution. Recognizing the growth and change in people, ongoing
connection implies a process of attunement to change, that is, staying
"current" in relationship. Western society discourages this possibility.
It highlights and encourages separation and individuation, does not
emphasize the importance of ongoing connection, and has not given
enough support or educational experience to the skillful engagement
of differences, conflicts, and powerful feelings in relationships. As a
result, this relational pathway of development is obscured; its potential
remains unacknowledged and undeveloped. This obscuring of the
relational pathway particularly affects women, especially in their
efforts to build adult forms of connection in which mutual strengths
can be activated, experienced, validated, and sustained. We need a new
language to describe adequately the change and transformation of
connections throughout life.

In the Stone Center Colloquium Series, we have often talked about
the problems for women related to the incongruities between their
early relational, connected self-experience and later societal definitions
of maturity that stress independence, self-sufficiency, and individuation. In particular, girls in this culture undergo a major period of
discontinuity at adolescence. The discontinuity of adolescence can
leave women feeling disconnected from their own experience of trust
and power in relationship, in the affective connotations and interactions between people.

Carol Gilligan (1982) has described this as the loss of women's
voice, the inability to find a language and system of logic to represent
our experience. The "dis-ease" of feeling and living this incongruity
has profound implications. As Gilligan says, these inconsistencies
become "raised as personal doubts that invade women's sense of
themselves, compromising their ability to act on their perceptions" (p.
49) and their ability to be empowered through the creation of and
reliance on mutually empowering relationships.

What is required is a recognition that relationships are the source of power and effectiveness, not of weakness or inaction or a threat to effectiveness. Because this kind of power transfers effectively to movement and action across many relationships, individual activity experienced in a context of shared activity can feel very powerful and sustainable. An appreciation of the enhancement of mutual power through relationship leads us to the next question: How to build empowering relational contexts for personal growth, learning, indeed all of our activities in life—whether in the family, the workplace, the classroom, or even the Congress? This is a very different question from the question usually asked in our psychological theories.

THE RELATIONAL CONTEXT

Building Connection through Dialogue

We have suggested alternative formulations to the separation-individuation model of human development (Surrey, Chapter 3, this volume). We have posited a relationship-differentiation process in which the motive for connection leads to increasingly complex differentiated networks of relationships, both within relationships existing over time and in new connections. Another descriptive term for this relational pathway could be "relationship-authenticity," reflecting the motivation for connection as contributing to the challenge to remain real, vital, purposeful, and honest in relationships. The challenge to "stay present with" and "responsive to" continues to create a mutually empathic context of dialogue which is the core of relational development (Surrey, Chapter 3, this volume).

An example of such a context is described by Kaplan, Klein, and Gleason (Chapter 7, this volume) in their discussion of the challenges inherent in the mother–daughter relationship at adolescence. In a study group formed to research the mother–daughter relationship, Wellesley students reported a strong desire to change and deepen their current connections with their mothers at the same time as they were engaged in creating new relationships. Their concerns and activity in this relationship are a good example of young women working toward building a relational context that deepens over time as more diverse and differentiated connections are made. Most students still saw their relationship with their mothers as one of the most important relationships in their lives. Daughters were struggling to clearly express themselves and their current experiences and perceptions. While they were concerned about the conflict they might create in this process, they desired authenticity and recognition. They wanted *more* connection and access to their mothers as adult persons, not just as their "mothers," and wished for more knowledge about their mothers' real feelings and experiences. They felt this would help them to understand both their mothers and themselves as they became adults. They desired increased mutuality, hoped that their own learning and change might contribute to their mothers' development, and expected even greater mutuality as they grew older and became mothers themselves. Daughters were also interested in hearing about mothers' new experiences and changes and worried about possible loss of contact.

This is hardly a picture of increasing "separation," but rather the desire for maintaining authenticity and connection and deepening the relational context to allow for new and potentially conflictual interactions in the movement toward mutual recognition and understanding. The underlying faith seems to be that authenticity can ultimately strengthen connection and mutuality. Early patterns of mother–daughter relationships must shift to permit the connection to deepen and to accommodate both participants as they grow and change and develop new relationships. Such growth occurs through the development of mutual empathy. This process may be fraught with anxiety and anger as well as satisfaction and pleasure, and it can be seen as a lifelong "conversation."

We have described how the ability to create a relational context for growth and empowerment arises out of early self-with-other experiences. Under optimal familial and social conditions, girls would be encouraged and challenged to develop larger and more complex relational contexts. The capacity to engage in such creative relational activity with a group of peers has been shown to have a major impact on women's empowerment. The consciousness-raising groups of the 1960s and the emergence of "support" groups for women in response to nearly every life situation and social problem attest to the power of such groups in women's lives.

Relational empowerment refers to the process of enlarged vision and energy, stimulated through interaction, in a framework of emotional connection. Movement-in-relationship refers to the alternations and fluctuations of figure-ground experiences moving toward mutual empathy and shared understanding. Both personal growth and intellectual development occur in this mode as described by Clinchy and Zimmerman (1985) and Belenky and colleagues (1986). They use the concept of "connected learning." Connected learning means taking the view of the other and connecting this to one's own knowledge, thus building new and enlarged understanding of broader human experience. The more numerous and diverse the perspectives one has connected with, the broader the relational context and the more enhanced will be the sense of being both connected to and empowered to respond to a larger "human" reality.

Not all human relationships develop in this way. When an important relational context cannot enlarge to allow for mutual experience and the movement of dialogue, women feel disempowered. If the connection feels severed there can be a sense of deadness, blackness, and even terror; some have described this experience as a "black hole." If the connection is only partially maintained, there can be a fragmentation of self. Here there can be feelings of stuckness, flatness, nonvitality, confusion, or blurred focus; one client calls this condition a "grey-out." Under these circumstances it may be necessary to acknowledge that the dialogue has stopped, at least for that moment. Relational empowerment also suggests the capacity to let go and come back to resume and maintain the process over a period of time.

The ability to be moved through emotion depends on each person's willingness and capacity to be open to her or his own feelings and to receive the feelings of others. Feeling together and moving together also involve thinking together and being open to new perceptions and ideas that arise in this affective, relational joining. One of the greatest sources of women's cognitive disempowerment is the sense of experiencing a split between feeling and thinking. As one woman in therapy said, "When I'm in the presence of someone who does not want me to feel—who will not join me at a feeling level—I can't think, everything dries up."

When the process of relational empowerment works in a group, the context is sustained and participants internalize the process as an increase in energy, power or "zest," and a sense of effectiveness based on their ability to contribute to everyone's greater awareness and understanding (Miller, 1986). A heightened sense of reality and a feeling of moving forward together occur. In this process each participant's voice is acknowledged, so that he or she experiences a heightened sense of personal clarity and feels affirmed and empowered as a relational being. The joining of visions and voices creates something new, an enlarged vision; the individual participants feel enlarged. Thus the sense of connection and participation in something larger than oneself does not diminish but rather heightens the sense of personal power and understanding.

The experience of mutual empathy and empowerment can be facilitated through the creation of growth-promoting relational contexts in any area—the classroom, the workplace, various political and social arenas, and, of course, the therapeutic relationship. When I refer to relational contexts, I mean both the structures we can easily see—that is, the number of people, the setting, the structure of the interaction—and the creative process itself, which includes the experience of an enlarged "space" that can stretch and grow to encompass developing perspectives, needs, and feeling states.

A Context for Empowerment

A 26-year-old woman, Marcia, whom I see in therapy, offers an excellent example of relational empowerment experienced in the context of a growth-promoting dyadic relationship. At the time Marcia began therapy, her close friend Laura was in the final stage of a 2-year struggle with leukemia. Marcia described their relationship as very special. Beginning in early childhood, the relationship had gone through many stages of closeness and distance and had weathered geographic moves, the addition of other relationships, and periods of great differences in interests and work. The two friends were now engaged in an intensive, nearly daily involvement as they struggled to come to terms with Laura's imminent death. They were reviewing their lives together and deciding what they wanted to take from and leave with each other as a way of both letting go and maintaining their connection beyond death.

Marcia describes the quality of authenticity in connection beautifully: "This relationship taught me what it means to be there, I mean really *there* as *myself*. I can recognize this in myself now in other situations—not disappearing or withdrawing because I'm afraid to say what I see or think, or feeling it's hopeless, or just getting angry."

In describing the relational context she says: "The most important thing was that I always felt that Laura would want to hear my experience. Even when we disagreed, I felt there was room for each of us to have her own viewpoint, and there would eventually be some way to come to see or understand the other person's viewpoint, although not necessarily to agree with it. Once, following an enormous disagreement, it took two years for us to fully understand each other's experience. Still I really felt that Laura wanted to hear what I thought, and I really valued her experience. We had some big disagreements and learned the ways we usually disagreed. This helped me to know myself better. The space and trust I felt developed into a faith in the power and endurance of the relationship. I never really felt this before. I feel my parents love and support me, but I don't feel they know me or share themselves with me in the same way."

In our discussion of her goals for therapy, she stated: "What I want help with now is: not losing this faith, and learning to bring myself to other relationships in this way. I'm especially concerned about not losing my sense of my self in my relationships with men. Laura used to get angry with me when I started getting confused, acting like a victim, what I call 'crazy angry' with my boyfriend. I guess you would say disempowered. I do know what it means now to be part of this healthy kind of relationship. Do you really think it's possible to have this again in my life?"

Throughout the relationship, and since Laura's death, Marcia has tended to see Laura as the more capable and insightful one. It will be important for Marcia to begin to see her own relational strengths, to see *herself* as strong and empowering in this relationship. As she recognizes her own part in creating the context and participating in Laura's development, she will begin to internalize this strength and competence and feel she is capable of bringing this to other relationships.

In the therapy setting, it is useful to explore and validate experiences of relational empowerment and to help the patient internalize this capacity and learn to establish new relational contexts in which strengths can be affirmed and new growth facilitated. The capacity to create such relationships is an important therapeutic goal. Marcia is beginning to learn that the creation of such a context is a mutual enterprise; both or all people grow in their ability to create and participate in this way.

This process is not limited to therapy. In all of life, the sense of being part of the growth and empowerment of the other develops through the process of seeing and feeling the other becoming "more of who they are" and simultaneously feeling this oneself. The ability to feel and move as part of such a "we" is the goal in other contexts. Many women have experienced the special quality of relationships between women in which both participants have grown and developed in their relational capacities. They are aware of the empowerment resulting from women standing in strength together, trusting in the continuity of the relationship. However, because we have all lived in a society supporting the "power over" model, such strengths have not yet been experienced openly and shared fully. It is essential that we learn to maintain and sustain our strengths through connection, and to do so we must learn to value and develop sustaining relational contexts.

Only as we value our connections and see that maintaining and deepening them are crucial to our development will we begin to take the risks necessary to empower our relationships. Growing and becoming empowered in relationship means being aware of our shared responsibility for mutual security and well-being through the aliveness and growth-supporting aspects of our relationships. It means learning how to open, create, repair, and let go in relationships with sustained awareness of how interconnected we are. This sustained awareness, in turn, will present a healthy challenge to the defensive need, based in part on contemporary Western culture, to feel self-sufficient and independent.

The power to create, build, sustain, and deepen connection does not mean always being strong, but it does mean being able to stay connected through periods of "strength" and "weakness" and through wide ranges of different feelings. It is rarely possible to experience a full spectrum of empowerment in one relationship. For most people, empowerment occurs through the creation of multiple and varied, although often overlapping, relational structures for personal, educational, work, social, and political development. As clinicians we need to foster consciousness of and competence in the building of empowering relational contexts.

CREATING AND SUPPORTING RELATIONAL CONTEXTS

I would like to move beyond both therapy and a two-person model to further examine empowerment in relationship. The dynamics of empowerment in "personal" relationships can be applied to activity in other arenas. Practical applications beyond the clinical context are important in themselves but they can also illuminate the therapeutic relationship.

Over the past year, I have been involved in the collaborative evolution of a day-and-a-half workshop designed to empower women to speak out for nuclear disarmament. The workshop is sponsored by Women's Action for Nuclear Disarmament (WAND), an organization founded in 1980 by Helen Caldicott and others to empower women to work with a singular focus for nuclear disarmament. This empowerment workshop, entitled "Our Vision—Our Voices—How to Speak Out for Nuclear Disarmament," offers a beautiful example of building a relational context that empowers women. It illustrates many aspects of empowerment through connection. Although, in this case, personal growth is not the primary purpose of the empowerment process, the workshop in fact does mobilize the strengths and energies of connection, shared vision, and shared activity. The workshop captures the essence of relational empowerment, generating increased energy, clarity, and commitment to action for all participants. It may serve as a useful model for efforts to create and support empowering relational contexts in other settings.

The workshop, which usually includes two leaders and 20 to 30 participants, begins with a graphic audiovisual demonstration of the arsenal of nuclear weapons currently in existence. Thus the real threat of potential world destruction is brought right into the room, demanding urgent attention. The first few hours are spent creating an atmosphere for the sharing of intense feelings and responses to this threat, including awe, terror, anger, grief, and helplessness. I personally experienced a tremendous sense of relief to finally have the opportunity to focus my feelings about nuclear destruction and to join with others in doing this. This experience suggests the reversal of what Lifton (1979) has called psychic numbing and what Macy (1983) describes as despair in her "Despair and Empowerment" workshops.

The framework of "looking together" provides the structure for the creative empowerment process. The opportunity to join together in emotional connection in a situation where people respond in free flow to each other's feelings and perceptions generates desires to care for and support each other. From the expressions of helpless rage, despair, and confusion, the group builds together to a sense of urgency and shared responsibility: We must do something.

Negative affects of helplessness, anger, fear, and confusion become transformed into the energy of positive movement. To call this process "just talking" or "sharing feelings" would be to trivialize and misrepresent it. As the movement or vision of the whole group begins to emerge, each person feels a heightened sense of authenticity, validation, and response/ability. The "I" is enhanced as the "we" emerges. Through building the "we," that is, "seeing" together through creating an enlarged vision, participants transform their personal self-doubt and confusion into clarity and conviction. The sense of powerlessness of the individual is supplanted by the experience of relational power.

Most of the work takes place in small groups of six to eight people, which meet three times during the workshop to provide opportunities for people to share more personally, to give each other feedback, and to compose and deliver a practice "speech" to an imagined audience. In the afternoon of the first day, there is a plenary session entitled "Women's Voices and Visions of Peace," which explores women's current and historical strengths as potential peacemakers. In this session participants directly experience their power to empower others through a guided exercise, performed in dyads, that evokes the creative energy of connected interactions. Participants carefully and attentively ask each other a list of prepared questions: "Why do you care?" "Why are you here?" "Have you ever felt that you don't know enough to speak out?" "What do you know?" "Where has this message come from that you don't know enough?" "What has kept you from acting?" "What has allowed you to act on your reasons for caring?" "What do you need to keep going?" Session leaders direct attention to the relational context created through addressing these basic questions together and to the sense of mutual empowerment that emerges through shared focusing on highly personal issues. This process acknowledges that participants need such a context both to initiate and to sustain action.

Participants' sense of connection arises from the intensity of the dyadic experience and then is extended, throughout the workshop, to the group as a whole, to WAND as an organization, and to women throughout history. This experience of different levels of connection parallels WAND members' growing motivation to extend this protection and care for closely related individuals, such as one's own children, to the entire human community. One technique for evoking widening ranges of connectedness is through the reading of emotionally evocative quotations from the writings of women speaking about the nuclear issue. An example is from Sally Miller Gearhart (1982):

> I believe we are at a great watershed in history, and that we hold in our hands a fragile thread, no more than that, that can lead us to our survival. I understand the rising up of women in this century to be the human race's response to the threat of its own self-annihilation and the destruction of the planet.

Quotations like this emphasize the ethic of care and responsibility, as well as the joy in courage and risk taking, in facing this threat together, and in creating a sense of safety and peace through awareness and experience of our connectedness.

The importance of building connections between women to create new understanding and new strategies of peacemaking is emphasized through the presentation and discussion of new research and theory on women's development. An example is a passage from Jean Baker Miller's *Toward a New Psychology of Women* (1976):

> Humanity has been held to a limited and distorted view of itself, from its interpretation of the most intimate emotions to its grandest visions of human possibilities, by virtue of its subordination of women.
>
> Until recently, "mankind's" understandings have been the only understandings generally available to us. As other perceptions arise— precisely those perceptions that men, because of their dominant position, could not perceive—the total vision of human possibilities enlarges and is transformed.

In response to the urgency of the nuclear issue, women in this workshop learn to operate from the source of their own power, which is staying centered and connected with each other in what we see, feel, and think. Toward this end the concept of a *paradigm shift* is introduced. A paradigm is defined as a set of assumptions, a mental framework from which beliefs and opinions are constructed. Throughout this workshop, exercises are designed to illustrate and elicit a paradigm shift. The goal of the workshop is for women to help each other shift from the paradigm of passive, helpless victim to a new paradigm of empowered, "related," responsible person; from the giving over of authority to the political and military "experts" to the taking of responsibility by concerned and caring human beings; from the valuing of technical or objective ("separate") knowledge to the valuing of personal and connected knowledge; and, finally, a shift from the emphasis on "public speaking" and debate to the emphasis on finding one's own voice and staying in dialogue.

Most participants in the workshop experience these paradigm shifts and understand how they lose their sense of power as peacemakers when they shift back into old paradigms. They perceive the necessity of staying connected with each other, that is, sustaining the relational context, to maintain these shifts. Finally, they perceive the power inherent in evolving new ways of entering the arena of the "experts" without losing touch with the source of one's own power. This is accomplished through both experiential and educational processes that examine the sources of relational disempowerment as well as empowerment and highlight the necessity of building relational contexts that support and sustain empowerment. For example, we play a tape of Elissa Melamed, a well-known peace activist, speaking to participants at the 1984 Denver WAND Speaker Training Workshop, saying:

> Basically, the barriers to being a good communicator are the fears that we feel and the ways that we disqualify ourselves and don't think we have a great deal to contribute as women. In addition to our own personal feelings of inadequacy that come from our own private histories there is a certain male norm of what makes for an effective speaker—and we are measuring ourselves by this norm and we are not stopping to ask how effective that model really is for what *we are* trying to do.

In the final session of the workshop, the whole group focuses on planning different modes of future action. People are asked to make specific commitments to concrete activities. Despite the overwhelming issue at hand, an enormous amount of energy, excitement, and joy are generated in this workshop. This is the "zest" or vitality experienced in feeling related, connected, and empowered together to work for what is truly important. This process can be acknowledged and built into strategies for initiating and maintaining activities of all kinds.

Inherent in the workshop is a respect for relational empowerment and for action at all levels, from the smallest personal change to the largest life commitment. Joining the group, sharing in the growing awareness, seeing and listening to others speaking about the issues are all important actions, as are movement and action in larger political arenas. Such a definition of action and activism is based on the understanding that individual and relational power are interconnected, grow simultaneously, and work synergistically.

Some people are moved by the workshop experience to change their lives dramatically, others in small ways. Some work collaboratively, while others work in solitude. Individual creativity or risk taking can be experienced as part of the larger relational context, just as can collaborative group work. For women especially, this sense of personal expression in action is often most meaningful when it is experienced as both intensely personal and related to the larger connection, the shared vision and commitment. This is what we mean by "action in a relational context."

Originally, WAND had followed the model of Physicians for Social Responsibility (PSR) in trying to develop a bureau of public speakers on the nuclear issue. PSR had trained medical doctors and other professionals to speak as "experts" on the facts and figures of the medical effects of nuclear war. It became clear that this "expert" training for public speaking was inappropriate for WAND. The "expert" model is based on an authoritarian model of power through debate, where the domain is scientific facts and numbers. WAND's evolving message is that it is precisely in questioning this model of authority that women reconnect to their own untapped power. Rather than becoming overinvolved with facts, figures, and technojargon, WAND offers the message that feeling and conviction are an appropriate and sufficient first response to this issue and form the most powerful basis for further education and action.

At the heart of the training is the recognition that it is insane to disconnect from feelings about the nuclear threat; rather, women must learn to speak out in an emotionally powerful and cogent manner. Women's power to empower others, and to use the power of their emotions effectively to move others to become involved and active, rests not on technical expertise but on personal authenticity and the energies released through emotional connection. The power of "listening" and "responding" from the heart is thus validated as forming a more valuable and lasting base for power than "speaking out" as an "expert." It is the building of relationship, the creation of the "conversation" that connects people, that is the core of women's powers and creative energies—and, potentially, men's as well. Accordingly, the workshop encourages connections with men. However, it also recognizes and addresses the ways that women can become disempowered when connections with men are fragmenting, that is, maintained at the expense of the deepest connections to self and other women. Thus women's connections with each other are seen as the first step in evolving a new relational structure for mobilizing, sustaining, and organizing information and activity. Men are welcome to work within this structure. Put another way, the workshop creates a more "realistic" and more total basis from which to gain and use our knowledge about the nuclear threat.

The workshop creates the initial setting for experiencing and validating relational power and for training in speaking out both formally and informally. It also provides information and structure for channeling this energy through individual, small-group, or organizational action on local, national, and international levels. The workshop helps participants move from positions of isolation, doubt, and confusion to a sense of connection, knowledge, and positive action together. This movement reflects a crucial aspect of women's moral development, described by Carol Gilligan (1982) as the development of an ethic of care, whereby the negative injunction against "selfishness" or hurting others can be transformed into the energy of positive responsibility for our mutual security, survival, and well-being.

The workshop experience has strengthened my own conviction that relational empowerment strategies are essential and relevant to women's empowerment in all arenas. We need to learn more about the tremendous creative power of moving and acting in relationship in order to better describe and facilitate it. Perhaps we ought to substitute "empowerment" training for assertiveness training. Further, this model of empowering the relationship may be the most fruitful way to study the process of growth and development in all of life—including psychotherapy. We will be exploring this proposal further in the Colloquium Series.

Based on a talk presented at a Stone Center Colloquium in January 1986.

10

The Construction of Anger in Women and Men

JEAN BAKER MILLER

Almost everyone agrees that our society has problems with anger. We often say that we have "too much aggression, violence, or hatred." While this certainly seems true, several questions can be raised about the postulate, particularly the basic thinking that leads to the quantitative term "too much."

In contrast, I would first like to suggest that we suffer from *constraints* that prevent us from expressing anger and even from knowing when we are experiencing anger—constraints that are different for members of each sex.

Second, even as the expression of anger is constrained, we live in a milieu that continuously produces anger—at the societal level and during the course of individual psychological development—for both sexes, but differently for each.

Third, there is a possibility that the very conditions that produce so much anger grow out of the reality that the expression of anger has been encouraged *differentially*—predominantly for one sex only.

Fourth, if the first three issues are valid, they may have influenced our very conception of what anger is and how it originates.

I shall begin this discussion with some observations on women's experience, then move to a few notions about parts of men's experience. Finally, I will return to reconsider these initial issues.

It is important to define the term *anger*, because there has been great variation in its usage. The topic has been studied by many workers in several disciplinary traditions. To sort the complicated lexicography, however, would take several papers in itself; as an alternative, I should like to formulate provisional definitions at the end of this paper. For the moment, let us start with the word *anger* and go along with whatever that word means to each of us.

WOMEN AND ANGER

In speaking about this subject, there is an immediate problem: One topic most people really do not want to hear about is women's anger! Our culture (and others) has a long history of surrounding this topic with dread and denial. Within psychological fields, there has been frequent use of such terms as *castrating women* and the like, but it is hard to locate any place at which women's anger enters as a "proper" phenomenon. It is virtually always seen as pathological.

Perhaps a description of a real person, whom I will call Anita, will help to make this more concrete. Anita was a married woman in her 50s who had spent her adult life contributing as well as she could to the growth and development of her husband and four children. At her first therapy visit she was depressed, and she cried almost continuously as she told of how inadequate and worthless she felt. She conveyed subtle hints of anger as well as clues that she was probably quite critical of several people, particularly her husband; but overtly she criticized only herself. At the same time, she clearly looked to her husband to provide affirmation and validation of her worth—and this is true for many women, even today.

In the past, I might have seen her anger as repressed and unreasonable, hence an indication of "pathology." Probably, too, I would have seen her as a woman who was "dependent" on her husband and therefore had problems with excess "dependency." I could have cited her need for her husband's affirmation as further evidence of her "poor sense of self." And all of this would have added up rapidly to a common diagnostic picture.

In a well-intentioned attempt to relieve Anita's depression, I might have thought it important to help her see her anger and its irrationality. I believe now that such a course is wrong, but that belief follows from a reexamination of women's anger.

We live in an androcentric (male-centered) society—that is, one that is organized in terms of the experience of men as they have been able to define it and elaborate on it. This elaboration is called "culture" and "knowledge." The society also is largely patriarchal, in that men (of a certain group) have held all of the legitimate leadership, power, and authority. But even if one does not feel familiar with all of the connotations of the word *patriarchy*, one can think of the conditions set in motion in any set of relationships that are structured so that one group is dominant and another is subordinate, whether the relationship is based on sex, class, race, or other characteristics. All historical evidence indicates that once a group is constituted as a dominant group, it behaves in predictable ways. Some of these are:

- It tends to act destructively to subordinate groups.
- It restricts the subordinate group's range of actions—and even reactions to destructive treatment.
- It does not encourage subordinates' full and free expression of their experience.
- It characterizes subordinates falsely.
- It describes this as the normal situation—usually the "natural" situation, ordered and ordained by higher and better powers, ranging from God to "biology. "

Subordinates usually are dependent on dominants economically, socially, and politically. Their experience and views are excluded from the culture and do not form the base for the construction of what is called "knowledge."

Obviously any subordinate is in a position that constantly generates anger. Yet this is one of the emotions that no dominant group ever wants to allow in subordinates. (No industrialist ever wanted the workers to be angry; no empire builder ever wanted the "natives to be restless.") Although the direct reasons for fear of subordinates' anger may seem obvious, this fear can become magnified in intricate fashion in the minds of dominants. In addition, the suppression of anger is reinforced psychologically in the minds of the subordinates in many ways. I will review just a few.

First, direct force has to be obviously available, even if it only lurks quietly in the background. For example, in this society we have only recently become more fully aware of the threat of physical violence that has always been exerted against women; but many women have known the private experience of beatings, rape, and other forms of brutality—or the threats of such force. The threat of social and economic deprivation is also a form of force, and, in general, men have controlled such resources.

Second, it is usually made to appear that subordinates have no *cause* for anger; if they feel anything like it, there is something *wrong with them.* They are uncivilized natives, dumb workers, sinful or unloved women,—or, in modern parlance, "sick," maladjusted, and the like.

Growing up, then, with the admonition to be "normal"—that is, to comply with the requirements of the situation—subordinates often develop several more complex psychological tendencies. These complicated characteristics often rest on a variation of some of the following inner beliefs:

1. *I am weak.* This can effectively stamp out hints of anger near their start, because to feel angry can produce immediate fear of overpowering retaliation. There is usually the accompanying belief that this weakness is inherent and that one is permanently incapable of developing greater strength.

2. *I am unworthy.* Harboring this belief, one then becomes afraid of having any anger, because it appears to mean that anger will only deepen her or his sense of self-denigration.

3. *I have "no right" and "no cause" to be angry.* This may be the most basic feeling of all; it underlies everything else. After all, if the whole world is said to be organized rightfully and properly, the subordinate person comes to believe that she or he certainly has no right to be angry. If the person feels any anger, that feeling can only intensify her or his sense of defectiveness, irrationality, and worthlessness.

The three characteristics are a few of the many that can arise for all subordinate groups. For women, there have been additional specific dimensions, particularly on the psychological level. These can be summarized by saying that women generally have been led to believe that their identity, as women, is that of persons who should be almost totally without anger and without the *need* for anger. Therefore, anger feels like a threat to women's central sense of identity, which has been called *femininity.* In recent years, Bernardez (1976, 1978), Lerner (1977), Zilbach et al. (1979), Nadelson et al. (1982), and Miller et al. (1981a, b) have written on this point and its several clinical manifestations.

A major exception may be noted. There is one place in which anger and aggressive action have been permitted to women—usually spoken of in terms of an animal metaphor—that is, in defense of her young, as a lioness defends her cubs. In such an instance, as in almost everything, the woman is allowed anger *in the interest of someone else.*

Many of the tendencies noted above follow from a basic point that underlies the interdiction of women's anger: Women are not supposed to use their own activity for their own self-initiated and self-defined goals or for their own development. From very early in life, women have been led to believe that their life activities should be for others and that their main task is to make and maintain relationships— relationships that serve others. This situation merits careful examination. Because of it, women develop many valuable psychological strengths, but that point warrants a long discussion (Miller, 1976; Gilligan, 1982). The problem is that these very valuable strengths have not developed in a context of mutuality, and they have not been complemented by the full right and necessity to attend to one's own development as well.

The situation complicates problems of anger. As Bernardez (1978) has written, to be angry can feel to women as if it will disrupt a relationship—at least it seems so in our culture. This factor alone exerts a powerful weight, making women afraid to feel the first stirring of anger. Once more, a stark reality is that most women live in relationships based on economic and social dependence, which leads to a realistic basis for fearing their disruption. There is great risk in disturbing the relationships that provide one's economic sustenance and one's whole psychological place in the world. Simultaneously, living in this kind of dependency continually generates anger.

All of these tendencies and their complications can lead to spiraling phenomena. For example, even small degrees of anger feel dangerous to a woman. Therefore she does not express the anger. Repeated instances of suppressing the anger can produce repeated experiences of frustration and inaction. The experiences of inaction and ineffectiveness lead to feelings of weakness and lack of self-esteem, which can increase the woman's sense of feeling unworthy and inferior. Feeling more inferior and unworthy makes a person more angry. Such spiraling situations can come to fill so much of a woman's psychological "space" that she can begin to have a skewed sense of herself. She begins to feel "full of anger," which then surely seems irrational and unwarranted. All the while this is really a false inner picture of her total psychological situation. But, very importantly, it is one that the external world—so-called "reality"—is only too ready to confirm, because any anger is too much anger in women. Indeed, the risk of expressing anger can appear grave and disorganizing. (Many women use a metaphor of a bottomless well of anger that they are afraid to tap. I believe that this frightening image offers a false picture.)

All this can end in a kind of self-fulfilling prophecy. If the anger is finally expressed, it often appears in exaggerated form, perhaps along with screaming or yelling, or in ineffective form, with simultaneous negations and apologies, or with various other untoward accompaniments. Such attempts can then be dismissed with a label such as "hysterical" and thereby discounted. Bernardez (1976, 1978) and

Lerner (1977) have given clear clinical illustrations of these points. I am sure many of us can add more.

Probably the most common occurrence, however, is that the anger is not conveyed at all. Instead, it is expressed, in the end, via the only remaining route—"symptoms," psychic or somatic, the most common of which is depression. This, I believe, was the case with Anita.

All of the issues I have discussed so far relate to another basic concept: The profound cultural fear of women's anger is probably connected to the fact that women have been the main "caretakers"— indeed, almost the only ones anybody can hope to have in this society. We have a culture that is not organized so that members of the dominant group really take care of each other. Men do not guarantee each other a bedrock assurance that they will look after each other no matter what, nor do they affirm that their development will be attended to with sensitivity and care. In fact, we have a culture in which men convince each other of quite the opposite. In this cultural context, the one person everyone believes should be there to do the caring, tending, and nurturing is a woman. Not only does everyone want to believe that women will do this, everyone wants to believe that women *want* to do it and want to do it more than anything else. It has been written often that this is the way women find the fulfillment of their ultimate motivations—their instinctive, hence biological, drives, which are said to be deeper than anything else. (Thus, if we are "letting them do that," how can they possibly have any rightful cause for anger?)

I believe that women do develop valuable psychological character-istics because they participate in and foster the development of other people (a description that is probably more accurate than "caretak-ing"). But again, this point would require a long digression.

As so far conceived, the image of the person who wants to provide total and always-present care has been made *incompatible* with a person who can experience the emotion of anger, except as pathological. It appears as if we have been unable to conceive of a person who has the need for and the right to anger, and who simultaneously could truly attend to and care for others. (It is amazing how directly this notion has been carried over into psychological theory.) Simplistic as it may sound, I think we have all been encouraged to believe in such a figure. Perhaps it has seemed important to keep such an image alive in a culture that does not include care of its people as an inherent part of its own workings. Perhaps there could not exist the ruthless economy of our "outside world" if we did not maintain the vision of the unreal madonna waiting for us in the "inside world"—that is, in inner psychological life. As an example, recent women writers have pointed to the amazing persistence or repeated reemergence of the figure of the Virgin Mary in the history of European civilization. She has no real power; she can intercede and plead for us, and she can comfort and care—and she is never angry.

To sum up this section, then, I have suggested that women have lived in the situation of being subordinate, a situation that continually generates anger; simultaneously women have been told that to be angry is destructive to their psychological being and sense of identity. Further, anger is seen as threatening to women's life work, for women have concentrated on upholding, maintaining, supporting, and enhancing other people's development as well as relationships between people—which is, of course, the place in which *all* development occurs.

In the face of this situation, there is only one way women's anger could go: into indirection and confusion. This path has had disastrous consequences for women themselves on the psychological level. But the situation has been part of (or more accurately, probably has been derived from) a larger societal history that has protected the dominant group from confronting its failure to incorporate care of its own members as a necessary, inherent part of the group's culture. In other words, the notion is perpetuated, for the dominant group, that care and provision for the development of all people does not have to be built into the system. It can be left to an "underclass." Members of the dominant group, then, do not have to feel the necessity to develop, as a *primary part of their personhood,* the conviction that they are, in a profound and real sense, responsible for each other. Indeed, they are forcefully *deterred* from developing such a sense of their identity, because it belongs to women. It is "feminine"—something men and a male culture should not want to be.

Meanwhile, the only human expression of anger that has had legitimacy has come from its manifestations in members of just one sex—men. This experience has formed the conception of anger that we all carry with us. Anger as we have known it, so far, may have taken on a particular shape just because it has existed within a context that allowed it to one sex only and, most importantly, to a sex that has not been engaged in the requirement to care for its own members.

In addition, men have had to live as members of a group engaged in upholding a structure of dominance, whether any individual chose that or not. It would seem that in order to maintain a structure of dominance, half of the species has been encouraged to take on certain "unnatural," or, at least, not inevitable, characteristics and to deprive itself of the development of certain others. So, for example, to maintain dominance, any group would tend to fear and deny, and therefore not really put into daily practice, its potential for such abilities as perceiving and "feeling with" the other person, sometimes called empathy, or for having a belief in and a great desire for the flourishing of the other person's resources and abilities. Thus, one sex has not been encouraged to engage in the activities that make for the growth and enhancement of other human beings simultaneously with one's self, or even to engage in the direct daily sustenance and care of sheer physical life. I believe that all of these potential, but as yet little-practiced, forms of activity actually *do* alter the way in which anger is experienced and made manifest. They create a different configuration and integration of all emotions, particularly in the inner construction about the nature of another person and one's relationship to her or him. To put it more concretely, the actual practice of life-enhancing rather than life-restricting activities makes a crucial difference in our inner mental constructions about what we can count on the other person to do with us—and *to* us.

MEN AND ANGER

I would like now to discuss briefly the effects of growing up as a member of a dominant group, mentioning only *some* of the influences on the boy in the family, as the family has been traditionally constructed, with the father as the head. But again, we must consider the larger context. Many scholars propose that the subordination of women was linked historically with the development of hierarchies of authority and power among males in society. That is, when men began to "own" women and children, men themselves had to be kept in their ordered places. Our culture has developed within a tradition, whatever its origin, in which men have been ordered in hierarchies. These dominant-subordinate relationships among men have been based on class, race, religion, or other factors. Therefore, the majority of men have lived in positions of subordination to other men. Whatever rightful anger men have had in response to that subordination has had to be suppressed, just as it has for all subordinate groups. Thus men, too, in their situations as subordinates, have not been allowed to express anger at the source and at the time and place when it may well be "appropriate" and could be appropriately handled.

Perhaps a preliminary definition of appropriate anger may be attempted here. Anger may merely be an emotion, an emotion that can be expressed in nonverbal and verbal ways. At its simplest, it tells us that something is wrong—something hurts—and needs changing. Thus, anger provides a powerful (and useful) recognition of discomfort and motivation for action to bring about a change in immediate conditions. It is a statement to oneself and to others. If it can be recognized and expressed, it has done its work. And, most importantly, others can respond. When I show my anger, you can know that something hurts me. There is a chance for back-and-forth action and reaction that leads to changing something between us, moving from what hurts to something better. If this possibility exists, the anger usually will dissipate. No one need be damaged. Problems begin and then become infinitely complex when anger is not allowed expression or even recognition at its source, in the immediate interaction.

In general, the societal hierarchical ranking of men has precluded the expression of anger in such a useful, productive, interactional mode. This same hierarchical patterning and the same preclusion of the interactional expression of anger is then replicated in the family structure. Here, of course, it affects the most intimate relationships between fathers and sons. In regard to men's psychological development, there is a good deal of evidence that the young boy, following the pattern of the larger society, is not permitted to express his anger directly and immediately, especially to the father, the historic "head" of the family. At the same time, however, the boy is stimulated and encouraged to be "aggressive," that is, to *act* aggressively. Boys are made to fear *not being aggressive,* lest they be found wanting, be beaten out by another, or (worst of all) be like a girl. All of these constitute terrible threats to a core part of what is *made to be* men's sense of identity—which has been called *masculinity.* And here we see how those simplistic divisions have come around to force men to define themselves *against* the definition of women, which is a falsity in the first place.

There is evidence that fathers, particularly, encourage boys' aggressive *action* (Block, 1978). Beyond that, however, some recent research suggests that fathers tend repeatedly to stimulate even very young boys from the ages of 1-1/2 to 2 years, or even younger, to anger and aggression and then do not tolerate the direct expression of anger back at its source, to the father himself. For example, Gleason (1975) found that upper-middle-class fathers, who think consciously that they love their sons, frequently sparred with the boys and called them names that are really "put-downs," such as "Little Dumbo" or "Peanuthead" and the like. But the men stopped "playing" and even punished the boys when they became angry and expressed their anger *to the fathers themselves.* The observers in these studies were shocked at the amount of hostility conveyed and the amount of anger provoked in the children. These observations confirm stories I have heard many times in clinical work.

There are complex ramifications of these points. Only one will be suggested here. It relates to the earlier point that men, in general, have not participated in daily close emotional interaction in children's lives and development; nor have they practiced this emotional interchange daily in relationships with adults of either sex. Consequently, many fathers have not built a base of exchange of many emotions with their sons (or daughters). This is important because at the time in which the boy's anger occurs, he usually experiences not only anger, but usually some combination of feelings—including hurt, humiliation, vulnerability, impotence, and, especially, isolation—being alone. But he is not encouraged to express these many feelings to his father, or indeed even to recognize them, to feel them for what they are. Instead, he is encouraged to translate them into action—aggressive action. Moreover, this aggressive action is not allowed to be directed to its source, the father. In general, even the young boy should not sustain and know a range of emotions for a short or long interval and then express them as directly as possible *as emotions*. Instead he is strongly encouraged to *act*—and act aggressively. This situation constitutes a powerful force beginning early in life and deflecting men from their *own* crucial experience. Here, it is men who are told that certain feelings are threatening to their identity and place in the world—all of this ending in various forms of denial of large pieces of reality. Incidentally, as women have begun to express their own perceptions in recent years, many women have observed that men do not seem able to talk about large portions of experience; they do not even have a conception of what the women are trying to talk about with them.

This, too, is very familiar clinically. And it is particularly common to find men acting most aggressively when they feel vulnerable, hurt, frightened, and alone.

This did seem to be the case with Anita's husband. When Anita began to voice even mild comments or questioning of him, he reacted with tyrannical anger and contempt, although he appeared on the surface to be a liberal, enlightened person. Anita now said that she had "sensed" this all along, although she could not have put it into clear formulations. I believe her husband felt, very basically, frightened of feeling alone and unsupported by Anita.

I am suggesting, then, that the boy's anger cannot be of the quality that merely states something like, "You have hurt me, and I want to tell you how hurt, humiliated, and frightened that makes me." Such a statement has to rest on a basic assumption of safety plus a belief that the other person will *be there* psychologically, will receive the message, and will respond in ongoing interaction. Instead, the boy has to feel something like, "I am angry at you and I must better you, so that there is no risk that you can hurt me again."

For obvious reasons, it is impossible to act on that feeling to a father, so the boy is encouraged to direct such action toward others—his colleagues and peers. (It is interesting to note the whole theory of the Oedipus complex and what an extraordinarily destructive scene it proposes. For those who follow traditional psychoanalytic theory, it is at this Oedipal period that the boy is definitively inducted into his culture and develops his morality. Some current developments in the theory propose that at this Oedipal stage the whole cultural symbolic system is incorporated—the language and thought that constitute the total way of being and thinking in the culture.)

For present purposes, I would stress only that a boy is led to deflect his anger from its immediate object, the father, who need not be treating the boy that way in the first place. Further, in order to allow their sons (and daughters) to express anger usefully, fathers first would have to build a base of interchange involving many varied emotions. Also, such a base would permit fathers to become aware of their own unnecessary and exaggerated stimulation of the sons' anger and aggression.

It is said that as they go on from this early stage, boys "develop" because they learn to use and channel their aggression, which I would call their deflected anger. They learn in organized games. The games, and their later counterparts (or perhaps their historical origins), such as the military, train men to operate in the *games* of business, politics, and power and thus to run the world. The key factor is said to be that boys learn to play by the rules (Gilligan, 1982). Indeed, some current writers propose that women's troubles in the world stem from the fact that we do not know how to play by these rules.

But what does learning to play by the rules mean? Some very interesting material is now emerging from scientific investigations of such games (Gilligan, 1982; Luria, 1981). To focus on only one part of it, Gilligan (1982) points out that one learns that it is the *game* that counts, not the people or the personal relationships among them. Trying to beat the other, hitting as hard as you can, and the like does not mean you are hurting anyone personally; you are just playing the game. Likewise, the recipient should not take it personally; it does not really hurt. But as far as I can see, it does. Clinical work with men reveals that it hurts in many ways.

Then, as the game is carried over into adult life, it allows men to compete, win, drive out the opposition, even totally destroy them. The game is played with the pretense that no one really is hurt. The same mentality can be—and has been—applied to war.

In the course of these situations, it is not only anger that boys and men feel; there are many emotions, but few can be known or expressed for what they are. A recent novel, *The House of God* (Shem, 1978), portrays such experiences at one stage in life, that of young adulthood. The story of an intern at a prestigious teaching hospital, it illustrates how many emotions—fear, horror, sadness, isolation, and, especially, pain and hurt—are turned into aggressive actions, even sadism, and into depersonalized sex with the nurses.

In such a life course the participants are taught an amazing denial of reality. Each person learns he must deny his experience and attempt to act aggressively. If he can do that successfully, he can outdo the other—that is, he can win—in a situation, which in the end, occurs rarely for most men.

If there were space, there are many additional points that could be made. For example, there are class and ethnic differences in the style of aggressive action, with middle-class premiums on less obvious physical aggression and more controlled manipulations to gain status and power.

Also I have not covered many of the major points about female and male development, especially the interrelationship of anger and sexuality. One major point, however, should be reemphasized, even briefly: Many men report the feeling that their fathers abandoned them emotionally, and sometimes literally. They feel that their fathers were not emotionally "there," ensuring that they could go through a variety of emotions with the *respect,* or even with the psychological *presence,* of their fathers.

DELINEATION OF ANGER

The suggestion here, then, is that our cultural tradition has distorted men's experience and knowledge of anger and precluded its integration within a wide range of complex emotions. We have come to know anger as an aggressive, isolating, and destructive experience. Yet anger *does not have to be that.*

Here I would like to make a connection with what may be one of *the* most destructive psychological phenomena. This phenomenon is at the base of much past psychodynamic thought, and many women writers recently have underscored its importance. It is the suffering of an experience, but then not having the "permission" to truly suffer it—that is, not being able to go genuinely through the experience, know it, name it, and react with the emotions that it evokes. Such an experience is inevitably a social encounter; it occurs in interaction with other people. The trouble comes when powerful people surrounding you say that you cannot react that way and, more importantly, that *you do not have* the emotions and the perceptions that you, in fact, have.

It is this situation that can create profound psychological trouble. Not only do you suffer deprivation or attack per se, but you suffer the experience of complex emotions and the simultaneous "disconfirmation" of them—often followed by punishment for any attempt to express the feelings directly. Such experiences make it almost impossible even to know what you are experiencing. This is terrible and confusing for adults. It is even more so for children.

Several theorists—for example, Sullivan and Bion—have spoken about this in the past, using their own sets of terminology. I am adding the suggestion that there is a context in our culture that makes certain key experiences and emotions likely to be systematically and repeated disconfirmed, but in different ways for people of each sex.

I submit, therefore, that our problems with anger are due to insufficient *real* experience of anger and insufficient allowance for its direct expression at the time when and in the ways in which it could be appropriate—when it need not have the connotations of harm, abuse, or violence. For men, the deflection of anger along with the simultaneous repeated restimulation of aggressive action is the problem. For women, the problem is a situation of subordination that continually produces anger, along with the culture's intolerance of women's direct expression of anger in any form.

PSYCHOLOGICAL THEORIES

I would like to end by raising some questions about traditional psychological models of anger, and of all emotions. Psychoanalysts, for example, and some others speak of "infantile" rage as the worst kind of anger, assuming a linear model that links earliest with "worst." On the contrary, I think that you have to have lived a little to experience the worst kind of anger. You have to have experienced the kind of hurtful and simultaneously disavowed experience that I have tried to describe in order to acquire the kind of anger that has the connotations we usually associate with the most terrible and terrifying rage. Usually we call this "helpless rage."

By comparison to this terrible experience, an infant's rage probably is a different phenomenon. Infants and children do demonstrate something we label anger, and it may be vociferous. I believe, however, that it is a much more straightforward, readily dissipated emotion—until it becomes complicated by the kind of experiences I have described. Unfortunately, within our cultural conditions, the straightforward anger is *very likely to be complicated by such experiences.*

Following Freud's later formulations, the traditional psychoanalytic model has taught that people are born with something called aggression, with the suggestion of either a quantitative store of it or an inherent propensity toward it. This aggression is talked of as if it occurs in an almost "raw" state, without content. Through socialization, then, it is said to be "neutralized," "sublimated," "controlled," "modified," or the like.

It is possible instead that emotions as we have classified them so far are "developed" phenomena. They are "crafted" according to what the environmental—that is, the social context —evokes. They are then named, delineated, and conceptualized by that environment—that culture. In other words, infants have the ability to react strongly in a variety of ways, and something like "anger" is one of them. But this expressive reactivity is *not* the same as the kind of rage that can be culturally produced and then projected into the mind of the infant by adult theorists.

As Schafer (1974) has put it,

> By devising and allocating words, which are names, people create modes of experience and enforce specific subjective experience. Names render events, situations, and relationships available or unavailable for psychological life. ... Consequently, whether or not something will be an instance of ... activity or passivity, aggression or masochism ... or something else altogether, or nothing at all, will depend on whether or not we consistently call it this or that or consistently do not name it at all, hence do not constitute and authorize its being. ... There are no preconceptual facts to be discovered and arrayed. There are only loose conventions governing the uses and groupings of the words. ... And these conventions, like all others, must manifest values. (p. 459)

In short, my notion is that the kind of anger that we traditionally have postulated as most extreme is not *there* originally. Our environment has created it and shaped it into the form we know. Such anger, then, is not intrinsic or inevitable. The anger we know is developed by a cultural structure that first incites an angry response. It then compounds the problem by not allowing individuals to fully acknowledge and know that response or to act on their experience. There is no context of assurance that we will be respected or well cared for if we make a direct, honest expression.

Because we—women and men—cannot experience anger as adults, we cannot yet allow it to our children. We have neither the emotional practice nor the concepts that would allow us to do so easily and without fear.

I do not intend to minimize the problem of anger. Instead, I am suggesting that it may be very difficult to entertain the proposition that we have a cultural structure that produces anger as we have known it so far. This cultural structure then ascribes anger to an inherent, dangerous drive—ultimately making us all afraid of ourselves and unable to use our anger to work for a better structure. All the while, the culture actively encourages members of the dominant group to use their anger against each other and against subordinates.

I believe that our culture, and perhaps some others, will not be able to solve its problems with anger until we encourage each sex to examine and understand its own experience more fully and truthfully. I believe that, so far, neither sex has been able to experience, or to express, a sort of anger that may well be possible but that we are not yet able to perceive or conceptualize.

To end this discussion I shall return to Anita's situation. She had been led to believe that her life value should be conferred by her husband, and he was not conferring much. That was a reason to be angry. Further, when she tried to act more independently in a straightforward way, he punished her for it. That was a reason to be angry. She had worked for years to try to provide total care for her husband, and she wanted someone not to take care *of* her but to care *about* her and her thoughts and feelings. No one cared about her in that way. That was another reason to be angry—and that is not dependency. In the face of these factors, plus other matters too lengthy to describe, she had problems in finding a valued sense of self. And that is not dependency, either; but it is another reason to be angry. Anita had to struggle to understand her quest for self-worth, to transfer her anger into productive paths, and to deal with her various disappointments. However, she could shift to activities that brought her at least greater possibility of a better basis for self-worth.

A central point is that a revised examination of the origins and development of Anita's anger enables a clinician to begin with a different perspective. Her anger can be seen as a potential source of mobilization for action—a valuable potential—but with many obstacles to confront in the realities both within and outside her family, and within the constructions of her own mind.

If one can truly come to *feel* this way, I think it makes a critical difference. I think that this is very different from seeing her—even with the best of "sympathy"—as an angry, infantile, dependent woman.

I submit also that a truly respectful interchange based on the experiences of both sexes—especially when these are combined with the study of other oppressed people—can lead us along a path of enlarging dialogue. And I believe that such a dialogue is the only path to further understanding of the realities of psychological development and—in this time of nuclear threat—even to the survival of us all.

This paper was presented at a Stone Center Colloquium in November 1982.

11

Women and Power

JEAN BAKER MILLER

In recent conversations people have told me stories that raise interesting questions. For example, a woman came up to me after a meeting and told me that she was supervisor of a large number of salesworkers. She asked, "Can you tell me what to do with these women?" Then she went on to say that her company has a big meeting once a month in which all the leading salesworkers are recognized individually and asked to say a few words. In the past year or so, quite a few women have been among the salespeople who are recognized. The women get up and say things like, "Well, I really don't know how it happened. I guess I was just lucky this time" or "This must have been a good month." By contrast, the men say, "Well, first I analyzed the national sales situation; I broke that down into regional components and figured out the trends in buying. Then I analyzed the consumer groups, and ... I worked very hard, overtime three-fourths of the nights this month, and ...." The point is, of course, that the women were doing something like that, too, or something in their own style that was just as effective.

Another kind of example came my way when a woman was describing a project she had initiated. She said as she starts to work, she thinks (and colleagues and friends have told her) this work might be genuinely significant and good. "Maybe I'm really onto something here," she tells herself. And immediately, almost in the same second, she says, "This is nothing" or "Everybody knows this anyhow."

Those two examples, I think, point to the question of women and power. In recent years there have emerged some writings about women and power (see, for example, Janeway, 1980), as well as some meetings to consider it from several viewpoints and disciplines. But if we are really going to build the kinds of institutions and personal lives that allow women to grow and flourish, I believe that we must apply much more conscious, concerted, direct attention to women and power. At the same time I believe that most of us women still have a great deal of trouble with the whole area. The only hope, it seems to me, is to keep trying to examine it together.

I am not implying that men *do not* have trouble with power (just look around the world!), but their troubles are different from those of women at this point in history. As with other major topics, I believe women's examination of power not only can illuminate issues that are important to ourselves, but also can bring new understanding to the whole concept of power. It can shed light on the traps and problems of men, perhaps illuminating those things most difficult for men themselves to discover.

I shall begin this initial consideration by reviewing some fairly common occurrences for women, analyzing them from a psychological perspective derived from clinical work.

DEFINING POWER

There have been many definitions of power, each reflecting the historical tradition out of which it comes; also, various disciplines have devised their own definitions (see, for example, McClelland, 1979). An example given in one dictionary says power is "the faculty of doing or performing anything: force; strength; energy; ability; influence"; and then, follows a long string of words leading to "dominion, authority, a ruler"; then come more words, culminating in "military force." I think the list accurately reflects the idea that most of us automatically have about power. We probably have linked the concept with the ability to augment one's own force, authority, or influence as well as to control and limit others—that is, to exercise dominion or to dominate.

My own working definition of power is *the capacity to produce a change*—that is, to move anything from point A or state A to point B or state B. This can even include moving one's own thoughts or emotions, sometimes a very powerful act. It also can include acting to create movement in an interpersonal field, as well as acting in larger realms such as economic, social, or political arenas.

Obviously, that broad definition has to be further differentiated. For example, one may be somewhat powerful psychologically or personally but have virtually no legitimate socially granted power to determine one's own fate economically, socially, or politically. Also there is the question: "Power for what?" One may think in terms of gaining power for oneself, or one may seek influence for some general good or some collective entity.

WOMEN'S VIEW OF POWER

While more precise delineations are necessary, I think it is probably accurate to say that generally in our culture, and in several others, we have maintained the myth that women do not and should not have power in any dimension. Further, we hold the notion that women do not need power. Usually, without openly talking about it, we women have been most comfortable using our powers if we believe we are using them in the service of others. Acting under those general beliefs, and typically not making any of this explicit, women have been effective in many ways. One instance is in women's traditional role, where they have used their powers to foster the growth of others— certainly children, but also many other people. This might be called using one's power to empower another—increasing the other's resources, capabilities, effectiveness, and ability to act. For example, in "caretaking" or "nurturing," one major component is acting and interacting to foster the growth of another on many levels— emotionally, psychologically, and intellectually. I believe this is a very powerful thing to do, and women have been doing it all the time, but no one is accustomed to including such effective action within the notions of power. It is certainly not the kind of power we tend to think of; it involves a different content, mode of action, and goal. The one who exerts such power recognizes that she or he cannot possibly have total influence or control but has to find ways to interact with the other person's constantly changing forces or powers. And all must be done with appropriate timing, phasing, and shifting of skills so that one helps to advance the movement of the less powerful person in a positive, stronger direction.

As a result of this vast body of experience within the family as well as in the workplace and other organizations, I think most women would be most comfortable in a world in which we feel we are not limiting, but rather are enhancing, the power of other people while simultaneously increasing our own power. Consider that statement more closely: The part about enhancing other people's power is difficult for the world to comprehend, for it is not how the "real world" has defined power. Nonetheless, I contend that women would function much more comfortably within such a context. The part about enhancing one's own powers is extremely difficult for women. When women even contemplate acting powerful, they fear the possibility of limiting or putting down another person. They also fear recognizing or admitting the need, and especially the desire, to increase their own powers.

Frankly, I think women are absolutely right to fear the use of power as it has been generally conceptualized and used. The very fact that this is often said to be a defensive or neurotic fear is, I believe, a more telling commentary on the state of our culture than it is on women. For example, in current times one can read that women are not being strong enough or tough enough. Such statements overlook the incredible strengths that women have demonstrated all through history, and they usually refer to some comparison with men's operations in our institutions. I believe they tend to overlook a valid tendency in women—that is, the desire to enhance others' resources and to know, from actual practice and real experience, that it is an extremely valuable and gratifying life activity. On the other side of the picture, however, such statements reflect part of a truth—that women do fear admitting that they want or need power. Yet without power or something like it (which may eventually be described by another term) on both the personal and political level, women cannot effectively bring about anything.

WHEN WOMEN CONFRONT POWER

Now I would like to focus on women's fears in confronting power, using individual examples that will further illustrate what may have been going on in the women I described briefly at the beginning of my remarks. I will highlight some women's inner, or intrapsychic, experiences.

Power and Selfishness

Abby was a low-paid worker in the health field who sought therapy primarily because of her depression. She had spent much of her adult life enhancing her husband's and her two children's development— using her powers to increase their powers. She then started work and did an excellent job, largely because she approached her patients with the basic attitude of helping them to increase their own comfort and abilities and to use their own powers.

After much exploration, Abby recognized that she tended to become depressed not when things were clearly bad but when she realized that she could *do* something more—for example, better understand and effectively act on a situation. She felt this especially when she wanted to act for herself. For example, she knew that she was actually better at some procedures than the doctors were—not just technically better, but *totally* better, for she helped patients to feel more relaxed, more in control, and more powerful. She began to feel that she should get to do more of the interesting work, get higher pay, recognition, and so forth. She also realized that almost at the same moment she felt this way she became blocked by fear, then by self-criticism and self-blame. This seemed to be a complex internal replica of the external conditions. The external conditions clearly blocked her advancement; she was a woman who worked in the lowest ranks of the health care hierarchy. But the internalized forces created even more complex bondage. Initially, for Abby, as for many women, there was the big fear of being seen as wanting to be powerful. This provoked notions of disapproval, but more than that, at a deeper level, it evoked fears of attack and ultimate abandonment by all women and men.

Further exploration unearthed several more sticking points. One was that the prospect of acting on her own interest and motivation kept leading to the notion that she would be selfish. While she could not bear the thought that others would see her as selfish, it was even more critical that she could not bear this conception of herself. I find this theme to be extraordinarily common in women—often women in surprisingly high positions and places—and, by contrast, a rare theme in men. With this theme for Abby there usually would come the notion that she was inadequate anyhow. She felt she should be grateful that anyone would put up with her at all, and she should best forget about the whole thing.

Eventually, this inadequacy theme gave way to yet another stage in which she felt that she indeed did have powers and could use them, but doing so meant, inescapably, that she was being destructive. For Abby, this stage was illustrated by thoughts, fantasies, and dreams indicating destructiveness.

Power and Destructiveness

Another woman, Ellen, was at a different point in dealing with the same problem. She felt able to work and to think well so long as she worked on her ideas and plans in her own house. She could not bring them into the work setting. As she used to put it, "If only I could bring my inside self outside." Eventually, she said that this fear seemed to stem from the experience that as she went into the outside world or to work, she immediately became attuned to the new context, readily picking up its structures and demands. She felt she could not help but respond to that context and those demands.

Again, this kind of feeling is common in women, and again it reflects a very valuable quality. Historically, a woman's being attuned to and responding to her context and to the needs of everybody in it has been part and parcel of helping other people to grow and helping a family to function. Women can bring a special set of abilities to many situations because they *are* able to attune themselves to the complex realities that are operating. (This perhaps is the essence of what mental health researchers have tried to describe in characterizing mothers' contributions to infant development (Winnicott, 1971).)

But consider the other side. Ellen felt that she could not get her own perceptions, evaluations, and judgments moving from inside her to the outside, although she had important contributions to make. To bring her ideas and action into the outside context she had to overcome her ready tendency to be only responsive.

But that was not all. She felt to do so would disrupt the whole scene. In other words, she would be destructive—and that was not a way she felt she should operate.

In each person such a theme forges its specific expression from the individual's history, but the basic theme occurs regularly in many women: To act out of one's own interest and motivation is experienced as the psychic equivalent of being a destructively aggressive person. This is a self-image that few women can bear. In other words, for many women it is more comfortable to feel inadequate. Terrible as that can be, it is still better than to feel powerful, if power makes you feel destructive.

Let me emphasize this thesis: Any person can entertain the prospect of using her or his own life forces and power—individually motivated, in a self-determined direction. In theories about mental health, this is said to bring satisfaction and effectiveness. But for many women it is perceived as the equivalent of being destructive. On the one hand this sets up a life-destroying, controlling psychological condition. On the other hand it makes sense if one sees that women have lived as subordinates and, as subordinates, have been led by the culture to believe that their own self-determined action is wrong and evil. Many women have incorporated deeply the inner notion that such action must be destructive. The fact that women have survived at all, I believe, is explained by the fact that women do use power all the time but generally must see it as used for the benefits of others.

Do not misunderstand me: Using one's abilities and powers for others is not bad by any means. It does become problematic for women and for men, however, when such activity is prescribed for one sex only, along with the mandate that one must not act on one's own motivation and according to one's own determinations. In most institutions it is still true that if women do act from their own perceptions and motivations, directly and honestly, they indeed may be disrupting a context that has not been built out of women's experience. Thus one is confronted with feeling like one must do something very powerful that also feels destructive.

Power and Abandonment

Another woman, Connie, illustrated this dramatically: She had difficulty finishing her work. But she discovered that she would become "blocked" not when she was really stuck but when she was working well, streaming ahead, getting her thoughts in order, and making something happen. At those times she would get up from her desk, start walking around, become involved in some diversion, talk to someone, and generally get off the productive trajectory. Further exploration of why this happened led eventually to her saying that if she let herself go on when she was working well, "I would be too powerful and then where would I be . . . I would not need anyone else." For Connie, the prospect was that she would be out in some scary place. She said she would feel like some unrecognizable creature, some non-woman. She spoke of the prospect as if it signified the loss of a central sense of identity. Her sense of identity, like that of so many women, was so bound up with being a person who *needs* that the prospect of *not needing* felt like, first of all, a loss of the known and familiar self.

On the one hand, it was an unnecessary fear. On the other hand, Connie touched on a sense that is present in many women—namely, that the use of our powers with some efficacy and, even worse, with freedom, zest, and joy, feels as if it will destroy a core sense of identity. One feature of that identity, as reflected by Connie's statement, demonstrates how deeply women have incorporated the notion, "I exist only as I need." Again, I think women are reflecting a truth that men have been encouraged to deny—that is, all of us exist only as we need others for that existence—but cultural conditions have led women to incorporate this in an extreme form. Along with it we women have incorporated the troubling notion that, as much as we need others, we also have powers and the motivation to use those powers, but, if we use them, we will destroy the relationships we need for our existence.

THE TROUBLESOME EQUATIONS

With these examples I have outlined some of the inner experiences women have related to me as they confronted the issue of power. They include the following:

- A woman's using self-determined power for herself is equivalent to *selfishness,* for she is not enhancing the power of others.
- A woman's using self-determined power for herself is equivalent to *destructiveness,* for such power inevitably will be excessive and will totally disrupt an entire surrounding context.
- The equation of power with destructiveness and selfishness seems impossible to reconcile with a sense of feminine identity.
- A woman's use of power may precipitate attack and *abandonment;* consequently, a woman's use of power threatens a central part of her identity, which is a feeling that she needs others.

It is important to emphasize again the many sides of all of this. On the one hand, most women are keenly aware of the essential truth that we all need others, need to live in the framework of relationships, and also need to increase the powers of others through our activities. On the other hand, most women have been encouraged to experience these needs as a predominant, central, almost total definition of their personalities. And their experience tells them that change can occur only at the cost of destroying one's place in the world and one's chance for living within a context of relationships. I believe this reflects accurately the historic and cultural place, and the definition, of women.

THE CHALLENGES AHEAD

The examples I have cited not only tell about individual neuroses but also reflect characteristics of many women. Right now I think it is important for women to recognize that we do need to use our powers. Many times, I think, women have done things that eventually proved to be destructive, often without being fully aware, because we actually felt so much pain and reluctance even to think about the topic.

Also, we need to help each other in several important ways. First, we can give sympathetic understanding to ourselves if we recognize the weight of the historic conditions that have made power such a difficult concept for most of us. Second, we can consider seriously the proposition that there is enormous validity in women's *not* wanting to use power as it is presently conceived and used. Rather, women may want to be powerful in ways that simultaneously enhance, rather than diminish, the power of others. This is a radical turn—a very different motivation from the concept of power upon which this world has operated.

Out of this, we can see that women already may have a strong motivation to approach the concept of power with a different, critical, and creative stance. Once admitting a desire and a need for power, women can seek new ways of negotiating power with others in personal life, work, and other institutions. Certainly this is a large and difficult prospect. It can appear naive or unreal even to talk this way. But the fact that it sounds unreal must not stop us. Once we recognize the undeniable truth that the world has been explained so far without the close observation of women's experience, it is easier to consider that seemingly "unreal" possibilities can become real.

Bear in mind these truths that have not been taken into account:

- Women's experience is usually not what it has been said to be.
- It is not men's experience. It does not necessarily operate on the same bases, the same motivations, or the same organization of personality.
- What we find when we study women are parts of the total human potential that have not been fully seen, recognized, or valued. These are parts that have not therefore flourished, and perhaps they are precisely the ingredients that we must bring into action in the conduct of all human affairs.
- Certainly these emerging notions must be used for the benefit of women, which is reason enough to pursue them, but they must be used also for the ultimate benefit of everyone.

This paper was presented at a Stone Center Colloquium in November 1981.

12

The "Self-in-Relation": Implications for Depression in Women

ALEXANDRA G. KAPLAN

In 1978, Arieti and Bemporad, two distinguished writers on the subject of depression, described a personality pattern commonly found to be associated with depression.

> The necessity to please others and to act in accordance with their expectations . . . makes him unable to get really in touch with himself. He does not listen to his own wishes; he does not know what it means to be himself. . . . When he experiences feelings of unhappiness, futility and unfulfillment, he . . . tends to believe that he is to be blamed for them. (p. 139)

The authors append this description with the footnote: "As is customary in English, I refer to the general patient as he and consider him and his male role. However, women with this type of personality are more numerous than men."

Language aside, the authors suggest, but do not address or elaborate upon, the possibility that there is a *reason* that the cluster of dynamics they describe is more frequently found in women than in men. Depression, as has been well documented now, is overwhelmingly a women's disorder. Twice as many women as men undergo depressive episodes, and one in ten women can expect to have a serious depression in her lifetime (Weissman & Klerman, 1979). But even beyond the more severe syndrome of depression, depression as a mood or a symptom seems to be a specter that haunts women, a mode of experience with which all women seem able to identify. As I was describing this paper to a woman whom I see in therapy, I explained to her that I would, in part, be contrasting responses of depressed and nondepressed women to an interview protocol. She looked at me with complete sincerity and asked, "So you mean you were really able to find women who were not depressed?" This woman spoke for many women's fears, if not felt reality, of the relationship between women and depression.

Indeed, the frequency of depression in women suggests that depression may not be an "illness" superimposed on an alien or indifferent personality structure, but rather may be a distortion—an exaggeration of the normative state of being female in Western society. This paper will develop the position that an understanding of the frequency of depression in women requires a recognition of the fundamental overlap between central dynamics of *depression* and key dimensions in the nature of *women's psychological development*. From an examination of this overlap, many points of inquiry follow, only two of which will be pursued here. The first is to illustrate how new perspectives on depression in women, qua women extend, expand, and refine key aspects of existing theories of depression. The second purpose, which I will cover much more briefly, will be to examine the extent to which the existing literature on depression supports our speculation that the features of depression we are describing are especially true of depressed *women*.

Locating our inquiry in the realm of the underlying personality structure of the class of people who are most likely to become depressed places us within one of the current directions advocated for the study of depression. Salzman (1975), for example, suggests that "the underlying personality in which a depressive episode occurs may be the key issue" (p. 44). Similarly, Chodoff (1974) argues that "the task for researchers, then, is to find ways to test hypotheses about predisposing personality factors or to initiate imaginative investigative forays which will provide new hypotheses" (p. 68). We could not have put it any better, except to clarify that while these writers are focusing on *individual* personality structures, we are arguing that the first step is to consider personality structures that may be common to the *group* of people most likely to become depressed, that is, women.

In looking at the broad sweep of underlying personality structure as it evolves within a social context, we will, by necessity, not review many important specific contributions to the study of depression in women. These include major works on sex differences in depression, such as those by Weissman and Paykel (1974), Hammen and Padesky (1977), and Blatt, D'Afflitti, and Quinlan (1976). In addition, we will not examine important studies of the social conditions that influence women's relative vulnerability to depression (Belle, 1982; Brown & Harris, 1982; Radloff, 1980). Finally, we will not explore the possible role of biochemical factors. Rather, as a preliminary inquiry, the focus will be on underlying personality factors as they evolve within a social context. These appear common to women in general, and exacerbated for depressed women.

A NEW MODEL OF WOMEN'S PSYCHOLOGICAL DEVELOPMENT: THE SELF-IN-RELATION

A discussion of depression in women in light of women's psychological development requires a developmental theory that validly reflects women's experience. It is generally accepted now that existing theories are rooted strongly in the male experience, with women understood in terms of what they are missing when measured against the male paradigm (Gilligan, 1982; Miller, Chapter 1, this volume). An alternative theory constructed to reflect women's development has been evolving at the Stone Center at Wellesley College. More complete statements of this theory can be found in Surrey (Chapter 3, this volume) and Miller (Chapter 1, this volume). I can present here only the basic parameters, referring the reader to the other articles for a fuller elaboration.

In brief, we are arguing that while existing theories posit some form of autonomy or separation as the developmental path, women's core self-structure, or their primary motivational thrust, concerns growth within relationship, or what we call the "self-in-relation." By relation we mean much more than is indicated in interpersonal or object relations theories such as those of Sullivan (1953) or Fairbairn (1962). What we are emphasizing, in contrast to these theories, are the key aspects of attaining a capacity to be attuned to the affect of others, understanding and being understood by the other, and thus participating in the development of others. Thus relationship is a two-way interaction, at its best a mutual process wherein both parties feel enhanced and empowered through their empathic connection with the other.

Connection with others, then, is a key component of action and growth, not a detraction from or a means to one's self-enhancement, as is implied in other theories. Further, what is important is women's sense of taking an active role in the *process* of facilitating and enhancing connectedness with others. Engagement in this process in turn fosters the gradual evolution of a differentiated self, a self with its own clear properties, wishes, impulses, and so forth—but a self that achieves articulation through participation in and attention to the relational process. Thus the growth of the differentiated self is commensurate with the growth of one's relational capacities and relational network, from the earliest parent–child dyad to an increasingly complex, multifaceted web of being with others that can ebb and flow in response to social conditions.

In reality, the extent to which women can act and feel empowered by their relational capacities is highly dependent on the extent of societal and individual valuing of these strengths. As Miller (1976) and others have argued, our society not only does not value these attributes, but tends to interpret them as weaknesses. This powerful denigrating of relational qualities has restricted the vast majority of women to less than the full use of their own resources, too often limiting their actions—at home or in the workforce.

We will now attempt to demonstrate that when women are severely constricted in the full development of their relational capacities, and when women are strongly discouraged or punished for self-expression, the conditions are established that can lead to depression. To illustrate this point, we will first document some of the key features in depression across varying perspectives and then show how extreme forms of curtailment of women's normative developmental patterns create the very intrapsychic conditions that are recognized as the hallmarks of depression.

KEY ELEMENTS OF DEPRESSION

1. *The experience of loss.* The experience of emotional loss, whether due to the actual disappearance of a significant person through death or desertion, or through the experience of emotional disconnection, is at the heart of many accounts of the origin of depression, especially psychoanalytic. It was introduced by Freud in his early writings (1917) and then elaborated upon as psychoanalysis moved on to develop its structural theory and then its ego psychology. More recent cognitive and behavioral theories and some research studies also cite the experience of emotional loss as a common precursor of depression (Beck, 1972; Seligman, 1975).

2. *The inhibition of anger and aggression.* This concept, again, figures prominently in psychoanalytic accounts of depression. As first

described by Freud, early relational losses cause the person to turn both her or his love for, and anger at, the failed love object back against the self. That is, the disappointing other is not rejected from one's emotional life, but rather is "internalized" so that feelings directed toward the other become directed toward the self. Thus, the angry reactions caused by the behavior of the other are now experienced not as anger at the other, but as an attack on the self.

3. *Inhibition of action or assertiveness.* The inability to act, immobility, is a characteristic diagnostic sign of depression (Spitzer, 1980). Inhibition of action and movement is noted in psychoanalytic accounts of depression (e.g. Bibring, 1953) in which it is explained as a powerless ego state. Beck's (1972) cognitive theory identifies such inhibitions as the behavioral result of negative cognitions about the self, the world, and the future, while Seligman (1975) links a decreased motivation to act with the condition he labels "learned helplessness," which comes from not having control over the consequences of one's behavior.

4. *Low self-esteem.* This concept is also at the heart of all major theories of depression. It is, in effect, the end result of the above three conditions, and in turn it contributes further to them. Feelings of grave injury to the self through emotional loss, suppressing anger, or turning it against the self are all said to contribute to the pervasive feelings of worthlessness and extreme inadequacy that comprise what we think of as low self-esteem.

Each of these aspects of depression is discussed in the literature without consideration of how their development and/or manifestation may be influenced by gender-based, normative developmental prescriptions. It is as though the way one handles anger, the capacity to act in the world, one's sense of being validated by societal norms and expectations have nothing to do with whether one is a woman or a man. And yet we know from many bodies of research that this is not at all the case. More specifically, there are even times when descriptions of the depressive syndrome are difficult to distinguish from the female experience. Listen again to the quotation with which I began this paper, but replace, now, the author's "he" with "she.": "The necessity to please others and to act in accordance with their expectations . . . makes her unable really to get in touch with herself. She does not listen to her own wishes; she does not know what it means to be herself. When she experiences feelings of unhappiness, futility and unfulfillment, she . . . tends to believe that she is to be blamed for them." Is this just a description of depression, or could this be a description of one aspect of the modal experience of being a woman in society?

DEPRESSION AND WOMEN'S PSYCHOLOGICAL DEVELOPMENT

We can now reexamine the four parameters of depression outlined above to explore how they relate to women's development and to examine how they can be distorted in ways that then characterize the depressive experience. Our own theoretical position will be illustrated by vignettes from women with whom I have worked in therapy and women who responded to an open-ended interview format that we have developed to explore more precisely some of our hunches. The interviews have been held with both women who were identified by their therapists as depressed and with women who had not been so identified. These vignettes are presented as anecdotal illustrations of the points we are making, not yet as confirmation of our speculations. As a group, those quoted are all white, single, heterosexual women ranging in age from their mid-20s to their 50s, college educated and currently in pursuit of additional education or engaged in a professional career, although for the depressed women not nearly in the manner nor to the extent that they would like.

Vulnerability to Loss

Self-in-relation theory suggests new understandings of the term *loss,* as it is used in the depression literature, that highlight its applicability to women. From our perspective, women, if not deflected, seek to maintain connection with others in an empathic mode that validates their own capacities as a relational being. Yet social values, as embedded in the construction of work and family roles, all serve to make this a difficult quest at best. The devaluing of relational qualities (e.g., when connection is interpreted as "dependency" on the one hand or "smothering" on the other hand—see Stiver, Chapter 8, this volume) can lead women to doubt or fail even to recognize the value of their own endeavors. But more, to the extent that women seek mutuality of understanding with others, they are often disappointed, especially but not only in relationships with men. This can leave women in a constant state of felt loss. Moreover, this is more than "object loss" as it is usually discussed. It is, instead, the loss of confirmation of their core self-structure as one that can facilitate reciprocity and affective connection in relationships.

For women who become depressed this pattern is greatly exacerbated. In the case of loss through death of a parent there is, of course, the ending of an important avenue for relational connection. There is also the possibility of a prolonged grief or even depression of the surviving parent, which could severely limit the availability of that parent to serve as a new or additional source of affective relatedness.

More typical, however, would be the loss the depressed woman can experience throughout her lifetime from the sustained state of profound disconnection from a parent who is affectively not available to her, or who responds to her impulses and attempts at contact with disdain, ridicule, or outright hostility. Such experiences, accumulated over the years, can generate in the child a pervasive sense of her utter inability to sustain relationship or please the other, which is tantamount to a major disconfirmation of her core sense of self-worth. Further, such rejection conveys to the child the sense that her basic wishes and impulses are inherently harmful to others. Thus the ultimate loss in many depressed women's history is not so much the loss of gratification from another, but the major loss of confirmation of their core self-structure.

This cycle is illustrated by the words of one of the women I interviewed. Much of her childhood was dominated by her attempts to forestall the loss of her father, who was constantly threatening to leave the family. "The thought of his leaving would devastate me—so I kept trying so hard to be responsible and mature and smart, and to anticipate what he was going to want. I think this happened at the expense of being a child. Everything went into that. When I was growing up, my father was my life line. The fear of him leaving was constant. I invested tremendous energy into pleasing—so that he would *love* me and not leave. He *had* to love me."

Inhibition of Action and Assertion

As women in general experience failure or frustration in their attempts at affective connection with others, they themselves take responsibility for the relational failure, assuming that if they were "better" they would not have such problems. In a somewhat paradoxical mode, then, failure at relationship stimulates further attempt at connection in the hope that renewed efforts will succeed where past attempts have failed and, thus, confirm the core self-structure. But the residue of self-doubt is played out in the inhibition of other forms of action. This leads them to curtail endeavors that, under more affirming relational conditions, they would be apt to pursue. Such inhibition of action directly embedded in a relational context is beautifully expressed by Emily Dickinson (1861/1960):

Why—do they shut Me out of Heaven?
Did I sing—too loud?
But—I can say a little "Minor"
Timid as a Bird!

Wouldn't the Angels try me—
Just—once—more?
Just—see—if I troubled them—
But don't—shut the door.

Oh if I—were the Gentleman
In the "White Robe"
And they—were the little Hand—that knocked—
Could—I—forbid?

For women who become depressed, the profound fear of major disruption of relational ties and the concomitant basic threat to the integrity and authenticity of the core self-structure can constrict seriously a large range of activities and modes of expression. But, as is the normative model described above, the constriction is not total. That is, there is a distinct *selective* inhibition that applies strongly to actions that further one's own goals, and not nearly as strongly, if at all, to actions that support or enhance someone else.

This pattern of women severely inhibiting their own strivings and actions so as to preserve relational ties emerges over and over again in clinical work with depressed women. One woman, for example, currently is working in a mundane job under a kindly boss who is nonetheless relentless in urging the workers to devote much more time than necessary to their work. This woman is grieved by the fear of letting her boss down, and she struggles to meet the boss's demands. Yet this commitment deprives her of any time to pursue her considerable talent in her chosen but nonlucrative field. Knowing that she is wasting her most productive years, she still sees disappointing her boss as a weakness in herself in that she would see it as putting the pursuit of her own interests over the needs of another.

Another woman who put tremendous effort into supporting her husband's career aspirations was paralyzed in doing the same for herself. On a few occasions she finally gathered up the courage to approach someone who might help her. If the initial response was negative, she would meekly reply "OK, thank you" and leave. In retrospect she is appalled at her lack of "courage" and full of ideas of things she could have said to try and change that person's mind. This same woman, a vibrant and lively talker in most instances, described to me a recent important career accomplishment in words so soft I had no idea what she was saying. I drew her attention to this, and she noted that "there I go again" as we both had a good, confirming laugh. In contrast to these examples is the experience of one of the nondepressed women, who, while describing herself as "very introspective," knows that she "likes to be in control of what's going on around me." She states that "I'm very aware of how people respond to me—and I can adapt to that, but I feel that I still have a definite personality that comes across regardless of my adapting to people's needs. I'm still very much me."

Inhibition of Anger and Aggression

Miller (1976, Chapter 1, this volume) argued that women inhibit their expression of anger out of a fear—often confirmed—that such expression will disrupt important relationships. But, she added, holding back anger is disempowering and leaves one feeling constricted, ineffective, and perhaps wrong for even feeling angry. Thus women's goal of mutually empathic relationships is felt to be thwarted by their anger, even though anger—directly and validly expressed— can be an affirming and bonding experience between two people if it occurs in a context of mutuality. Feelings of powerlessness in turn generate more anger, but this anger also is constricted, leading to further feelings of ineffectiveness until the anger may explode in ways that may be greatly exaggerated or "off target."

For women who become depressed, this pattern, again, is greatly exaggerated. Similar to their feelings about action on their own behalf, anger is associated with "destructiveness." That is, their inner sense of "badness" generates the fear that expressed anger would be explosive, out of control, and devastating to the receiver. Depressed women are sometimes aware of and in touch with their feelings of anger. And yet the fears of the consequence of this anger are severe because these women experience their anger not as a valid sign of strength but rather as a confirmation of their bad and worthless selves. The struggle to contain their anger, however, further contributes to the inhibition of action as described above.

Fears of the destructive consequences of their anger were expressed by many of the women. For one woman, this fear arose regarding her feelings of intense anger at her mother and sister. Having fought with them, she would then feel "devasted" and go off alone to her room to cry. "My fear," she reported, "was that if I really let them know how angry I was, I would kill them." Another woman spoke about her inability to act on her rage at her husband. This woman, less able to act on her immediate anger than the woman just described, projected her feelings and fears onto her husband. She could not leave this difficult marriage, or even present her grievances, she recalled, because she was convinced that if she did so, her husband would kill himself, for which she would hold herself fully responsible.

Another woman, who had a difficult and conflictual relationship with her mother, had for years struggled to please and care for her, efforts that were consistently rejected. She had, by adolescence, long linked her angry feelings toward her mother with strong feelings of responsibility for their difficulties because of her "badness." This was illustrated poignantly in adolescence, beginning with her mother's insistence on giving her a fancy birthday party, something that she did not want because she was "so undeserving." Yet the party occurred, after which the mother suffered a serious heart attack. The young woman was devastated, feeling herself responsible for her mother's infirmity and seeing the illness as direct confirmation of her inherent "destructiveness."

These situations can be contrasted to the account given by one of the nondepressed women. She recalled being with two men friends riding in a small car and driving too fast on a dark and poorly paved road. She was furious because it was a new car and they were not used to it. She had begged them not to make the trip at all in that car, let alone recklessly. She knew that if she became angry and asked them to slow down, they would not. Instead, she found another strategy. She said something like, "Well, this is not fair. I have not had my turn to drive yet." In response, the driver did pull the car over.

Low Self-Esteem

Women's general sense of low self-esteem is both the end result of and a contributing factor to the conditions described above. The felt responsibility for failures in evolving mutually affirming relationships can leave women doubting the value of their own relational worth. To reemphasize this point, we have suggested that women's sense of self-worth rests heavily on their sense of their ability to make and build relationships. Further, women are limited in the gains to self-worth that could come from the free expression and confirmation of their own wishes, a freedom that they fear—or know—will threaten connectedness. Yet it is precisely this freedom of expression in pursuit of one's own desires that receives the strongest cultural support, especially when it is exhibited by men. Thus, for women in general, there lingers a certain sense of inadequacy (especially when they measure themselves against culturally valued masculine norms) that is directly translated into lowered self-esteem.

Again, the pattern is much the same for depressed women, only more extreme. Early and continuing emotional disconnection from others, marked often by punishment or withdrawal in response to their attempts at sustaining relationships, contributes to a basic sense of personal worthlessness and futility of action. The profound sense of responsibility that depressed women assume for these failures creates a core sense of their own "destructiveness." This inner sense in turn severely inhibits those actions that are not directly in the service of facilitating the growth of others. This inhibition of action further fuels their sense of worthlessness, and so the cycle continues.

These themes of one's inherent "badness," the fear of harming others even as one is reaching out, and the sense of personal inauthenticity appear repeatedly in therapy with depressed women. This is reflected in even relatively minor areas of everyday life. One woman felt terrible because she had failed to look up at me when I had entered the waiting room to get her, feeling that she had seriously insulted me. Another woman described her intense fear, even when she dials a wrong number, that she might say the wrong thing. At such times she would have a true anxiety reaction with sweaty palms, heart palpitations, and a sense of being frozen. Her only recourse was to become able to predict what the other person would say and to prepare a proper response. What is striking about these examples is that these women not only feel diminished in self-esteem by relatively minor actions, but come in time not to trust, or even be able to recognize, their own impulses, which then feeds into the inhibition of action discussed above.

Another situation reflects a more extreme instance of how fear of harming others contributes to a devastation of self-esteem. In this instance, a woman cried at length about something she had done that was so terrible that she could not tell me, but that left her feeling grievously destructive and damaging to another. This action finally was discussed, and it turned out to be her failure to submit my bill to her insurance company at the proper time.

By contrast, one of the nondepressed women, who did feel bad about herself when relationships with others were not going well, was then able to act so as to better the situation. "When I'm not feeling good about myself and keeping up with my friendships, I'll force myself to go out with a person and lend them my time and understanding and then I'll definitely feel better about them and then about myself."

CRITIQUE OF EXISTING THEORIES OF DEPRESSION

These new formulations about women's experience of depression can be used now to refine and extend the concepts of vulnerability to loss, inhibition of action, inhibition of assertion, and low self-esteem as they are constructed in the more traditional models of depression. In general, our formulations provide major new interpretations of dynamics described in existing theory by illuminating more clearly women's experience of depression. Even our basic starting point, although in line with psychoanalytic concepts of depression, differs from them in important ways. That is, in the psychoanalytic literature, relational (i.e., interpersonal) factors are seen to play a key role in the developing personality of depressed people. As Salzman (1975) puts it: "Depression is something that is happening to a person in reaction to others." But the traditional analytic construction of these relational factors is different from the use suggested by our model. Both our theory and analytic theory link relational precursors of depression with some form of emotional loss or the vulnerability to loss. But psychoanalytic theory locates the impact of this loss on the loss of something that would be given to the individual—in their terminology, "narcissistic supplies." Included in that idea are both the absence of gratification of oral needs and relational disappointment in terms of rejection or disappointment from others. Note that within analytic theory, the loss occurs in one interpersonal direction—from the "external supply giver" to the self. Gratification is being withheld, needs remain unmet. Analytic theory, then, posits that this loss of gratification has a devastating effect on one's self-esteem. Again, this effect is put in relational terms, but not as we would. The emphasis remains unidirectional; low self-esteem is seen as coming directly from feelings of being wounded, hurt, or neglected in a relationship with another. In general, Kohut (1971) continues in this line of thought.

Self-in-relation theory provides important refinements in the understanding of this process. Rather than putting our emphasis on the one-way loss from the so-called giver to the so-called receiver, we would emphasize much more of a two-way, mutual process. As our theory stresses, psychological development, especially for girls, is based on mutual understandings and reciprocity of affect. It is the flow of empathic communication and mutual attentiveness from one to the other that not only permits the child to feel cared for but begins to develop in the child a sense of herself as a caring being, as one who derives strength and competence from her own relational capacities. Thus, in our theory, what is ultimately lost is not just something that should be provided by another but, importantly, the chance to take part in a mutually affirming relationship—to be affectively connected with another and thereby confirmed in the validity of your own self as a person-in-relationship. And it is the absence of this capacity for connecting with others—the denial of the opportunity for full development of one's relational goals—that would be the hallmark of the effect of loss.

Findings from recent research studies also point to the general importance of relational factors for depressed women. Relationship loss figures prominently, according to some studies, in the childhood experiences of women who become depressed as compared to women who do not become depressed (Brown & Harris, 1978). Relatedly, the presence of an intimate confidante has been found to be a major barrier against depression under stressful life circumstances (Belle, 1982). Other studies found that the majority of women who sought therapy for depression had experienced a relational loss within the 6 months just preceding the onset of their depression (Weissman & Klerman, 1979; Schwartz & Juroff, 1979). Similarly, depressed women more than depressed men sought help from others as a means for countering their depressive states (Padesky & Hammen, 1981). In all of these research studies the point is usually made implicitly or explicitly that the loss of gratification from another is responsible for the connection between loss of an important relationship and depression. We would not disagree that this sort of loss does have an impact on the development of depression. But, again, we would add that women in addition suffer the loss of confirmation of their relational self-structure, the opportunity for contributing to the relational process. The absence of intimacy is experienced more centrally as a *failure of the self*, even if in conjunction with failure of support or love from another.

Self-in-relation theory also enriches understanding of the process of the inhibition of action and assertion as described by others. Seligman (1975), for example, offers an explanation for such inhibitions under the rubric of "learned helplessness." He argues that depression results from the loss of control over the modes of reinforcement for one's behavior. That is, depression can result if one feels unable to anticipate or predict the consequences of one's behavior, prediction that is necessary for one to feel able to act so as to produce change. In the absence of such control, one in a sense "gives up," with concomitant feelings of helplessness and futility. This framework is consistent with what we are saying, but only to a point. For one thing, Seligman does not speak to the impact of this "loss of control" on one's core self-structure; it is not only helplessness but self-blame and responsibility that we would posit as the key issue here. For another, Seligman does not distinguish between relative degrees of "helplessness," depending on the kind of action involved. We would argue, as described above, that depressed women are not equally inhibited in all modes of action. Rather, this inhibition would be especially marked in actions felt to be selfish or destructive in a relational context and much less marked in actions felt by the woman to be especially facilitative of others. In fact, as Miller (1976) has pointed out, depressed women can be very active if they see their actions as occurring within the "proper context."

ON THE COMPARISON OF DEPRESSION IN WOMEN AND MEN

Having demonstrated some key dynamic links between major features of women's psychological development and central aspects of depression, it now behooves us to consider whether the qualities we are describing are indeed more true of depressed women than of depressed men. Are they qualities that are linked generally to depression or more specifically to depressed women? In either case, the link we have demonstrated would be instructive. Indeed, even if depressed women and men followed essentially the same dynamic pattern, the greater fit between this pattern and women's, more than men's, normative developmental trajectories would provide one important explanation for the greater incidence of depression in women than in men.

However, the depression literature does provide some clues to the possibility that there may be differential patterns of depression in women and men. These are merely hints, and they come from two sources. The first source are those instances in which researchers note, but do not elaborate on, an empirical finding that specific patterns of depression are more common in one sex than in the other. The second comes from identification of several different patterns of depression within a research population, one of which conforms closely to women's developmental characteristics and the other to men's (this is, however, typically not pointed out). A few examples will illustrate these tendencies.

Arieti and Bemporad (1978) provide one such distinction. They describe, for one, the "placating personality," which I have excerpted in earlier quotations. Briefly, you will remember, this description focuses on elements of an inability to listen to one's own wishes, the need to please others, and feelings of self-blame if things go wrong. This description is very similar to some of the key elements we have highlighted about women and depression. These writers could have "gotten it," but they stopped short of exploring the *implications* of their finding that this pattern does indeed occur more often in women than in men.

Arieti and Bemporad contrast this portrayal to a second type of predepressed personality, which may be prototypical of men's experience. It is consistent not with a core self-in-relation but with a self-in-advancement, a "performing self." In the words of Arieti and Bemporad, this type of person is characterized by

> the pursuit of a significant goal and gradually becomes haunted by this dominant goal. The dominant goal is omnipresent—and as a rule is grandiose, like winning the Nobel prize or becoming the chief of the firm, and the actions of the patient can be interpreted as being motivated by the attempt to attain what his grandiose self-image demands—the attainment of the dominant goal seems motivated by a thirst for glory. Unconsciously, the patient feels that he will be worthy of love from others or from himself only if he succeeds in achieving the dominant goal. (p. 141)

While both of these personalities are oriented to a search for love, the paths they take are diametrically opposed. For the first, the search occurs within a relational process with the feelings and self of the person altered and shaped so as to preserve connectedness for which the person holds herself responsible. For the second, the search occurs via the path of self-aggrandizement, which secondarily may promote connection with others. Others should love the person for what he has *done for himself,* while his own actions reflect no contribution to building connection, nor does his self-esteem lie in his capacities to forge this connection.

A similar dichotomy can be found in the writings of Grinker and colleagues (1961). Based on an intensive interview study, he identifies several major factors in depression, two of which are of interest here. The first, which is consistent with our portrayal of depression in women, is characterized by feelings of sadness, shame, and guilt that derive from a basic feeling of unworthiness. This bad self in turn leads to self-punishment and a pervasive feeling of low self-esteem. The second factor, which they found to be significantly higher in men, is characterized by an almost complete concern with external problems, most notably material loss and a sense that their inner state could be changed only by the outside world's providing something for them. While this portrayal is more delimited, it still suggests a basic dichotomy between failings as being either internal or external and responsibility (and blame) as being located in the self in the first instance and in the external world in the second.

CONCLUSION

We are arguing that the field of psychology needs to make fundamental revisions in its thinking about the dynamics of depression in women and, indeed, about women's psychology in general. Such thinking would center on a developmentally grounded understanding of women's core self-structure as it is enhanced and as it evolves through growth-in-relationship—and as this growth is thwarted by social denigration of relational capacities. This line of thought would permit an understanding of many women's sense of inadequacy in the face of barriers to the kind of relational goals that they seek. Such validation would be an important counter to women's current tendency to place responsibility for their failures on themselves. A lessened sense of self-blame could, in turn, free women for more effective action that would be consistent with their relational goals.

Some of this work can be done in psychotherapy, although individual solutions cannot be an adequate response to a pervasive social problem. But therapy under the proper conditions can provide a corrective experience to the downward spiral of worthlessness and immobility that is so often described in women. But "proper conditions" are crucial. Most importantly, women's inner state needs to be understood in terms of its relational meanings and relational goals. Without this, there is a too-easy link between women's self-reports and clinicians' labels of "dependency" or "neediness," terms that highlight women's "weaknesses" and belie the active relational strivings behind their situation. Without a relational frame, women may hear in therapy that they are trying to do "too much," that they should lower their aspirations and look more to others for assistance. (Indeed, this is a direct derivation of the depressive condition that we suggested *might* be consistent with the male, but not the female, experience of depression, where depression was linked with failure to achieve a "dominant (performance) goal." This, in turn, suggests that while many clinicians have made observations that tend to show different types of depression, their therapeutic actions are often those that fit the more "male" kind of depression, despite the fact that the majority of depressed patients are women.

The quality of relationship between client and therapist would also be a central component of the proper conditions for therapy. In essence, an empathic bond between client and therapist is essential for the therapist to hear and validate the client's own experience as she, not the therapist, constructs it. In the absence of an empathic mode of communication, women's fears or feelings of realistic sadness or inadequacy may be brushed off or "pathologized" by the therapist, especially as these feelings fit a therapist's expectations of women, again, as overemotional, dependent, or the like. Therapy can be a place for a mutually empathic relationship to thrive. I experienced this anew as I prepared this paper and sought permission from my clients to include parts of their stories. They were pleased that their experiences contributed to my understanding of depression, just as I was gratified that my understanding could be of benefit to them.

Beyond psychotherapy, there is of course the ultimate "corrective experience" in terms of changed life conditions. But there is also an important intermediate step, which is sharing these new ways of knowing and thinking with other women. Knowledge is indeed empowering. A lot of the work that is currently done in therapy with women probably could be done as well, or better, by women being with other women, especially when given access to appropriate models for understanding and validating their experience. Women have not had such access to date and, worse, what models they did have served often to invalidate their own experience. We hope that recent writings on women and relationship are providing a contribution in this direction.

This paper was presented at a Stone Center Colloquium in December 1983.

13

Work Inhibitions in Women

IRENE P. STIVER

Two studies illustrate some of the facets of women's work problems. In one, Ruth Moulton (1977) surveyed 200 psychoanalysts—150 men and 50 women. They were asked the simple question: "Would you refuse an invitation to speak publicly?" Fifty percent of the women said they would refuse to speak, contrasted to 20% of the men. This seems particularly surprising because the subjects were women psychoanalysts who were presumably sophisticated and self-aware. In another study (Crandall, Katkovsky, & Preston, 1962) with latency-aged boys and girls, it was found that the brighter the boy, the better he expected to do in the future and the more he thought his good scores were a result of his competence. In contrast, the brighter the girl, the less she was apt to think her good performance was a reflection of her own capacity, and she did not expect to do better in the future.

Despite such observations, women rarely come to therapy with a presenting problem around work. Men who have difficulties at work seem to see them as a legitimate reason for entering therapy. Women more typically come into therapy because of a concern about a personal relationship, and it is only as the therapy progresses that work issues come into focus.

When the work problems emerge, it is striking to see how frequently and pervasively women still experience conflict and varying degrees of distress in their jobs. Some women experience so much anxiety about entering or reentering the work arena that they do not try to get a job, even though they may have a strong interest in doing something that would use their talents and abilities. Other women, working out of economic necessity and feeling dissatisfied with their jobs, often feel hopeless about their ability to move into work which might be more meaningful. Then there are those women who do pursue work interests and prepare for a career but get stuck at some point and cannot go further—for example, a graduate student who does well up to the point of writing the doctoral dissertation and then becomes blocked and cannot complete her work, or a woman in industry who reaches the middle management level and then sabotages her own chances to move ahead or does not take advantage of opportunities for advancement. Even women workers who are clearly successful, effective, and competent often feel privately that their horizons are limited significantly by the kinds of anxieties and difficulties they experience in their work situations.

I believe that some of the recent writing on this topic has given us fast explanations that have not probed many deeper realms. Some of these answers have even attained notoriety in the popular media, where they have taken on an almost sloganlike repetitiveness. The major effect has been, I believe, to make women feel worse. In this discussion, I will address several facets of women's work experience. In some instances, this means raising issues with the explanations currently offered in order to highlight the problems in these explanations. Perhaps we can move on to a more complex and appropriate exploration of work issues with which women struggle without reducing them to additions on the list of "problems women have."

Are women's problems about work different from men's—and if so, how? What is immediately apparent is that for men, work has been a means of enhancing their experience of themselves as men, supporting their identities as men, and work has always been an important source of their self-esteem. The successful man is perceived as more masculine than the man who is less successful. Many women, on the other hand, experience considerable conflict between their sense of self at work and their sense of self in their personal lives. Typically for women, work has not been a source of self-esteem. But it is important to say here that these remarks refer to white women. Black women, for example, integrate work into their sense of self and self-esteem in a different way—a way that also differs from the experience of black men (M. Malson, personal communication, February, 1983; B. Nelson, personal communication, February, 1983).

To understand women's work in a full and appropriate way, we would have to understand the structure and forces of our economic, cultural, and occupational institutions. Many writers are illuminating these today. I will not attempt to review that large body of material but will limit this discussion to some of the problems women tend to bring to us as workers in the psychological field.

In the current literature about women and work such problems are discussed, but the suggested resolution usually involves helping women learn more about competitive situations called for at work—for example, how to take more power, be more competitive, become more task oriented, act more impersonal, develop more invulnerability to feedback, and think more analytically.

I question this strategy for resolution because I believe it contains some of the very problems with which women are struggling. Therefore I shall begin by listing a number of areas that come up frequently when women talk about difficulties at work, describe them, and speculate about what might be behind them.

SELF DOUBTS

It is noteworthy how often women express enormous doubts about their abilities and their competence. Repeatedly I am struck by the degree to which women still minimize and negate signs of their effectiveness, what they know, and what they can do. They minimize their intellectual worth and their inner ambitions, and they work hard to hide their abilities. Occasionally their intelligence and conviction overcome their discretion and they speak up, but they begin to ruminate afterwards about whether they made fools of themselves. They worry whether they were too aggressive; should they have said that, should they have said this; perhaps they should not have spoken so long or so little or so much. If somebody recognizes them for saying something worthwhile, they are gratified at the moment; then they begin to worry about how they fooled so-and-so, how they are phonies and frauds, and someday people will find them out. While women are often aware that they do this and are annoyed with themselves for doing it, they do believe that they are fooling people or they do not know as much as other people think they know. And women typically also attribute their successes to chance events—they say that they happened to be at the right place at the right time, or they were just lucky.

What I find particularly interesting is how much women resist changing such attitudes about themselves in the face of contrasting information and other dynamic interpretations (Applegarth, 1977).

When women talk about their sense of inadequacy, it often is in the context of how defective they feel. They usually overvalue men, undervalue women, and feel that they are lacking something. Responding psychoanalytically, we might say this is a reflection of penis envy or envy of men's power position, at least in the work situation. But such interpretations are no more effective in changing the women's attitudes than other kinds of interpretations.

We must ask, then, why women hold on to the sense of themselves as inadequate, helpless, and not knowing very much.

In a recent book called *The Cinderella Complex*, Colette Dowling (1981) angrily accuses women of using their helplessness and dependency, waiting for the strong man to come and rescue them. She also says that since he never will come, women must become "independent," "strong," and "self-reliant." Certainly there is some truth to the idea that our culture supports a woman's assuming a dependent role and presenting herself as helpless—with the seductive promise that she will be taken care of, even though it typically is disappointing. This seductive fantasy may itself be so gratifying that women hold to a helpless position even though it is damaging to their self-esteem. I believe, however, that this formulation is deceptive and oversimplifies the meanings of women's "dependency."

In our culture we too readily equate a need to be related to other people with dependency. In the last colloquium on empathy and women's sense of self, an important formulation was emphasized and expanded. It holds that a woman's sense of self is a *relational* one (Gilligan, 1982; Applegarth, 1977; Surrey, Chapter 2, this volume) and that a woman's need to feel related to others is a crucial aspect of her identity. I believe that women's attempts to form relationships are often mislabeled as expressions of dependency. But it is also true that assuming a dependent position has been the only mode available to many women, particularly in relating to men.

It is fascinating to note the degree to which the term *dependent* is used pejoratively in our culture, which I believe is related to the tendency to see dependency more often as a female than as a male characteristic. Yet it seems to me that both men and women are vulnerable to regressive pulls and seductive promises of being "taken care of." Women acknowledge it more because it is more permissible. But, paradoxically, men live it out more in marriage, for emotional dependency needs are more often gratified by wives than by husbands. Women are better trained to be nurturant caretakers. In other words, the successful man gets cared for, and the successful woman is considered to be someone who can take care of herself.

ASSIGNING PRIORITIES

Another area I hear about when women talk about work is how one assigns priorities to tasks. Again, the literature tells us that women have all sorts of blind spots about recognizing opportunities and challenges. We learn that women rarely seek opportunities for advancement; indeed, they often experience such opportunities as burdensome obligations and feel resentful rather than grateful.

A good example of this kind of thinking is cited in *The Managerial Woman* by Hennig and Jardim (1977). In the authors' investigation of how women function in industry, they surveyed women in business settings and sat in on numerous meetings. In the book the following anecdote was offered to illustrate how women fail to recognize challenges that are right in front of them:

> In a meeting where a young, up-and-coming woman executive presented an impressive plan, the Vice President of the organization responded very positively, saying, "I am going to meet with the President this weekend. Would you prepare a draft of this for me on Friday?" She replied, "Friday? I can not possibly present it on Friday; I have to go to a conference out of town."
> "Then I won't object if you have it in my hands on Thursday."
> "Thursday? I have all these visuals to prepare. I have to go out of town early."
> "Then I'll accept it on Wednesday."
> "But I'm going on Tuesday, and I have to clear my desk, etc., etc."
> As they left the room she said to the authors, "Did you hear him? Drop everything! Put that first priority!" Then they explained to her that she had a great opportunity to be heard by the President, and she blew it. She said, "Oh my God, I never saw that!" (pp. 27, 28)

As I read this account, my heart went out to the young woman, and I felt furious at the Vice President. Nobody asked the woman what her priorities might have been. The assumption was that she was some poor fool who had not seen something rather obvious in front of her. No one thought that maybe the President could hear about it a week later. It just seemed to be assumed that her advancement should come first and that nothing else mattered. One has to raise questions about that idea itself.

Is it as simple as the authors of *The Managerial Woman* suggest? Are women more naive in the working world? Have they not been trained sufficiently as competitors? And do they have blind spots about recognizing new possibilities? I think the answer lies elsewhere. In the first place, women continue to carry significant household responsibilities even when they are working—and despite the changes in some households where men have assumed more domestic responsibilities. Also women's involvement in the family tasks often is not understood sufficiently.

Family tasks are more than the sum of hours required to execute the tasks. We already have stressed the importance of relationships to women, and I believe that the emotional bonding, and the intensity of the bonding, with those "at home" involves significant emotional energy. Thus the "wrenching away" from home to work and from work to home takes more of a toll on women than men. Because of this struggle, women often develop a precarious balance between what they do at home and what they do at work. If anything occurs to threaten this balance—for example, one more demand at work—many women experience enormous anxiety and begin to feel they do not have things sufficiently under control. Every new obligation and every new task carries the potential of creating a disequilibrium in that balance.

Also, women are taught that they should do for others before themselves. Consequently, if they do something for their own advancement ahead of something for other people, they feel selfish and opportunistic—an uncomfortable self-image.

Another factor is that women's self-doubt and sense of inadequacy makes them much more timid about risk taking and moving into new areas. This is important, because women can also feel resentful when they are bypassed and miss opportunities. These are only some of the factors that come to mind in response to the *Managerial Woman* vignette. There are others.

"PROFESSIONAL" BEHAVIOR

Another thing one often hears when women talk about work is their concern that they behaved "unprofessionally" or a discussion about other women who behave "unprofessionally." The men I talk to who are successful in work almost never worry about whether somebody did something that was unprofessional. Why are women continually stewing about that? And what do they mean when they say someone behaved "unprofessionally?" I think they mean that the person did not behave "like a man." The fantasy is that men move through every work situation strong, confident, self-sufficient, and clearly not emotional, because to be emotional is the worst kind of unprofessionalism.

Recently a woman who has a high administrative position said to me, "I have to separate my professional from my personal opinions." When I asked why, she was startled and replied, "That's what men do." But is that what men do? I believe men do act on their "personal opinions" in work situations. I also believe that men and women differ on the type of personal concerns they allow to influence their decisions. I think what the woman meant goes something like this: "I have to separate my objective appraisal of employee performance from my opinion about whom I like and do not like. I cannot make liking or not liking someone influence my job decisions." Men, however, give much more legitimacy to the entry of personal considerations into their decisions, and it feels all right to them when it involves issues of power, competitiveness, or even vindictiveness. I heard a man say recently when he was about to fire someone: "He does not accept my authority." Well, that is pretty personal—hardly a measure of the person's competence—yet he felt perfectly comfortable in thinking it was a perfectly good reason to fire an employee. I truly believe it would be very hard for a woman to allow a personal feeling such as that to influence how she made a decision.

Many bright women seem to think there is a set of polarized characteristics—feminine on one end of the continuum, masculine on the other. Masculine characteristics are "good" at work, feminine are "bad," and they must be kept separate. To show too many feminine characteristics at work is a precursor to failure. It is the concern about being "unprofessional"—if one's feelings somehow escape, one's head will stop working, or people will expect it to stop working.

In this connection, I think that one of the greatest fears a woman has—the worst "unprofessionalism"—is to cry on the job. I heard from a friend about a work situation where she was one of the few women in a meeting. She was feeling scapegoated, tears welled in her eyes (which made everybody nervous), and the man who was running the meeting ended it prematurely. As the participants were leaving, one man turned to her in a patronizing way and said, "Are you all right?" "I would have been a lot worse if I had not cried," she said. He was a little startled with that.

We must raise the questions about exactly which feelings are and which are not "allowed" in the work environment. Consider the nature of communication in our lives: When women communicate with a strong emotional tone, they often are called "hysterical," and the message is quickly discarded. Yet the expression of feeling can be as much a communication as the content of what one says. I think this is something that is generally easy for women to do but hard for men to hear.

Again, I will illustrate with a vignette: Recently I was talking to a male colleague about something I considered to be extremely important. I needed his support, and I was talking with a good deal of feeling. He minimized what I said and downplayed its importance. I could not agree, and I was getting more and more exasperated. He kept saying, "Well, it is really not that important" or "Let's wait and see." Finally, in a kind of apathetic way, I said quietly, "Well, there is this, this, and that. . .," enumerating the points again, but this time without any feeling. He said, "Oh, why didn't you say that before—instead of coming on like a witch on a broom!" At first I was hurt, then I thought further—I tried to tell him something and let him know it was important, but he could not hear me. My intense expression of feeling made him too anxious to hear the message, yet I felt that my feelings were just as important to the communication as the words. The point is that women are made to feel they need to curtail such feelings, as though one cannot harmonize cognitive effectiveness with affect (Jordan, Chapter 2, this volume). But one can be strong about convictions and emotionally expressive; can be involved in tasks, master them, and be concerned about people; can be analytic in problem solving and be intuitive. None of these qualities have to be polarized.

COMPETITION

Another troublesome area for women is competition. We know that, compared to men, women are more likely to avoid competitive situations, less likely to acknowledge competitive wishes, and not likely to do as well in competition. Again, the assumption is that to be as competitive as men is a good thing—it is the American way. And, again, the writings on women and work say that women should learn to be more competitive and become more skilled at it. I found only two exceptions to that position—specifically, in Jean Baker Miller's (1976) book *Toward a New Psychology of Women*, and Helen Block Lewis' (1976) book *Psychic War in Men and Women*. Those are the only writings I know that address the value of "feminine" characteristics in work situations.

For several reasons, it is difficult for women to be competitive. First of all, when a woman is openly competitive, she frequently experiences herself as aggressive and destructive. Fearful that others will perceive her that way, she feels that the worst thing she can be called is a "castrating woman." But it goes deeper than labels other people give. Women are trained to be concerned about other people and to be empathic, so that it is very hard to enjoy vanquishing a rival if one is at the same time empathic with that rival.

There is another problem surrounding competition that is more complicated for women than for men: Whom do you compete with? Interestingly, although women are not given the permission to compete the way men are, women are allowed—and even encouraged and groomed—to compete with other women for men. Men struggle in competing with men—perhaps a symbolic competition with their fathers over their mothers, in which success may carry fear of retaliation, guilt, and anxiety. Accordingly, some men have difficulties with work and fears of success.

For women there are many more complications. When they compete with men, several problems arise immediately. First is the danger of being considered unfeminine, aggressive, and destructive— and potentially being called "castrating." Second, because some women need to idealize men and see them as stronger and more powerful for the sake of the "rescue fantasy," it is too threatening to "do better" than the man one wants to idealize. Yet when women compete with women, they also are competing with the very people they want for support. Also, they are competing symbolically with their mothers, and that raises other complications, in terms of guilt and anxiety, which are different from those of men with their fathers and mothers.

SEPARATION FROM MOTHER

Perhaps the most important area I want to address is the issue of identification with and separation from mother as women move toward work and a career. For many reasons work issues highlight the ways women identify with their mothers. For many women these issues reveal their struggle against identification with mothers who are seen as devalued, and the women often feel alone and lost.

I will give you two examples. One woman, a physician, told me that, as a resident, during rounds, she made a rather dramatic correct diagnosis. People were surprised and impressed by her ability to do this. Clearly, she had made quite a coup. She was exhilarated, yet she suddenly experienced enormous anxiety, had to retreat to her office, and felt acutely alone and isolated. Another woman who had recently returned to her career in her 40s had been timid in work situations, but began to speak up more and more. At one conference where she expressed her thoughts more fully, her contributions were appreciated, and she felt encouraged and pleased. But that night she had a nightmare in which she was lying in bed, helpless and immobilized, calling out desperately for her mother. Her mother had died about 2 years earlier.

In order to understand such problems, I believe it is necessary to explore differences between the types of attachment men and women develop with their mothers and the ways they mature and change that relationship. Current theory speaks of this process in terms of "separation." It says that little girls in growing up are not encouraged toward separate strivings, nor are they encouraged to achieve a separate identity from their mothers, as little boys are. A paper by Janet Surrey (Chapter 2, this volume) discusses the ways mothers bond with their daughters and how they teach their daughters mothering behavior with some expectation of mutual caretaking and mutual empathic interactions. It is not surprising, then, that girls continue to experience a strong attachment to their mothers, with a much deeper sense that they must be *like* their mothers and truly take care of their mothers *psychologically*, with all that implies. Women, consequently, have different kinds of problems than men do in separation from their mothers.

Mothers, in turn, often feel the need to continue their role as mothers. It has been an integral part of their female identity, and they often can continue to play the role more comfortably with daughters than with sons. While mothers feel they need to help their sons to separate and develop more independence, they can fulfill their needs for more direct interpersonal connectedness through maintaining attachments with their daughters. The more positive aspects of the mother–daughter bond, however, are countered by the mother's tendency to project feelings of inadequacy onto her daughter. While this may give the mother more license to hold on to the daughter and to "mother," it contributes to the highly ambivalent aspects of mother–daughter interrelations. Thus, mothers may express their ambivalence by holding on to their daughters at the same time they are quite critical of them. Also, mothers can become competitive and fearful, as well as gratified, as they see their daughters move forward in a positive and competent fashion. And daughters, as one often hears in psychotherapy with women, often struggle to defend against their identification with their mothers, whom they see as critical, devalued, and unhappy. Yet these same women fear betraying their mothers and experience considerable guilt if they move ahead and demonstrate "differences" from their mothers. In attempting to break this bond, the women may feel that the only alternative is complete independence, which is again an attempt to identify with the more valued masculine goal. But the woman is left feeling absolutely alone in the world, without any support and with a significant sense of loss in disconnecting from her mother. A woman's attempts to resolve this dilemma by looking for a strong man who will take care of her results frequently in considerable disappointment. In other words, efforts to gain vicarious gratification through identification with the powerful man only leaves a woman with longstanding resentments and low self-esteem.

Another area highly relevant to the issue of women and work is the conflict women face between having children and having a career. It is such a complex topic, however, that it would require a separate paper even to begin exploring all the pertinent issues. It is clear that women face harsh difficulties in this area, and I do not think one can overemphasize the degree of anguish women experience in their struggle to resolve the conflict. They sometimes tend to minimize the struggle because it seems so impossible, sometimes overstate one side of the conflict and understate the other.

FEAR OF SUCCESS

The influence of the notion that success jeopardizes women's femininity and attractiveness to men cannot be overestimated, but it also merits reexamination. Again and again women report the feeling that a successful woman alienates herself from both women and men. And single women often feel that the more successful they get, the narrower will be their choice of acceptable men.

The literature suggests that women who have very supportive fathers typically are more successful (Hennig & Jardim, 1977). But in my clinical experience, when the chips are down and there is a struggle between personal and professional lives, these fathers suddenly stop being very supportive. Here is an example: A woman whom I was seeing in therapy was very successful in her work, and her father had always been supportive, encouraging her to pursue her career and taking pride in her success. She had earned an important promotion in her job with increased obligations and responsibilities, so she was bringing work home on evenings and weekends. She also had trouble with her marriage—the original reason for her coming into therapy a year earlier. After the promotion, the marriage had become more troublesome, and she finally talked to her parents about her marital difficulties. Her father became enraged. He told her that the recent promotion had been too much, that she was putting work ahead of her family, and her husband should come first. Further, if she stopped all this nonsense and put her energies into her marriage, not into her work, things would be different. She was devastated. Her father's reaction was unexpected, and it confirmed her belief that her personal life was compromised by her getting ahead in her career.

The notion that "fear of success" jeopardizes women's personal lives is part of the thesis put forth by Matina Horner (1972). Working with high achievement women, she talked about the anticipation of success in competitive activity countered by the anticipation of negative consequences—for example, social rejection, disapproval, not being liked, and loss of femininity.

I will conclude by raising some important questions about this thesis when it is used to explain why women eschew success.

Women certainly do have difficulties with success. I believe, however, that "fear of success" is primarily the fear of not being related to another person, since success for women often carries with it a threat to feeling connected with others. But we need to ask these questions: Is success, as defined by our culture, such an admirable goal? And is the way of reaching that success something that women should emulate? I will describe two clinical vignettes that point up some problems inherent in those questions.

Susan is a woman of 35, divorced, with two young children, who during the process of psychotherapy completed the requirements for a bachelor's degree, which she had postponed for more than ten years. It was around that time, too, that she was able to divorce her alcoholic husband and apply for graduate school. After finishing a master's degree, she was encouraged by faculty to pursue a doctorate at a much more prestigious university. She did this with some trepidation, still feeling unsure of her ability to juggle the responsibility of running a one-parent home and becoming part of a very competitive program. Nonetheless, she entered the program and began a strenuous course of study. During this time she also became involved with a man who was already an established professional in the field. He, too, was divorced with two children. Since his wife had custody of the children, he lived alone in a bachelor-type existence, hard working and ambitious. This relationship was especially significant, for it was her first truly intimate relationship with a man.

In one session, she reported that over the past weekend her ex-husband had taken the children, and for the first time in a long time she had unlimited free time to catch up on her work. However, she and the man with whom she was involved typically spent weekends together, since the weekdays were so busy for each of them. She knew he expected them to relax and enjoy each other. He had had quite an unencumbered week devoted entirely to work, but she had gone to class, run errands, visited her daughter's school, stopped in on her mother who was ill, helped out a friend in distress, and so forth. She wanted to tell him that she could not spend all the weekend playing but felt this would seem selfish and too ambitious. Still, she mustered her courage and did tell him. His reaction was surprising. "Of course," he said, "work would always come first with me." He was very accommodating, helping her use much of the weekend to do her work.

The other case is somewhat different. About one year after Joanne had terminated therapy she returned to see me about a crisis at work that had caused her considerable anxiety and obsessive preoccupation. She held an executive position with a company she had been with for 12 years, and she supervised a large staff. I knew she had given birth to a baby 6 months earlier, because she sent me an announcement, but she spoke only of the issues at work. She was troubled by the hostility she felt from the junior staff, and she thought it centered on her having recently been given more responsibility in the company. There was so much upheaval that she feared the corporation president would see her as unable to do her job effectively. She expressed considerable anger at members of the junior staff, whom she felt had always been her friends, and she was quite upset at the thought that they disliked her now. After two sessions of talking about this, I noted that she had hardly said anything about her new son. Even she was startled by how little she had mentioned him, since she had intense feelings about him and about dividing her time between home and work. What soon emerged was that the complaints from her staff were that she had become aloof and uncaring—in sharp contrast to her style before her son's birth. She became aware that she had considerable difficulty leaving her baby to come to work, as well as proving she could combine motherhood and a career. At home she had almost handed over the care of her son to a housekeeper and to her husband. At work she curtailed her nurturing, sensitive feelings toward her staff in order to prove her ability to continue her career after having the child.

These two women illustrate different facets of the problems addressed here. Susan wanted to be responsive to the man in her life and at the same time to be able to put herself forward without feeling she was hurting or harming him—a common dilemma for women. To act for herself made her feel she was being selfish and destructive to the other person. Although she was relieved at his response, she felt she could not fully accept that value for herself, and one would have to question whether this made her a less effective person than the man. Joanne felt she had to suppress her concerns for others to prove that she was effective and, in fact, became less sensitive to her staff and less effective as a consequence.

So what is the goal for women? Is it to become president of the corporation and climb the ladder of success at any cost? Is it to relinquish the values women truly cherish if they interfere with achieving higher status? It seems to me there might be other goals: to achieve freedom to pursue work interests; to use talents and power to develop other people's abilities for getting the job done; to be affirmed as an effective person and still maintain relatedness to others, with all the richness and complexities that relatedness encompasses. Women need to feel entitled to pursue their work interests without feeling held back by beliefs that the needs of others are inherently always more important and valid, and without feeling selfish and destructive. In the end such feelings add to women's resentment and interfere with their ability to respond effectively to the needs of others.

A paper by Lois Hoffman (1972) says, "Driving a point home, winning an argument, beating others in competition, and attending to the task at hand without being sidetracked by concern with rapport are all hurdles women have difficulty jumping, no matter how innately intelligent they may be." Is this what we have to accept? Or are there alternate ways for women to deal with work situations and gain gratification without experiencing so much guilt, shame, frustration, and alienation?

Doing psychotherapy with women about work issues has taught me that it is important to validate the intrinsic conflict between success, as defined in our culture, and the qualities that women value for themselves. It is crucial to help women see how deeply they have internalized assumptions, attitudes, and stereotypes of what is better, worse, valued, and not valued, based on a masculine model of success—which may sometimes be destructive and often inhumane.

Women need help to feel that it is indeed important that they affirm their more person-directed, empathic qualities. If these interfere with attaining higher status and more power, the basic problem is not in the woman. And women need to be encouraged to pursue their career interests and realize their intellectual and creative potential. If they perceive this as selfish, the basic problem, again, is not in the woman. My hope is that women can learn to experience these conflicting attributes as less alien to their sense of themselves both as women and as competent, effective human beings. There are reasons for these conflicts. They seem to be inherent in just being a woman today and therefore are all part of women's sense of self. Let us continue to explore these struggles, rather than to accept them or to offer simplistic solutions that continue to devalue women.

This paper was presented at a Stone Center Colloquium in March 1982.

14

Eating Patterns as a Reflection of Women's Development

JANET L. SURREY

Food, weight, eating patterns, and body image have become intense preoccupations in many women's lives today. As clinicians and teachers, we find these topics are important in our personal lives and relationships as well as in our professional roles. Of special concern is the apparent increase in the number of young women suffering from serious, even life-threatening disturbances of eating patterns that are diagnosed psychiatrically as "eating disorders." The *anorexic* and *bulimic* syndromes are characterized by extreme preoccupation with achieving ideal body weight, attempts at rigid control over food intake, disturbances in maintaining body image, and cycles of extreme dieting or fasting followed by severe binging and purging through vomiting, use of laxatives, or compulsive physical activity. The scope of the problem, however, is not limited to these extreme instances (estimated very roughly by surveys to affect 10% of the current young female adult population). Rather, for this paper, the examination of the severe disorders may be suggestive in enhancing our understanding of the "normal–abnormal" eating patterns characteristic of many women today.

Let us look briefly at some current national statistics. It has been estimated that 20 million Americans are currently on a "serious diet" for weight reduction. Ten billion dollars a year are spent on the diet industry in America, including books, health spas, diet groups, and so forth (Millman, 1980). This is an anomaly in human experience, where hunger and starvation haunt much of the world population. It has been viewed as a function of an affluent society—overfed, overstimulated by food, physically inactive, nutritionally unbalanced, and stressed. Truly the obsession with dieting is a national problem. More discouraging are the reports suggesting that 90–98% percent of those on "successful" weight-loss diets will regain the lost weight or more when a careful 2-to 5-year follow-up assessment is made. Frankly, the picture represents a major cultural *denial* of reality.

Looking at the statistics in further detail, we can begin to see the implications for women. Although there are few good epidemiological studies, a Nielson survey in 1978 showed that 56% of all American women aged 25–54 were "dieting" (Nielson, 1978). According to current medical definitions (as reflected in life insurance tables) more than 50% of American women are considered overweight. Self-report studies indicate that between 50% and 75% of American women consider themselves to be overweight (Nielson, 1978). There is some variation by ethnic and age group and in the degree of concern over reaching ideal body weight. Further, the degree of preoccupation, the attempts at serious dieting, and the disturbances of self-esteem associated with perceived failure to meet ideal body weight vary significantly for individual women. However, if 50–75% of American women are living with day-to-day worry about weight control, I believe it must taken as a *norm*. Those of us who are concerned with understanding the psychological development of women in this society must give serious attention to the implications of such a widespread phenomenon.

ADOLESCENCE—A TURNING POINT

It appears that puberty and adolescence are critical times for the developing preoccupation with body weight. The adolescent growth spurt, the normal tendency to gain weight, and the significant increase in body fat relative to overall weight associated with pubertal development in girls are important factors (Wooley & Wooley, 1980). This weight gain and the experience of the body as "getting fatter" seem to initiate the psychological disturbances in body image and the tendency toward attempts at weight reduction in affluent countries where thinness is highly valued. Careful studies in the United States, the United Kingdom, and Sweden suggest an increase in eating disorders among the young adolescent group. The mean age for onset of anorexia is thought to be between 17–19 years of age. Nylander (1971) did an excellent survey of all adolescents (2,370 subjects) in a

Swedish town in 1970. Most girls reported feeling "fat" at some time during this period. Of 14-year-old girls, 26% reported feeling fat; by age 18, the proportion was about 50%. In contrast, 7% of the boys "felt fat" at age 18. For the girls, the percentage attempting to curtail their food intake was 10% of 14-year-olds and 40% of 18-year-olds. In contrast, boys seldom reported dieting.

For boys, puberty brings an increased percentage of muscle to overall body weight, and this is viewed by the culture as highly desirable—again, a contrast to the normal adolescent changes in women's bodies. Normal adolescent boys generally experience the changes associated with the growth spurt as positive, self-affirming events. Clearly, much more research is necessary to understand the subtle interactions of genetic predispositions toward a probable variety of body weights as well as other physiological, psychological, and sociocultural factors necessary to explain the incidence of severe eating disorders that develop in adolescent and young adult populations. We know that eating patterns and associated psychological disturbance originate most often during the teenage and young adult years, and it appears that this is a critical period for researching the physical and psychological development of young women in today's cultural context.

CONCERN ABOUT WEIGHT IS THE NORM

I would like to mention a few more important studies that indicate the degree to which concerns about weight and disturbed eating patterns are the norm today. Rosenbaum (1979) studied a sample of 30 normal girls aged 11–17. When asked to describe what they did not like about their bodies, the leading concerns were related to weight. When given three magic wishes for anything they wanted, the number-one wish of most girls was "to lose weight and keep it off." Garner and Garfinkel (1979) devised an objective test of anorexic eating behavior, the Eating Attitudes Test. When other investigators gave the test to a college female population, a large group of normal subjects received extremely high scores on the test, as high as anorexics in the clinical population. The authors concluded that anorexic-like behavior seemed to be the norm in many apparently well-functioning college women (Thompson & Schwartz, 1981).

In a pilot survey of eating patterns at Wellesley College, conducted in the spring of 1982, a small sample ($n = 106$, or 5% of the student population) was studied (Surrey, 1982). The research conclusions were the following.

On the average, there appears to be a significant level of concern about weight issues. Sixty-four percent of students judge themselves to be overweight, and 72% express moderate to extreme concern about reaching their ideal body weight. Thirty-six percent of students are "significantly" or "extremely" concerned about their eating patterns. Yet the questionnaire also suggested that the average student is within 5–10 pounds of her ideal weight, and eating patterns are generally within normal limits. This suggests an exaggerated level of psychological concern relative to the actual weight loss desired. Although 58% of students reported significant weight gain in their freshman year, by their senior year 72% reported no weight fluctuation through the year. This survey suggests that although there is a considerable population (22%) of students who may have a problem of "serious concern about weight," there is a not an "epidemic" of eating disorders on campus. However, the data also indicate that there is a small group of students with severe eating disorders.

The overall level of concern and preoccupation with eating is striking. More than 25% of the students indicated that their present weight negatively affects their self-image to a large degree. One-third of the students said that they were always or almost always preoccupied with controlling their eating, and more than half expressed the wish that they could get help in changing their eating patterns. Half of the students surveyed expressed "fear of being overweight," "feeling guilty after eating," and "giving too much time and thought to eating." The young women reported particular difficulty in controlling their eating at night, when alone, and during periods of emotional or academic stress.

A NEGLECTED AREA IN THEORY AND RESEARCH

It is clearly time to begin an in-depth exploration of this current "crisis" in women's self-image related to weight control. New data from biology, physiology, anthropology, and sociology must be integrated into our understanding. But I believe such data must be gathered within the framework of our evolving theories of women's psychological development, so that we may learn new strategies for education, prevention, and intervention. Until recently this apparent "crisis" for young women has been underestimated, trivialized, and personalized. Individuals have been made to feel personally inadequate for failing to achieve ideal body weight; they have been judged, and have judged themselves, as weak willed, passive, and "unconsciously" self-destructive or "rageful."

There are a number of important reasons for such a characterization. First, the medical model for understanding obesity and weight-loss diets was based on male body types and physiology. Dr. Barbara Edelstein (1977) was the first to begin to point out that the old diet models, which posit lower caloric intake and carbohydrate avoidance, simply are not appropriate for women's metabolic, physiological, and psychosocial situation. It is also interesting to note the degree to which our whole cultural "fat phobia" reflects the interpretation of fatness as a voluntary state, chosen by the individual, either due to "not caring sufficiently" or as indicative of a psychological profile of a weak-willed, docile, passive, dependent individual, unable to control "oral" impulses. Could it be that these traits are highly correlated with many of the same traits generally considered to be more "feminine"? In the classic study by Broverman and colleagues (1970), these are some of the same characteristics judged by clinicians to describe healthy adult functioning. Has the lack of research validating women's experience been another instance of viewing women through inappropriate medical and psychological models, where women become defined as "deficient"? Has this silence in research reflected the fact that food and eating have been predominantly a "female" domain? As James Hillman (1981) has pointed out, "food is so fundamental, more so than sex and aggression, or learning, that it is astonishing to realize the neglect of food and eating in depth psychology." Could it be that it has been trivialized and neglected because, until recently, women have not begun to speak out? In particular here, I wish to mention my gratitude to five women—along with the works they authored—who have begun to break this silence: Marcia Millman (1980), *Such a Pretty Face: The Experience of Being Fat in America*; Barbara Edelstein (1977), *The Woman Doctor's Diet for Women*; Susie Orbach (1978), *Fat Is a Feminist Issue*; Hilda Bruch (1973), *Eating Disorders*; and Kim Chernin (1981), *The Obsession: Reflections on the Tyranny of Slenderness*. Although I do not necessarily agree with all of these writers, I am greatly indebted to them for opening up the subject for more critical feminist analysis.

Second, the mental health professions certainly have been deficient in bringing adequate attention and serious concern to the subject of eating disturbances in "normal" young women. A recent anthology, *Female Adolescent Development*, edited by Sugar (1979), has only one article on body image and no references to dieting and weight concerns as serious problems. In her chapter, Rosenbaum (1979), who found weight to be the most frequent concern for adolescent girls, makes the following statement, which clearly invalidates the real meaning of these concerns.

Many of my female patients express anxiety and conflict *in terms of* concerns about their bodies. There is the preoccupation with various body parts and with asynchronous growth; there are many questions about normalcy and the innumerable concerns that come under the *guise of* weight control. (Emphasis added)

This reflects a tendency within the clinical profession to underestimate, invalidate and interpret these real concerns as masking "deeper" psychological problems.

Last, the issue of diet and weight control is so embedded in the current dominant values of our culture that it is very difficult to see the magnitude and reality of the problem with a critical eye. Edelstein, who has clearly recognized that women have unique bodily issues related to weight control, still wrote in 1977 the following advice for dieting:

The middle teens are an excellent time to attempt a *serious* diet. Growth in the female is usually complete. Menstrual irregularities have usually straightened out, and fluid retention is not yet a problem. Motivation is often strong, especially if there is an interest in boys. Stubbornness, so characteristic of adolescence, can be harnessed to the service of vanity and become a useful adjunct in diet therapy. (Emphasis added)

SOCIAL AND DEVELOPMENTAL INFLUENCES

I would like to begin an attempt to describe the current preoccupation with body image and body weight as a major cultural disturbance, or cultural "disease." It is extremely important to examine the underlying meaning of disturbances in eating patterns and to see them as communications about the experience of growing up female in this society (Steiner-Adair, 1986). In the context of current ideas about women's psychological development in this culture, there are a number of important issues to be raised.

The Cultural Pursuit of Thinness as a Cause, not Symptom, of Problems

The prevailing norms and standards of what constitutes female attractiveness warrant careful examination. In many cultures, the standards of female beauty suggest the glorification of fullness, plumpness, and roundness, where the female body reflects a symbol of fertility and abundance. Our cultural norms reflect a value shift to extreme thinness, flatness, and smallness in all areas (except the bust)—a body type reflective of a preadolescent girl or young man.

Perhaps we should wonder if this "fat phobia" in our society reflects a cultural debasing or devaluing of the full development of the adult woman. Perhaps the new cultural body ideals reflect the current cultural obsession with more traditionally male values, stressing linearity over fluidity, definitive ego boundaries over more permeable and flexible boundaries, and the discomfort with, and avoidance of, certain basic human needs for nurturance and contact. The hatred of "fat" seems to reflect a cultural conflict around oral issues, issues of emotional and physical needs, and dependencies.

Standards of ideal body weight, set by U.S. insurance company tables, recently have been adjusted upward, based on research showing that a certain degree of so-called overweight is predictive of greater health and well-being in the overall population. But a study done by Garner, Garfinkel, Schwartz, and Thompson (1980) reviewed the norms for Miss America contestants and *Playboy* magazine centerfolds over two decades and found support for the impression of an evolution in our society toward a thinner ideal shape for women. Thus, while the medical profession has recently corrected some of the overvaluing of "thinness," at least in its standard tables, the general public's standard for ideal body size has decreased significantly. This suggests that the "ideal" weight encouraged for most young women may be set at a level lower than what is normal or healthy for proper functioning of their bodies.

New research on "set point" theory suggests that appetite and metabolic function are "set" at certain physiological levels of weight and fat/lean body ratio for each individual (Polivy & Herman, 1983). If this is true, many young women at puberty may be beginning a lifelong struggle against the needs of their bodies to be comfortable at slightly higher weight (Wooley & Wooley, 1980). This may explain some of the discomfort and obsession with weight control seen in many apparently "normal"-weight women. But even worse—for those who are unable to achieve this so-called ideal weight—a psychological syndrome of low self-esteem and chronic sense of deficiency may become basic to the young woman's sense of self. This may be reflected and projected in many other significant aspects of her life, with negative consequences for her overall psychological functioning.

The Magic Number Syndrome: The Attempt to Meet External Standards

One of the important issues is the shift from internal to external standards. As the emphasis on meeting rigid and extreme external standards increases, there can be a very serious diminution in awareness of and a lack of attention to one's own inner experience. Hilda Bruch, in her brilliant analysis of anorexia, points to this phenomenon as a basic definition of anorexia nervosa—the girl's loss of ability to be aware of her own inner hunger states. Current research indicates that hunger mechanisms may be very delicate and precarious for all human beings following starvation or any tampering with metabolic function. This shift in young women may reflect the tendency for women to be highly responsive to meeting the standards and norms expected by important people in their lives. Pleasing others or giving to others may become more important than learning to listen to oneself. *The loss of the inner voice, of the awareness of one's own needs, desires, or interests in the effort to respond to external expectations is a crucial issue in understanding basic aspects of women's psychological development.* The push toward rigid and chronic dieting, as well as the emphasis on meeting culturally defined standards, may be an important factor in this critical loss of a basic sense of self. It is reflected in the focus away from inner sensations and perceptions that are the basis of self-knowledge and healthy self-expression. The ability to feel "alive" inside, to feel connected to oneself, is important in all human functioning. Its loss or diminution is central to understanding problematic eating patterns as well as other common occurrences—for example, vulnerability to depression.

Further, the ability to feel "connected" in this way, to feel and enjoy bodily pleasure, may be partially a function of healthy enjoyment of food, since food is so basic to life. One of the dangers of increasing fear and guilt related to eating may be a decrease in the capacity to experience eating as a simple pleasure. I suspect that with less "permission to eat," hunger mounts to an unbearable tension state, and eating or bingeing becomes a response to this state. Such a pattern then institutes a serious basic bodily shift; it makes the ingestion of food or particular foods more like drug-taking behavior than food ingestion. This may contribute significantly to the development of severe eating disorders.

Dieting as a Way of Life

For many women, growing up female today means becoming a "good dieter." A friend of mine related recently that his 8-year-old daughter (of normal size and weight) announced that she was no longer going to eat potatoes, which had formerly been her favorite food, since they are "very fattening." Competition and comparison among women may become related to the degree of thinness or success at dieting. This creates a "deprivation mentality," where self-esteem becomes equated to how well one is doing in controlling food intake. Being "good" means staying on a diet, and being "bad" means violating the diet. Thus, in a more general sense, self-esteem becomes bound up in controlling and curtailing one's own appetites, instincts, and needs. A sense of effectiveness or agency becomes related to control over one's eating, which then becomes an important index of overall self-esteem. This connection between inner control, sense of agency, or effectiveness, and self-esteem reflects an arena for the expression of a basic and somewhat hidden aspect of a more general aspect of self-esteem in women. Effectiveness comes to represent the ability to *control* oneself rather than to *express* oneself.

Clearly, the ability to control impulses is a valuable human quality. When there is no emphasis on balancing this control with the expression of needs, however, the situation becomes tilted in an unhealthy direction. Moreover, this pattern sows the seeds for periods of "loss of control," since the women are attempting a form of inappropriate food control that is slated for failure. This may lead to increased rigidity in setting standards, followed by diminished self-esteem when the controls fail, as they are clearly destined to do. Cycles of overcontrol (dieting and fasting) are followed by periods of overeating and/or "binging," which may then be followed by further artificial means of weight control (vomiting or purging by use of laxatives). Such cycles may become an arena for self-definition that provides important insights into the psychology of self-esteem in women. In this model, the whole arena for the development of a healthy awareness and expression of one's own needs becomes diminished and dissociated, leading to unrealistic and confusing self-images and an inability to express one's own needs openly and clearly. Here I am again suggesting that disturbances in eating patterns represent both a vulnerable arena for the expression of psychological conflicts *as well as the actual cause* of more serious emotional and physical problems.

The index of agency defined as self-control is supported by the culture. Historically, there has been a great fear and sense of danger associated with women's acting directly on their own impulses. Consider the myth of Eve, whose temptation leads to eating the apple, the fruit of the tree of knowledge, often described as knowledge of self; this act was responsible for the fall of all humankind from the Garden of Eden.

The Relational Self in Women

The basic connection between women and food reflects a deep and universal theme in the psychology of women—connection with the mother and connection with the self. The whole expression of the mothering role is reflected in women's relation to food throughout the life cycle. The ability of the woman to mother, to sustain life, to be present and empathically responsive to the physical and emotional needs of the child is actualized and symbolized in the provision of food. Psychologically speaking, this basic theme is reflected in the development of values of intimacy, caretaking, responsivity to others, and the maintenance of close, empathic connections between people (Bruch, 1973; Gilligan, 1982).

At a former colloquium session we discussed the importance of the development of empathy for women's self-development. For women, mutually empathic relationships are essential for a sense of overall well-being and for promoting healthy growth and development. Such relationships are constructed through mutual understanding, emotional support, and the commitment of all individuals involved to the development of each individual and the collective unit. We have described this core self-structure in women as "self-in-relation," that is, the "self" is discovered, experienced, and expressed in the context of human bonds and relationships. Theorists have posited "separation-individuation" as the goal and direction of healthy male development and have described this line of development through the boy's movement from early attachment to differentiation from the mother. We have defined the female line of development as relational and the goal of development as "relationship-differentiation." In this model, other aspects of development (competency, agency, initiative, industry, and so forth) progress within the context of relationships. The "oral stage," then, for women is not "split off" in early childhood but remains as a basic pathway for female development, and the development of empathy proceeds along this line with further emotional and cognitive elaboration. Without the male-defined Oedipal stage, girls maintain a closer, comfortable level of relationship and identification with their mothers throughout childhood. It is in this early mother–daughter relationship that the core self-structure is defined for women. Identity is based on positive identification; connectedness is based on open, physical, and emotional sharing plus the early mutuality of caring that is found in healthy mother–daughter interaction.

The complex journey of feminine development is only beginning to be understood, but I think such understanding is essential to our analysis of the "disturbances in eating" described as "normative" in young women today. Disturbance in women's basic relationship to food and eating, then, can be viewed in the larger context of the lack of validation and attention given to the importance of relationships to others that women confront throughout life. The basic healthy expression of the need for this connection is met with conflicts and obstacles as girls grow into adolescence and adulthood in this culture.

If the culture is not in basic resonance with fundamental self-structures, attempts at "adaptation" will be disturbed and conflictual. I believe that disturbances in eating patterns reflect critical aspects of discontinuity for women between early childhood self-development and the demands and values of the current cultural milieu through the years of adolescence.

I will mention briefly only two of the major inconsistencies that I see as fundamental.

First, *there are discrepancies between the preadolescent mother–daughter relationship and the postpubertal mother–daughter relationship.* The ease and comfort of the early mother–daughter relationship is disturbed by the emergence of sexuality and the growth spurt responsible for weight gain. Mothering adolescent daughters today means beginning to help the daughter move into the adult female role, where physical attractiveness, thinness, and the inhibition of drive states become important tasks. In my opinion, "separation" issues and sexuality are often less conflictual today than the conflicts around food and eating. Mothers often become active in young girls' attempts to meet rigid standards of cultural attractiveness. The result is conflict, mutual blaming, and severe relational discord. Nearly all the women I have seen who have any difficulty around weight control report serious, painful conflicts with their mothers, with whom they basically report loving and caring interrelationships. I do not believe this is just a metaphor for "separation" and "boundary" issues, but a real and critical problem. There is little help or accurate understanding of this in the culture at large. Clinicians do not help when they continue to blame the mothers for "overinvolvement," enmeshment, and failure to tolerate separation, and when they continue to define the major task of adolescence as "separation-individuation."

Second, *there is a significant cultural inconsistency between the pathways of relational self-development for young girls and the current cultural values, which stress self-development through academic self-sufficiency, autonomy, "assertiveness," and competition.* For example, a young woman in distress felt she needed to talk to her friends, but it was during exam period and the norm at her college was that academic demands override all other needs. The "new assertive woman" or the "new managerial woman" is supposed to be self-reliant, confrontational, "looking out for Number One," able to compete in a man's world. Emotional openness and sharing, cooperation, attention to and concern for the needs of others, and participation in others' growth are not of direct value in this world. When these basic relational needs are not valued or given outlets for development, there is a sense of being out of touch with oneself, disconnected, and unsupported. Psychologically we could say that the internalized mother–daughter relationship is disrupted, and food becomes an important arena for acting out this disruption. Eating becomes an attempt to reinstate the sense of connection. However, for many reasons, the surrender to these impulses is highly conflictual and tends to create progressive disturbance and disruption, especially in individuals who are physically or psychologically vulnerable to developing more serious disorders.

PREVENTIVE AND THERAPEUTIC APPROACHES

I have attempted to sketch an outline of the psychological background necessary for our understanding of eating disturbances in young women today. This is just a beginning. The need to address these problems with new theories and creative solutions is pressing. The physical and psychological tolls such disturbances may exact are only beginning to be researched. Certainly education and prevention programs are needed, because the problem does not originate in the individual.

It is important to validate and explore the importance of eating habits with all female clients, even those not presenting with serious eating disorders. As clinicians, we have been delinquent in failing to take up these matters in a serious and thoughtful way with our clients.

For treatment programs, more understanding of the psychology of women will help suggest creative and innovative strategies utilizing women's particular strengths and adaptive capacities. It is clear that "dieting" approaches and/or traditional psychoanalytic psychotherapy have not been very helpful. The fact that 64% of Wellesley students indicated that a "personal support network" would be useful in helping them with their eating patterns as opposed to a "diet group" suggests that treatment approaches need to offer in-depth understanding of the complexities of the problem and to utilize relational strategies. An example would be to employ mutual empowerment techniques such as those found in self-help recovery groups. There is a need to stress relearning how to eat without fear and guilt, *not* how to perpetuate the diet syndrome. In the Boston metropolitan area, I recommend Overeaters Anonymous (OA), Anorexia Aid Society (ANAS), and "Feeding Ourselves," along with new and creative programs now being developed in settings primarily dedicated to the overall health and development of women. Similar groups exist in other cities. Importantly, these organizations have taught us about the deeper meanings of eating disorders, as well as the effective forms for immediate action that are derived from listening to women themselves. We urge that women continue to build research and action programs that are informed by their life experience and by further analysis of the larger societal forces at work.

This paper was presented at a Stone Center Colloquium in 1983.

15

The Meaning of Care: Reframing Treatment Models

IRENE P. STIVER

At first blush the connection between caring and psychotherapy seems obvious, and yet for many of us trained in the traditional model of therapy, caring about one's patients often is seen as something that may get in the way of effective treatment. The maintenance of distance between therapist and patient as well as general prohibitions against the expression of caring can be attributed to two major assumptions underlying this traditional model. The first assumption is tied to a broader model of treatment in which the treatment of the patient requires that the treater be objective, nonemotional, and relatively impersonal in order to be most helpful to the patient; it involves a kind of caretaking through, for example, the prescription of medication, the administration of appropriate treatment strategies, and so forth. Personal qualities of warmth and kindness are certainly seen as important assets, but they should be monitored carefully lest the therapist become "too involved," that is, perhaps care "too much" for the patient.

Let me say a few words here about the complicated meanings of "caring." I believe one needs to distinguish between "caretaking"—the giving of care which implies a more parental and, if you will, unequal relationship—and the concept of "caring about," which suggests more of an investment of feeling in the other person, with no implication about status or equality. While both types of caring are considered suspect in the process of therapy, I believe that "caretaking" is relatively acceptable as an attitude of the treater, indicating the intent to do what is in the patient's best interests, while "caring about," with the possible *expression* of caring feelings, is seen as more threatening to the therapeutic process. Later I will explore some of these distinctions in more detail.

The second assumption is that growth and change can occur only if the therapist does not gratify the patient. The experience of frustration and learning how to tolerate and respond to deprivations in therapy are seen as valuable and therapeutic. This assumption also would argue for the need for the therapist to be relatively neutral and objective. The earlier and more extreme view of the psychoanalytic model in particular emphasized the need for the analyst's neutrality, and personal reactions to his or her patients were often labeled as "countertransference," which needed to be analyzed away.

While this model has been modified through the years, with the role of empathy and concepts such as the "holding environment" gaining importance in the therapeutic process, there are still strong prohibitions against more open expression of therapists' feelings toward the patient. Let me make myself clear at this point. I am not advocating that therapists become emotionally involved with their patients, either in the service of gratifying their own needs or through misunderstanding their patients' needs. I am, however, raising serious questions about the all-encompassing discomfort experienced by many therapists about having and expressing caring feelings about their patients.

In this paper I will be examining the model of therapy in which objectivity and distancing play such an important part. Specifically, I believe that this model is essentially a masculine model, since it reflects a style much more congenial and familiar to men than to women, that is, objective, nonemotional, impersonal attitudes, and so forth. For precisely this reason, this model does not seem to work very well with women, and perhaps not with some men either. The need to erect barriers to create distance from patients may also then reflect countertransference reactions among male therapists toward their female patients, who are different from them in important ways. Later, I will trace some significant differences in male and female experiences of self and in the pathways each sex has taken developmentally, which will help in the understanding of the nature of such countertransference reactions.

While there are various therapeutic strategies that contribute to distancing in therapy, I will be addressing the ways in which the formal and informal language of diagnosing and labeling contributes to the barriers between therapist and patient and both maintains and reinforces a state of inequality between them.

A brief vignette describing the experience of a colleague and friend perhaps can illustrate both concretely and symbolically some of the issues I have been outlining so far. My friend, whom I will refer to as Alice Smith, is a clinical psychologist in her 50s, highly regarded and respected in her profession. At the same time that she has managed to be active and productive in her work, she has also suffered for years from profound and debilitating depressions. Several years ago, after many trials on various antidepressants, she responded very positively to a new drug and reported that she had never felt better. During this time she was in psychotherapy with a woman psychiatrist, also an analyst, who felt that since she was not sufficiently familiar with the field of psychopharmacology and since medication had proved to be so important with my friend, it would be best to refer her to another psychiatrist who specialized in pharmacology. He would monitor and prescribe medication, concurrent with the ongoing psychotherapy. This was certainly acceptable to everyone, and things proceeded well.

About a year later some physical problems emerged. After experiencing back pain, my friend was diagnosed as suffering from osteoporosis. At times she became quite debilitated, but amazingly her spirits remained reasonably good. And then another blow occurred, when breast cancer was diagnosed. She handled this extremely well; she did not become significantly depressed but arranged for several consultations and second opinions and finally decided to have a lumpectomy and radiation treatments. During this period of radiation treatment, she often felt quite ill and also continued to experience back problems, so that she was frequently in significant physical distress. Her therapist caringly noticed what a physical effort it was for her to get to her appointments and suggested that until she felt better they conduct their therapy on the telephone. My friend was most relieved at this suggestion and accepted it enthusiastically. In this instance the therapist was able to be flexible and apparently did not find her concern or caring about her patient to interfere with the effectiveness of therapy. It then occurred to my friend that perhaps she could arrange something similar with the psychopharmacologist she also was seeing. When, however, she asked him for phone consults instead of office visits for a while, he became angry and accused her of "acting out" to get special treatment, since he felt that she could perfectly well come in for the appointments and also that it was important to maintain an objective stance and not to gratify his patient for her best interests. She, however, was hurt and felt very misunderstood; but she accepted the situation. At some later date she had to call to reschedule an appointment. When his secretary asked who she was, she said, "Dr. Smith" and was put through to him immediately. When he heard who it was, he became very angry and told her she was being manipulative in trying to get him to talk with her on the telephone instead of leaving a message. My friend was most upset at this angry outburst and asked, "Why are you so angry?" to which he replied, "You should have said you were a patient."

What I want to highlight about this story are two major observations: (1) Such terms as "acting out" and "manipulative" are often used as pejorative labels to talk to and about patients in ways that maintain both distance and a certain balance of power in therapeutic relationships and that significantly interfere with the process of caring; (2) I believe that the psychopharmacologist's anger at his patient for "getting through" to him reflected the anxiety aroused in him because she had crossed the barrier he needed to erect between him and her (and perhaps his other women patients) in order to maintain the distance for *his* comfort in the relationship.

Thus, the typical standards of "care" in general psychiatric settings and in psychotherapy, which often support both explicitly and implicitly the need for barriers between mental health professionals and patients, may function to contain the anxiety of the treaters more than the treated. Yet as we have seen, some of the barriers erected have been developed with a rationale about how psychotherapy works best, which justifies them as serving the best interests of the patient.

Let us now examine those barriers created by the formal and informal language used in "diagnosing" and evaluating patients. I hope to show how they result in uncaring rather than caring in psychotherapy. The belief that women are more readily victimized by psychiatric labeling was the major theme of Chesler's book *Women and Madness* (1972), and also was illustrated dramatically in the classic study of Broverman and colleagues (1970). Broverman's study demonstrated a double standard of mental health, since clinicians set standards for healthy men and adults different from those set for healthy women. Among the terms used to describe healthy women were that they were "more submissive, less independent, more suggestible, less competitive, more excitable in minor crises, more emotional, and more concerned about their appearance" than either healthy men or the generic healthy adults. Chesler felt that the other side of this double standard of health was the labeling as pathological of those women who were seen as too passive, too dependent, and overemotional. She felt that this simply represented an overconformity to feminine sex-role stereotypes, a caricature of those "female" behaviors that were labeled healthy in the Broverman study. Chesler noted that pathological labels were also assigned to those women who were nonconforming to such sex-role stereotyping and were called aggressive and castrating. Thus, women have to walk a thin line between being too feminine—that is, histrionic, dependent—or not being feminine enough, as described, for example, in a paper entitled "The Angry Woman Syndrome" (Rickles, 1971). Men, on the other hand, need only to conform to the male sex-role stereotype in our culture to be identified as healthy and in fact are labeled as unhealthy primarily if they display characteristics that are seen as stereotypically female, that is, dependent, passive.

In a recent paper entitled "A Woman's View of DSM III" Marcie Kaplan (1983) illustrates the degree to which masculine biased assumptions about what behavior is considered healthy and what unhealthy are codified into diagnostic categories, which in turn influence evaluation and treatment. *DSM III* (1980b) is the third edition of the diagnostic manual, created by the American Psychiatric Association, that is the standard used throughout the mental health professions. The author notes that such bias is reflected primarily in the codifying of personality disorders, which, according to *DSM-III*, entail "significant impairment in social or occupational functioning or subjective distress." Kaplan's analyses of the Histrionic Personality Disorder and the Dependent Personality Disorder are of particular interest. Although Chesler and Broverman published their ideas and data over a decade ago, their observations about diagnostic labeling of women are still alive and well in both these categories. Thus the items listed to warrant a diagnosis of Histrionic Personality Disorder include ones similar to those Broverman and others reported that clinicians used to identify the normal healthy female, such as "overreaction to minor events," "vain," and "dependent." Also included are those items that would represent what Chesler called the overconformity to the female stereotype or caricatures of female behaviors, for example, behavior that is "overly dramatic, reactive and intensely expressed" (1980). The Dependent Personality Disorder is defined as: "Passively allows others to assume responsibility for major areas of life because of inability to function independently and subordinates own needs to those of persons on whom he or she depends in order to avoid any possibility of having to rely on self" (p. 324). Since women are generally seen in our culture as more dependent and less mature than men, and since they are encouraged to put others' needs ahead of their own, they would readily be vulnerable to such a diagnosis. And indeed the manual reports that both the Histrionic and the Dependent Personality Disorder are found more frequently in women than in men. I believe the very descriptions of these diagnostic categories reflect a misunderstanding of the behaviors involved, which I hope to demonstrate more fully later. Kaplan (1983) points out, however, that *DSM III* scrutinizes the ways in which women express dependency but not the ways men express dependency. For example, men do rely on others to maintain their homes, care for their children, respond to their emotional needs, and so forth. More important, however, is Kaplan's observation that neither the earlier *DSM II* nor the current *DSM III* addresses those male behaviors that are caricatures of masculinity, behaviors which could be seen as impairing social functioning and, if not producing subjective distress in the men themselves, may provoke it in those with whom they live. In following this line of thinking, Kaplan indulges in some fantasy and develops two fictitious categories to be included in *DSM III*.

One she called the Independent Personality Disorder and the other, the Restricted Personality Disorder. Here are some of the criteria she lists for the Independent Personality Disorder: "(1) puts work and career above relationships with loved one, e.g., travels a lot on business, works late at night and on weekends; (2) is reluctant to take into account the other's needs when making decisions, especially concerning the individual's career or use of leisure time, e.g., expects spouse and children to relocate to another city because of individual's career plans."

Her Diagnostic Criteria for Restricted Personality Disorder include:

"A. Behavior that is overly restrained, unresponsive and barely expressed, as indicated by (1) limited expressions of emotions, e.g., absence of crying at sad moments; (2) repeated denial of emotional needs, e.g., of feeling hurt; (3) constant appearance of self-assurance; (4) apparent underreaction to major events, e.g., is often described as stoic.

"B. Characteristic disturbances in interpersonal relationships as indicated by (1) perceived by others as distant, e.g., in individual's presence others feel uncomfortable discussing their feelings; (2) engages in subject changing, silence, annoyance, physical behavior or leave-taking when others introduce feeling-related conversation topic; (3) indirectly expresses resistance to answering others' expressed needs, e.g., by forgetting, falling asleep, claiming need to tend to alternate responsibilities" (pp. 790, 791).

The bias reflected in these formal classifications of mental illness is even more dramatically evident in our informal language. Such terms as *manipulative, seductive, controlling, needy, devouring, frigid, castrating, masochistic* and *hysterical* have been used pervasively, primarily to describe female patients, with the clear implications that such patients are hard to tolerate, and almost impossible to treat and that if one does not manage them carefully one will be taken over, fused with, devoured, and so forth. Even when the perception of the patient is more benign, the labels of "dependent," "seductive," and so forth are at best patronizing. The end result of such labeling is that the patient is not understood and not cared about.

Let me share with you a brief clinical example. I was asked to consult about a young woman who had become anxious and depressed enough to require rehospitalization after a period of fairly good adjustment. She is a young, attractive 19-year-old honor student at an Ivy League college, and is highly intelligent, very sensitive, and articulate. She talked readily to me on several occasions about the anguish she often experienced in a world that felt unreal to her. When I approached one of the administrative psychiatrists to discuss the case, he told me immediately that she was "very manipulative" and was going to be "a handful." I was a bit surprised, since she was always well mannered and quite cultivated with me and I asked him what he meant. "Oh, when we do rounds, if you look around at the group talking to her, everyone looks tense and uncomfortable." As I mused about this curious definition of "manipulative," I thought about what her major concerns were—she was always afraid that her ability to put up a good facade, to be so well socialized and so successful at academic pursuits, and so forth, would hide what she called her "true self," the self that was so terrified, so uncertain, and so confused. Her concern was that she would be misunderstood. I was often very moved in her presence by her unusual capacity to communicate the power of her frustration and pain. I could imagine her "performing" at rounds, while at the same time being vigilant about how others would respond to her, and feeling helpless and even desperate if they did not see what was underneath the facade. I also know that once she felt the other person did not understand her, she gave up trying, with a deep sense of disappointment and underlying rage. That her anxiety and anger at being misunderstood were communicated to those conducting rounds must have contributed to feelings of discomfort among them; I also believe they needed to ward off the intensity of her underlying feelings. The labeling of her as manipulative also created a climate that kept her at a distance and cut off the possibility of understanding her or of engaging with her in a meaningful way.

Male patients certainly may be misunderstood, but I am focusing here on the specific kinds of language that affect women. I would like to suggest that when the language is pejorative and serves to maintain distance between the therapist and the patient, women are more likely to be victimized in the process than are men. We know that the greater number of patients in therapy are women and, among therapists, men represent a significantly higher proportion than women. But it is not even that simple. Women who enter this profession have largely been taught by men (and treated by men) and in order to survive in their careers have often needed to adapt to the standards and values that have been associated with their professions; thus most therapists, male or female, may be very much influenced by those standards classifying mental health and illness that reflect the masculine model of therapy described above.

Recent writings on the psychology of women by Miller (1976; Chapter 1, this volume), Gilligan (1982), Surrey (Chapter 3, this volume), and others have brought to our attention the extent to which women are seen as lacking and defective when evaluated according to masculine models of personality theory and developmental psychology. These models fail to recognize the unique qualities of female development and experience. Gilligan noted that women were seen as lacking in moral development only when compared with data gathered on all-male samples collected by Kohlberg; in examining the female experience of morality, she demonstrated how much it is organized around issues of responsibility for other people within the context of investment in relationships. In the same way, current developmental theory has stressed the process of separation and individuation and the achievement of independence and autonomy as the hallmarks of maturity. This model, however, seems more applicable to male than female development in our culture. When this model is applied to women, they are seen as relatively immature and dependent, since the model overlooks the power and significance of human relationships for women and ignores important differences in the developmental paths followed by men and women.

There is, in fact, a significant asymmetry when one compares the process in men and women as they move from their earliest relationships with their mothers and fathers through adolescence into adulthood. Since mothers experience their daughters as more like and continuous with themselves, there begins a particular relationship between mothers and daughters that includes expectations of mutual caretaking and mutual empathic interactions and interdependency. Daughters can then experience more continuity with their past relationships, such as early dependency on their mothers and others, without seeing it as a threat to their growth and maturity. The dynamic of the mother–son relationship follows another developmental path. Mothers experience their sons as different from them and are under both inner and outer pressures to affirm this difference. The cultural expectations of how boys should be are internalized by mothers; they believe that in order to help their sons develop a strong masculine identification they need to encourage aggressive behaviors and separate strivings. These pressures continue to exert a powerful influence on males to be separate selves in their journey toward adulthood.

A recognition of these different lines of development and careful attention to the experience of young female children and adult women have led to a new understanding of women, a "self-in-relation" theory of development. In particular, the writings of Miller (1976), Surrey (Chapter 3, this volume) and Jordan (Chapter 4, this volume) have attempted to trace the ways in which early mother–daughter relationships have enhanced the development of empathy, the range of affective experience, and other relational skills.

Miller, in writing about the development of the self in women, describes the dynamic nature of the process of connection with the main caretaker (usually a woman). The connection is not with a static figure but with a person who is involved in an ongoing relationship. Thus, the internalization of the mother reflects what is happening between people and is represented in a relational mode. The evolving self is one which cares both about others and about the relationship itself between two or more people. Surrey describes the early representation of self in girls as being a more open sense of self with more permeable boundaries in contrast with the more limited and boundaried self characterizing boys. Miller notes also how often women's involvement in relationships is misunderstood, either in pejorative fashion by labeling women as dependent or in apparently more positive fashion by referring to women as altruistic. But the latter description also misses the point when it suggests a sacrifice of a kind of self-interest, when in fact women engaging in relational interactions experience them as a source of great pleasure, gratification, and as self-enhancement.

While it is not the purpose of this paper to elaborate in great detail this new conceptualization of female experience, I believe it can serve as an important context in which to talk about how women often are evaluated and compared to standards that are not relevant to their experience. I am suggesting, too, that countertransference issues evoked in many male therapists who treat female patients contribute to a misunderstanding of women that is maintained through this process of labeling and diagnosing.

Miller (1976), Stiver (Chapter 8, this volume), and Surrey (Chapter 3, this volume) have raised questions about the ways in which the emphasis on separation, individuation, and "becoming one's own man" have had a negative impact on the development of self in men, often resulting in a rigidifying of boundaries between self and others and interfering with the development of their relational selves. This theme is more fully developed in Bernardez's (1982) paper on "The Female Therapist in Relation to Male Roles." "The contradictions," she writes, "between the advantages in the social realm and the impairments in the emotional and psychological realms inherent in the male role have not been examined by psychotherapists" (p. 440). In particular, Bernardez observes that the very factors involved in rearing men for independence may also lead to "suppression or underdevelopment of qualities of nurturance, empathy, affiliation, cooperation, affective awareness and expressiveness" (p. 441).

In tracing the socialization process for men, she notes as especially important the extent to which males in our culture are pressured to separate and give up very early their strong connections with their mothers. But she also believes that the nature of these early connections with the mother contributes to the development of highly ambivalent attitudes in men toward women. On the one hand, the mother is certainly experienced as a very powerful figure, since she so often is the primary caretaker; on the other hand, her position in the social world is secondary and often devalued. As a consequence, men are both threatened by women's apparent power and contemptuous of their apparent inadequacy. This early loss of connection with the mother, and the social pressures that prohibit the little boys' continued open dependency on the mother before these longings can naturally be resolved and reorganized, lead men then to deny and defend against their longings for dependent, affectional ties with others.

According to Bernardez, this premature separation from mother leaves little boys with a feeling of abandonment and vulnerability to loss that is hidden behind a more independent exterior. The underlying rage that many men experience toward women is understood by her to be in large part related to this sense of abandonment and to feeling cut off from a more continuous close connection with their mothers as valued figures in our culture. Thus, men do not typically have sufficient opportunities to develop their self-in-relation because of the enormous pressures placed on them to perform and achieve in independent fashion, and they are denied a fuller participation in a growing relationship with their mothers, with all the emotional richness that this implies.

How can we understand the relationship between these processes in masculine development and our conceptualization of female experience and development as occurring in a relational context, in which emotional expressiveness, interdependency, and mutual empathy are encouraged? If men have to deny these qualities in themselves to defend against the strong connection with their mothers, which is prohibited and devalued, they might indeed find threatening the expression of these qualities in women. Indeed, as Miller (1976) has pointed out, men's need to control women is in part a reflection of their need to control the *feelings* that women "carry" for men.

If one reviews the descriptions of pathology in *DSM III* (1980b), there are some interesting differences between those categories reputedly found more often with women than those more often found with men. The Histrionic Personality, the Dependent Personality, and also the Borderline Personality all have characteristics that involve interactions with others and intense expressions of affects. In contrast, those types of pathology more typical of men, such as Paranoid Personality and Antisocial Personality, involve symptomatology that reflects distances from rather than engages with others, for example, the paranoid's suspiciousness and the sociopath's exploitation of others. Thus women are apt to express their conflicts and concerns more in emotional, relational terms, and men need to defend against the intensity of their own feelings and yearnings for connection. The result is that traditionally trained mental health professionals use techniques that create distance between them and their female patients. Their male patients already have distanced themselves by the very nature of their symptomatology.

A relevant observation is the way medication can be used as a distancing strategy. Women are reported to receive a disproportionate number of drug prescriptions for both mental and physical conditions (Fidell, 1973). Women are also more likely than men to have their depression and anxiety treated with drugs (William, 1974). I was supervising a male resident who, in the service of caretaking, quickly offered to prescribe antidepressant medication to a female patient he was treating when she began to cry about an abortion she had had only 3 days previously. As he and I talked about it, it was clear to me that he could not tolerate the intensity of her pain and sadness, which he warded off, distanced, through offering medication.

Men's need for distancing, however, is often coupled with intense anger at women, both from a sense of abandonment early in development as well as from envy of women's freedom to express feelings. The quality of the descriptions used to identify female psychopathology suggests that intense anger must fuel these descriptions. In reviewing the literature, I found no titles about male pathology that compare with such titles as "The Intractable Female Patient" (Houck, 1972) or "The Angry Woman Syndrome" (Rickles, 1971)—with the exception of more pejorative labeling sometimes used to describe those males guilty of violent and destructive behaviors who more often end up in prisons than in mental health facilities.

Take as an example the description of the diagnostic classification of the "Hysteroid Dysphorics" by Klein (1972):

> They are fickle, emotionally labile, irresponsible, shallow, love-intoxicated, giddy and shortsighted. They tend to be egocentric, narcissistic, exhibitionistic, vain and clothes-crazy. They are seductive, manipulative, exploitative, sexually provocative, and think emotionally and illogically. They are easy prey to flattery and compliments. Their general manner is histrionic, attention-seeking and may be flamboyant. In their sex relations they are possessive, grasping, demanding, romantic and foreplay-centered. When frustrated and disappointed, they become reproachful, yearnful, abusive and vindictive and often resort to alcohol. (p. 152)

While Klein recognizes that this rather histrionic description may be considered misogynistic, he states that it is consistent with a caricature of femininity in our culture. If I may quote again, he notes that "women with a normal range of emotional responses utilize a wide variety of exhibitionistic and seductive social tactics with discretion and accuracy. The hysteroid dysphoric patient is a caricature of femininity because her pathological sensitivity to rejection drives her to attempt to repair her dysphoria by an exaggeration of the social, seductive and exhibitionistic tactics allowable to women in our society" (p. 152).

In a paper by Houck (1972) on "The Intractable Female Patient," a type of "borderline patient" is described as particularly troublesome. The author quotes from the dictionary definition of "intractable" as best illustrating the kind of female patient he means—"not easily governed, managed or directed, obstinate, not readily manipulated or wrought, not easily relieved or cured—unruly." He also finds these patients in therapy to be "assertive and manipulative." His formulation is essentially that these women simply want to take flight from responsibilities at home and that they use the hospital as an escape. Thus he recommends that the hospitalization be short that therapy be supportive only, and that "the woman's attention needs to be firmly fixed on home, family and adult obligation." Most important, however, the author says, is the "aggressive work" that needs to be done with the spouse, who is seen as passive and without ability to "dominate" his wife.

The anger evident in these descriptions of female pathology underlines my contention that the countertransference attitudes many male therapists have toward many female patients contribute to the need to achieve distance in therapy and to erect barriers between therapists and patient, which in turn maintains the therapist in a position of power and control.

This brings me to the sexual issues that further reflect this theme in psychotherapy. In a paper on dependency (Stiver, Chapter 8, this volume), I have noted that for reasons related to how men are socialized, they often search for intimacy primarily through sexual experience. For many men, one of the few settings in which they can give expression to their needs to be given to and cared for, and can experience deep feelings and still feel manly, is the bedroom. I believe that male therapists' experience of caring for their female patients often takes the form of strong sexual feelings, which are often projected onto the patients; then the female patients' needs to engage with their therapists, to be accepted and valued, are consequently misunderstood and misidentified as "seductive." I am not unmindful of women's propensity to sexualize relationships, but I believe for many women to be "sexual" is also a way of "being" and relating with a man. It is the therapist's responsibility to understand not only women's particular way of incorporating sexuality as part of their total way of being but also the distorted aspects that occur because women are still seen, and react to being seen, more totally as sexual objects. Bernardez (1982) believes that men's tendency to sexualize relationships serves to ward off loving and tender feelings and is often a disguised expression of anger. For some male therapists it is a significant struggle to ward off sexual feelings toward their female patients, and this may contribute to even greater distancing. Other male therapists act out their impulses directly in sexual contact with their female patients. While there are more data about the greater incidence of such acting out than was available before (American Psychological Association, 1975), we continue to hear about female seductiveness and very little about men's needs to sexualize relationships.

A brief clinical example is illustrative. I was seeing a woman in therapy who was in her 40s, quite conservative and diffident but also friendly, with good social abilities. While in general conventional, the one area in which she expressed some zest and creativity was in her dress. She wore clothes that were unusual but always modest and tasteful; she wore bright colors, unusual fabrics, and so forth. Before she started to see me, she had been in treatment with a male psychoanalyst for 3 years. She liked him and was aware of warm and affectionate feelings toward him, since he seemed caring and interested in her. After about a year of treatment, he told her she was dressing up for him, accused her of being seductive, and urged her to talk about her sexual feelings for him. She was hurt and felt that there was, after all, something bad about how she dressed—one of the few areas in which she felt good about herself before—but she also felt she had failed as a patient since she was not aware of having the feelings she presumably was supposed to have. As the therapy moved toward termination, her therapist told her that his marriage was foundering and he wanted to establish a different relationship with her after the therapy ended. This was very traumatic for her. It felt as if all the work she had accomplished was undone and that her sense of his caring was all in the service of his sexual interest in her—the precise feeling she had had with her husband. This was the impetus for her coming to see me. I might add, she continued to dress with a flair with me—which I valued and appreciated and saw no reason to challenge or interpret.

I would like here to attempt in the most general way, because of limits of space, to take some of the female behaviors so pejoratively labeled by our diagnostic categories and translate them into terms more meaningful from the point of view of the self-in-relation theory of female experience and development.

Let us consider first the behavior of the "hysteric." Most noteworthy is the intense expression of emotions associated with this classification. The criteria which indicate that such expression occurs "in reaction to minor crises" suggest that it is relatively unprovoked or unexplained by the social context. I would suggest, instead, that women's efforts to be heard and truly listened to are often experienced as intensely frustrating when the other person seems emotionally impervious. The result for the woman is often an escalation of intense feelings with increased loss of focus and defusion of intense affective expression. There is a tendency for women, particularly when in trouble, to present a kind of self that often feels unreal in the service of desperate attempts to persuade the other person to relate and engage with them in an emotionally meaningful way. This presentation may take the form of an exaggerated expression of affect in order to be heard, attended to; it is also a reflection of the woman's compliance with the expectation of how she needs to be, to engage the other to respond to her in some fashion—even if it be in an angry and uncaring way.

Next we will look at the Dependent Personality Disorder, presumably so characteristic of women. In a paper on "The Meanings of Dependency in Female–Male Relationships" (Chapter 8, this volume), I took the position that the term *dependency* has acquired a pejorative connotation precisely because it is seen as a feminine characteristic. But most important, I believe that women are not basically more dependent than men. They have, however, an investment in presenting themselves as dependent as a means of becoming engaged with others, and it has been the established mode of relating to men in the expectable direction. Men, we know, have their investment, too, in seeing women as being more dependent than they are. I suggested also in the earlier paper that pathological dependency is not being "too dependent," as the literature suggests, but rather is a function of the underlying rage about unmet needs. Those who are called "too dependent" are often those who ask for help in a way that makes it very difficult to respond because of the communication of underlying rage at both self and others. Thus it is not the asking for help, the dependency on the other person, which is problematic, but the ease and comfort with which one is able to identify what one wants and then to ask for help. I do not think women have any more trouble than men do about that.

Another diagnostic category found more often in women than in men that needs reexamination is "depression." Why it is found more in women than in men has been explored by others with developmental, social, and biological explanations offered (Arieti & Bemporad, 1978; Bart, 1971; Weissman & Klerman, 1977). What is of particular interest are the marital differences in incidence of depression. Among the single and widowed, men are more likely than woman to become depressed, while women are more likely than men to become depressed during marriage (Radloff, 1975). That marriage is more stressful to many women than to men has been noted in the literature (Bernard, 1971). I would like to suggest that the depression found in women who are married may reflect the frustration they experience in making the kinds of connection they want and often cannot get. As Kaplan points out in Chapter 12, depression in women cannot be seen solely as deprivation or loss of psychological supplies; it is also a result of the lack of an adequate relational context. Thus some women experience a continuous sense of loss when they are in relationships in which there are limited opportunities for mutual empathy and mutual empowerment. I also believe that since women need to deny their own needs in the service of being unselfish and attentive to the needs of others, they develop underlying resentments—which they turn inward, considering the degree to which our culture prohibits more open expressions of anger in women (Miller, Chapter 10, this volume).

Let us now look at the characteristics of the Borderline Personality Syndrome, which evokes the most pejorative labeling of all diagnostic categories and is also more frequently diagnosed in women. If one reviews the major characteristics used to identify this diagnosis in DSM III (1980b, p. 322), again they include affective, relational features— "inappropriate intense anger or lack of control of anger, affective instability with marked shifts in mood and patterns of unstable and intense interpersonal relationships." Impulsivity, identity disturbance, and physically damaging acts are also mentioned. Again, I believe the relational needs of such patients are not recognized adequately by these designations. In my own experience with such patients, I have found them highly attentive and vigilant to the other person's reactions to them, but because of disturbances in early relationships with caretakers, so much anger is aroused that it interferes with more accurate perceptions of others and in fact significantly distorts them. Instead, one sees a repetition compulsion of maladaptive attempts both to reaffirm and repair the early pathological relational experiences, which then get played out, lived out in therapy. Thus, the patient feels caught in unhealthy relationships that keep re-emerging and lead to an escalation of emotions similar to the process described in hysterics, as well as pathological dependency, since there is an inability to believe that anyone can be helpful.

A few words about the "Masochistic Personality Disorder," no longer a legitimate category in *DSM III*. In a recent paper entitled "The Myth of Women's Masochism," Paula Caplan (1984) takes serious issue with the ease with which masochism is applied to female behaviors that are presumably self-sacrificing and altruistic—when both attitudes are encouraged and valued in our culture. Caplan analyzes the concept of unconscious masochism and demonstrates how one can offer less pejorative alternatives for women and a more accurate understanding of behaviors otherwise labeled as masochistic. She notes that what is regarded as secondary to the motivation of males is focused on as primary and pathological in the motivation of females. To illustrate this point she uses as an example "the painful and dangerous occupation of professional football players," for example, "he spends many hours being brutally assaulted in the cold, the mud and the rain. He can count on frequent and serious injuries to his body in exchange for admiration and applause for his physical strength and willingness to experience pain and injury so that others may enjoy themselves."

The translation of behaviors to their underlying meanings brings us back to an understanding of the concept of caring and its role in the process of psychotherapy. Earlier I spoke about a distinction between "caretaking" and "caring about." "Caretaking" I referred to as a kind of caring that allows one to maintain a more objective, impersonal stance in the delivery of care and that contributes to an imbalance of power in the therapeutic relationship. "Caring about" I suggested is not tied to this kind of power imbalance and could be more egalitarian and also implies an emotional investment in the other person's well-being. I believe that what our women patients, and perhaps some men as well, want is to be cared about—but to be cared about in a particular way, that is, to be listened to and understood in a way which precludes the kind of distancing that exists in the more traditional models of therapy. The most powerful therapy sessions in my experience have been those in which I have been very deeply there in the relationships with my patient and have had a genuine sense of where my patient is at that time. In Chapter 4, Jordan demonstrates beautifully how cognitive and affective components harmonize in the empathic encounter—and clarifies the importance of flexible boundaries between therapist and patient. It is this notion of empathy that plays such a central role in "caring about" one's patients.

I think most of us, both men and women, are capable of relating to our patients in a "caring about," genuine way that involves our being present in the relationship as a real person and, I might add, that does not mean burdening the patient with personal data about the therapist, and so forth. But this requires a relatively nondefensive attitude and awareness of the differences in the socialization processes between men and women.

It is most important to note that styles of caring in therapy do not seem linked in a simple one-to-one fashion with sex of the therapist. That is, some women therapists have in a sense overconformed with the distancing, "masculine model" of therapy as a result of trying to survive, to be successful and adept in this field. On the other hand, I have known "caring" male therapists who are able to be flexible and responsive to both their male and female patients in a genuine, empathic, and nonauthoritarian fashion. We are all aware that selective factors operate that make it more likely that such men, rather than, if you will, hypermasculine, unemotional men, will enter this field. However, what I have also noticed is that often these men are apt to apologize for or hide this style lest they be criticized and devalued by their male colleagues.

Let me close with an example that nicely illustrates this curious dilemma. A woman psychiatrist told me about her termination with a female patient in her last year of training. She was leaving the clinic setting and moving to another city. Because she felt connected to this patient and sad about terminating, when the patient asked where she was going and if she could contact her, she told her, and added that she would be glad to hear from her. When she reported this to her supervisor, a male psychoanalyst, he told her she had been very seductive, had behaved inappropriately and was too involved with her patient. She felt bad and accepted his criticism. She was also terminating her own therapy with a senior male analyst. When asked if she could see him again when she visited Boston he said, "Certainly, I would love to hear from you." She felt vindicated and said, "What goes on behind closed doors! There are all these analysts secretly acting like human beings but nobody is supposed to know it!" I do believe that good caring treatment does go on behind closed doors, but it is time to take it out of the closet. Let us give legitimacy and value to a model of therapy that takes into account the unique aspects of female experience and development and that also allows a more egalitarian "caring about" our patients to become a matter of prime importance.

This paper was presented at a Stone Center Colloquium in January 1985.

16

Female or Male Psychotherapists for Women: New Formulations

ALEXANDRA G. KAPLAN

Should women see only women therapists? This question is provocative. An affirmative answer threatens the livelihood of many practitioners; a negative answer intimates that the sex of a therapist is irrelevant to therapy. The question stirs personal and economic fears that lurk behind the more academic issue of "gender influences in the process of psychotherapy," for it potentially implies that the majority of practitioners (men) may be unqualified to treat the majority of patients (women).

To advance discussion of this issue, this paper will emphasize several points. First, the focus will be the actions of the therapist, not the decision-making process of the patient. No one theory can predict to the individual situation; the final selection is an agreement between two specific individuals, not between an abstract "woman" and an abstract "man." Second, given the focus on the therapist, the question becomes not whether women or men offer the best therapy for women but, rather, what therapeutic conditions are most likely to facilitate women's emotional growth and how best can those conditions be established in therapy.' This loaded question in turn contains two subquestions: (1) Are there specific conditions that especially facilitate women's emotional growth? (2) If such conditions exist, how are they affected by therapist gender? To address these questions, I will integrate ideas from psychotherapy research and psychoanalysis with others from the study of women's psychology and development.

GENDER EFFECTS IN THERAPY

Answers to the question of whether the sex of the therapist has an effect on clinical work can be examined within two related but distinct bodies of literature—psychotherapy research and psychoanalysis.

Psychotherapy Research

In psychotherapy research, there has been a fair amount of attention in recent years to the effect of patient* and therapist gender (Brodsky & Hare-Mustin, 1980). The overall conclusion commonly drawn from studies of the psychotherapy process is that there is as yet no clear, replicable evidence of a strong and specific gender effect (Mogul, 1982; Zeldow, 1978). Typically, this is explained by noting that the sex of the patient and/or therapist is but one of many factors that influence the process of therapy. Consequently, it is argued, research methods must improve to incorporate multiple factors; the answer, then, is to be found in increasingly complex multivariate analyses. But the reduction of therapy to its component variables, however carefully operationalized and analyzed, cannot capture the subtle realm of inner and interpersonal experience in which gender probably has its most profound influence. The absence of replicable gender effects in therapy, in other words, may be more a function of method than of a real absence of potentially discernible effects. More intense, thematic attention to interactional elements in the therapeutic process might be a more fruitful—albeit more difficult—way to discern gender effects in therapy.

Psychoanalysis

The second major body of literature that bears on the question of gender effects in therapy is that of psychoanalysis. Although Freud (1931) suggested that the sex of the therapist may influence the psychoanalytic relationship, psychoanalysts rarely have explored the full implications of this possibility. This neglect follows from the general character of psychoanalysis as an interpretive discipline. Thus, bringing infantile conflicts to awareness took precedence over analysis

---

* Throughout this paper, "client" and "patient" are used interchangeably. We are not satisfied with either word, in that "patient" does not seem fully appropriate in speaking of psychotherapy, while "client" suggests a formal, legal relationship. It is noteworthy that there is no independent word for someone who seeks psychotherapy.

of the emotional interplay in the therapy hour. This pattern has been changing in the last few decades, however. Recent writings by Langs (1973), Gill (1979), and Stone (1981) highlight the critical importance for psychoanalysis of what can succinctly be called the "here and now." Analysis, as Stone observes, is in part an "actual adult relationship between patient and analyst." In that relationship the therapist, as experienced by the patient, plays a distinct role in influencing the transference that evolves.

While some psychoanalysts (Blum, 1971; Alexander, 1950) identify the sex of the therapist as one of the salient relational features of the "here and now" situation, few have explored the ramifications of gender-related issues beyond passing mention of "mother transference" and "father transference." This is at variance, however, with regularly reported findings in the social science research literature suggesting that gender is a "master variable" (Gore, 1977) in the construction of human interaction.

Male–Female Differences

There is increasing support, in a number of research areas, for the position that there are major and significant ways in which women and men live psychologically in "worlds apart": Men and women have different values by which moral reasoning is constructed (Gilligan, 1982). They vary widely in certain modes of communication, both verbal (Thorne, 1975) and nonverbal (Henley, 1977). They have different definitions and experiences of success and achievement (Horner, 1972). They have fundamentally different experiences in the home and in the paid labor force (Bernard, 1972). They differ in their expression of intimacy and sexuality (Safilios-Rothschild, 1976). And, finally, they may have fundamentally different courses of psychological development (Chodorow, 1978; Miller, 1976; Gilligan, 1982; Surrey, Chapter 2, this volume).

Across this range of experience and expression, two common themes characterize the gender differences: (1) When *status* is at issue, such as in verbal and nonverbal communication and in family and labor force roles, men's responses reflect and convey a position of dominance, while women's responses reflect and convey a position of subordination. The distinctions between these two positions and their psychological ramifications have been portrayed by Miller (1976). (2) In those areas of research that depend directly or indirectly on key aspects of *sense of self* (moral reasoning, roles at home and in the labor force, and self-development), women's responses typically portray the self as a relational being, while men's responses typically reflect an autonomous and separate sense of self (Gilligan, 1982; Miller, 1976).

Effects in Therapy

Given the breadth of experience in which gender differences in status and sense of self play a central role, it is reasonable to speculate that these same distinctions will influence the psychotherapeutic relationship (Kaplan, 1979). Both issues are crucial: Status is played out in the relative power and authority held by client and therapist. Appropriate recognition of the status differential is essential for a viable, trusting therapy relationship. The "nature of the self," in turn, may be considered the heart and soul of the therapeutic work. The therapist's own self-structure and concept of the healthy self will shape her or his presence with the client and the basic direction of their work.

In the most general sense, I am proposing that female therapists working with women bring to their role some sense of their core self (and, by extension, their patient's self) as a relational being, as well as some internalized experience of being in a subordinate position. By contrast, male therapists bring to their role some sense of a core self (for them and their patients) as a separate, autonomous being, and as well as an internalized experience of being in a dominant position. Wide variations exist, of course, in the degree to which members of each sex hold and reflect such postures. There also are wide variations in the extent to which members of each sex modify their personal positions through their own therapy and clinical training.

A woman therapist, for example, might be especially cognizant of present, interactional considerations in her clinical work and more receptive to the client's ongoing affective experience. She might be particularly apt to use herself as an empathic vehicle through which greater understanding of the client is reached. She also might be especially sensitive to the dangers of overstepping the boundaries of her authority, concerned about making arbitrary or capricious decisions, and likely to check out the meaning of her decisions for her client—or wonder if a decision was the best one.

A male therapist, in turn, might build less on affective connectedness and more on questioning or interpreting the client's remarks. Affect might be handled more in terms of its transferential implications and less as a process of mutual exploration within the ongoing therapy relationship. He would probably be comfortable with the dominant aspects of the therapist role, less apt to worry about overstepping boundaries, and less likely to weigh his decision-making process based on the client's reaction.

I offer these formulations as samples of hypotheses suggested by our knowledge of women's and men's personality development; careful research is required to assess their validity. There is now a great deal of evidence on gender differences in personality style in general, but whether, how, and when these are injected into the therapy hour remains to be demonstrated. Obviously we cannot afford to put treatment aside until all the evidence is in. Much of our clinical work, after all, is based on formulations that have yet to be tested. It is possible, then, to consider some likely effects on work with women clients if male and female therapists generally bring these different styles to their clinical work. The literature on psychotherapy outcome studies sheds some light on this question.

Therapist Gender and Success Rates in Therapy

As with other areas of psychotherapy research, the study of gender influence on outcome has generated inconsistent results, wide variations in operationalizing terms (most importantly of "success"), and different conclusions based on similar patterns of findings. However, while no definitive statements can be made, certain general trends have begun to emerge. Mogul (1982) has recently summarized the findings on therapist gender and patient satisfaction or benefit: "There appear to be some demonstrable trends, under certain circumstances, toward greater patient satisfaction or benefit from psychotherapy with female therapists and no studies showing such trends with male therapists." This situation does not apply equally to all male and all female therapists. Specifically, a gender effect is less apparent with experienced therapists than with inexperienced therapists (Howard & Orlinsky, 1979; Kirshner, Genak, & Hauser, 1978). The data presented by Howard and Orlinsky (1979) from a study of women outpatients are instructive. Based on ratings made by two independent clinical observers from intake data, therapists' treatment notes, and termination summaries, the authors rated each therapist along a 3-point continuum: (1) those for whom at least 50% of their patients were considerably improved, with the rest improved and none worse than before therapy; (2) those for whom at least 33% were considerably improved and fewer than 10% were worse; (3) those for whom fewer than 50% were improved and more than 10% were worse. Using these distinctions, no differences in therapist "quality rating" were found between moderately experienced (2–6 years) and very experienced (over 7 years) women therapists, both of which groups were equally as good as the very experienced male therapists. These three groups had rates of 4% worse and 41% considerably improved, with the rest improved. In contrast to these three groups—moderately and very experienced females and very experienced males—the moderately experienced males had at least twice the others' rate of worse and unchanged patients, and half the others' rate of considerably improved patients.

Howard and Orlinsky end their paper by stating: "The most pressing question that we are left with is: On whom are male therapists to practice until they become highly experienced?" Upon reflection, I would pose their question differently: "What do male therapists gain by experience that seems to be in place for only moderately experienced women therapists?" Here we need to turn briefly to general reviews of therapy outcome, such as those by Bergin and Lampert (1978), Dent (1978), Gurman (1977), Orlinsky and Howard (1978), and Strupp, Fox, and Lessler (1969). These reviews concur that, as stated succinctly by Orlinsky and Howard, "the positive quality of the relational bond, as exemplified in the reciprocal interpersonal behavior of the participants, is more clearly related to patient improvement than are any of the particular treatment techniques used by therapists." There is consistent evidence that relational variables are especially powerful predictors of outcome (Dent, 1978; Feifel & Eells, 1963; Gardner, 1964; Sloane et al., 1975; Strupp et al., 1964). The centrality of the relational bond has been found in studies of both psychoanalytic and behavioral therapies (Staples et al., 1976; Ryan & Gizynski, 1971) and seems to persist regardless of whether the source of data is patient accounts, therapist reports, or ratings by non-participant observers.

WOMEN'S PSYCHOLOGICAL DEVELOPMENT AND THE WOMAN PATIENT

We can now consider the critical relational bond as it interacts with the two modes posited to vary in the work of female and male therapists. What male therapists may gain by experience, and what women therapists seem to bring with them to their work, is a greater capacity to work in a way that fosters a facilitating relationship in therapy. Unfortunately, few have explored the quality of interrelationship between therapist and patient by which a relational bond has its effect. One key component would certainly be therapist empathy (see Jordan, Surrey, & Kaplan, Chapter 2, this volume). The term *empathy* suggests the capacity to take in and appreciate the affective life of another while maintaining a sufficient sense of self to permit cognitive structuring of that experience. This is a complex and multifaceted experience, requiring, at a minimum, an ability to understand the nuances of

emotional expressions, listen for their meaning to the person expressing them, and reflect them back to the person in a way that will confirm
and enrich her or his own experience.

If we turn to developmental theorists for knowledge about the
development of the capacity for empathy, or the more general capacity
for experience at the relational edge, there is little to aid us. Virtually all
existing "classic" developmental theories describe growth and maturation as a process by which sense of self is articulated through increasing
levels of distinction and separation from others. One learns who one is
by comparison with what one is not, and one becomes increasingly
competent to the extent that one is able to function autonomously.
While the capacity for love or intimacy is highlighted at particular
stages, there is little in the theories to suggest how one evolves such
capacities or how one becomes a relational being.

Understanding the possible roots of women's greater capacity to
weave a relational bond in therapy requires that we turn to recent,
preliminary formulations about self-development that derive from the
female experience. Recent writers—for example, Miller (1976), Gilligan
(1982), and Jordan, Surrey, and Kaplan (Chapter 2, this volume)—in
contrast to the "classic" theorists, argue that women's self-development and self-articulation centrally evolve via attention to their
relational matrix. Beginning early in life, daughters and mothers
experience a process of mutual identification whereby each responds to
the feelings and experience of the other in a mutually affirming way.
This process stimulates awareness of the process and quality of
interactions and focuses on connectedness *as a path of growth*—not as a
means toward the end of "separation." With increasing age, girls
continue to gain sensitivity to the affective states of others and to the
value for self development of maintaining relational bonds. Such
qualities, in turn, are validated and supported by others, and become
the cornerstone of women's self-image and sense of self. Thus, the core
self in women is best described as the "self-in-relation" (Surrey,
Chapter 2, this volume). It is a self whose growth and development are
fostered and enhanced by and through relationships and their
internalized meanings. Learning is enhanced by mutual activity, by
learning in context, and by the use of cooperative or collaborative
modes.

As the self develops, so does the complexity and sophistication of
one's relational matrix. Rather than becoming increasingly autonomous, one becomes *differentiated* from others, but *at the same time more
connected* to others in ways that enhance one's own development.
Similarly, the capacity to *facilitate the growth of others* becomes a
validating part of one's own self development. With age, there is also

an increase in the variety and nuances of relational modes. While connections with those from one's early years may be maintained and strengthened, other relationships form and develop as well. One's "relational repertoire" gains in complexity and breadth, as new ways of being in relationship evolve.

IMPLICATIONS FOR CLINICAL TRAINING

Within such a framework, psychotherapy becomes one specific experience of the more general pattern of self-in-relation. If this developmental formulation for women is valid, then a woman client would gain greatest self-awareness and stimulus for growth by experiencing the self *in relation*. This involves a genuine sense that the therapist has truly heard what she is saying and can validate her experience by an appropriate response. Comments and interpretations from the therapist that may even be "correct" dynamically may feel distancing or even damaging if they serve as barriers between the therapist and the patient's own experience.

We are far from knowing what qualities within the therapist can foster empathic listening in a way that can assure true engagement with the patient, but several dimensions seem critical. Assuming that all therapists work from some implicit or explicit theory of the nature of the self, the closer this theory comes to a correct formulation of women's relational self, the more likely it is that the therapist will be at one with the patient in identifying salient features of her experience.

To the extent that theory disconfirms women's experience, it can result in therapy that is useless or damaging to the patient. Even more important, the therapist herself or himself can be more or less open to "taking in" the nature of women's lives—"taking in" both the quality of their daily experience and the associated affect. This requires a capacity to be receptive to the state of another with minimal interference from one's own needs that would negate or disconfirm whatever the patients express. This phenomenon is broader than the usual concept of countertransference, or response to the patient based on the therapist's conflicts or feelings. I am speaking of the larger notion of the therapist's basic assumptions and preconceptions of women and men, of a fundamental way that she or he sees the world, of basic understandings about appropriate and meaningful ways of being.

When judging the extent to which a therapist's theories, attitudes, and beliefs confirm women's experience, one cannot make absolute distinctions between female and male therapists, but several observations are worth noting. The vast majority of recent documents on the psychology of women are written and read by women, and professional presentations bearing on women's psychology are attended by many more women than men. Thus it is likely that women, more than men, will practice therapy that is informed by important new understandings of the female experience. Further, men are less likely than women to be able to confirm the validity of their women clients' experience by direct reference to their own lives, and it is possible that women clients will report feelings and events that challenge or disconfirm a male therapist's own experience. This could lead to difficulties in the therapist's drawing on his own affective life as a basis for intervention. At one level, a male therapist could approach unfamiliar affect or experience warily, curiously, perhaps seeking to draw it out—but without a direct connection to the client's state. At worst, he could judge the client's response in terms of his own experience, and thereby interpret a viable (but different) reaction as something pathological. The therapist's reaction, in turn, might be to explore the historical or transferential implications of the client's comments rather than to build on his own empathic connection with the client's affective experience.

Men may have additional work to do, therefore, in preparing themselves for work with women clients. This speculation is supported by findings reported by Orlinsky and Howard (1978). In their study of the therapy experience of 118 female clients, those seeing male therapists reported more eroticized affection, anger, inhibition, and depression than those seeing female therapists. After therapy, the women with male therapists saw themselves as less self-possessed, less open, and more self-critical than did the women with female therapists. The male therapists were described by their patients as more demanding, less encouraging, and less expansive than were their female counterparts.

The Trainee's Experience

Unfortunately, few of these issues are regularly addressed in training programs of any of the major clinical disciplines. Standard training curricula tend to emphasize cognitive elements such as psychodynamic formulations and techniques of intervention, with much less attention given to developing a capacity for empathic understanding and opening oneself to the client's experience. The more conceptual components are, of course, necessary and important elements of one's learning. But training seems to stop at the point of translating these formulations into a way of being with the client that best facilitates genuine openness to and communication with the client. In early training experiences, one is more often judged by what one knows rather than by one's capacity to take in accurately the affective experience of another. Even the capacity to listen is at times reduced to specific techniques—for example, maintaining eye contact, reflecting back, developing "listening skills."

This situation is only partially remedied in supervision, the process where the most thorough exploration of ongoing clinical interaction could occur. By and large, supervision also tends to focus on cognitive formulations rather than on the immediacy of contact during the therapy hour. An entire supervisory hour can be spent on elucidating the client's history, identifying key intrapsychic dynamics, and evolving diagnostic formulations without exploring the clinical process of listening and responding. Again, diagnosis and dynamics are clearly important as the framework out of which the actual clinical work evolves. But they are the beginning point, not the entire process. More importantly, such an emphasis on cognitive formulations can work against the therapist's availability to the patient. The therapist who is focused on "conceptualizing" what the patient is saying is turning attention away from contact with the patient, away from sensitivity to the nuances of the client's experience, and away from empathic connectedness.

To the extent that relational issues are discussed in supervision, too often they are assessed in terms of their potential negative impact. That is, much more seems to be known about how a therapist can relate poorly than how a therapist can relate well. For example, there are the "problems" of "overinvolvement," "fostering dependency," and "being manipulated." All of these can and do occur in therapy, and they warrant attention and correction. But in the absence of knowing more beneficial modes of relating, the tendency may be to compensate by greater distance rather than by more accurate empathy. It is noteworthy that there are no parallel common terms for "underinvolvement," "fostering disconnectedness," or "not responding to the client's needs."

RELATIONAL ISSUES IN PSYCHOTHERAPY

The application of the theory of the self-in-relation to clinical work with women can be illustrated by the use of clinical vignettes. The vignettes have been selected to demonstrate how theory and interpersonal openness consistent with a relational formulation can facilitate therapy with women and, conversely, how theory and attitudes that are not relationally oriented can impede this work. Each illustrates how the use—or lack—of a relational framework affects progress in psychotherapy.

Communicating in a Way that Is Believable to the Patient

As Stone (1981) puts it, "I have not yet seen a patient who wholeheartedly accepted the significance of his [sic] neurotic or transference-motivated attitudes or behavior if he felt that 'his reality' was not given just due." This is simply another way of stating the importance of the therapist's ability—by virtue of her or his theoretical orientation and assumptions about mental health—to speak to and validate the patient's own experience. In a therapy dyad of woman patient and woman therapist, knowledge of women's relational course of development combined with resonance to attendant potential conflicts can provide one route to this "believability."

For example, an upper-middle-class, urban-raised, doctoral-level female therapist was working with a woman from an impoverished rural background who was currently employed as a clerical worker in a large company. The patient was subjected to frequent sexual and physical provocation from some of her male superiors, and she was unable to respond with anything but anxiety, self-blame, and withdrawal. In her own professional career the therapist had never experienced overt harassment, but she had undergone subtle instances of discrimination that had similarly led her to question her own competence. The therapist was working from a theory in which a reaction of self-doubt is "expectable," and she could respond to the patient based on their shared internal responses. Each woman knew the intense anxiety that muted the emergence or expression of anger, and each woman had experienced the basic sense that she was responsible for the problems she encountered. In the therapist's view, it was her recognition and validation of the patient's reaction, based on their shared experience, that was a key factor in consolidating their working alliance and moving toward positive change.

Identifying More with Someone in the Patient's Life Than with the Patient

Many of the problems that emerge in therapy with women concern their relationships with men—as friends, lovers, colleagues, bosses, subordinates and, frequently, as therapists. Racker (1968) has suggested that therapists should attend to the possible danger of their identifying not with the patient, but with one or more of the patient's "internal objects." This can be extended to include danger that the therapist might identify with present or past "external" as well as "internal "objects in the patient's life. If the therapist has more in common with others in the patient's life than with the patient, the likelihood of this happening will increase. Such a situation occurred with a woman patient in her mid-20s who was seeing a senior male therapist. The patient had recently become involved in a relationship with a man to whom she felt increasingly committed. She had been struggling with how to handle what she saw as the one major obstacle: his tendency to treat her "politely"—opening doors, carrying packages, and holding her coat for her. She did not want to disrupt the relationship or hurt him, but she felt strongly that such actions contributed to the subordination of women and therefore were symbolically wrong. She came to a session reporting an illuminating experience. She and her boyfriend did some grocery shopping, and when they were finished, he casually took the grocery bag (which was not heavy) from her arms. Suddenly she had an intense, pervasive sense of shrinking, as though her arms were physically being held down and her power being sapped from her. The sensation passed quickly but left a profound impact. "For the first time I could feel in my gut, not just understand in my head, that 'the political is personal,' " she reported to her therapist, somewhat anxiously but with great pride. "Now I know I have to discuss it with my boyfriend; if he doesn't mean to undermine me, he'll at least be open to talking about it." The therapist then asked, "Do you think there are other ways you might have responded?" Considered by itself, this is not a countertherapeutic, hostile, or defensive response and, under many conditions, could lead to some useful explorations. However, according to the patient's experience, this was not one of those times. The patient was primarily communicating a shift in her own thinking from a concern with the *consequences* of her behavior (Will I hurt him if I voice dissatisfaction with what he is doing?) to an emphasis on the central importance of making explicit her *own inner reaction,* even at some threat to the relationship. Within a relational framework, this was a major moment of awareness, requiring attention and exploration. By contrast, the therapist's comment served to direct attention not to her own experience of self or "self in relation," but rather to the external manifestations of her behavior. The patient became aware of this shift and tried to convince the therapist that it felt more salient to discuss her own reactions than her subsequent behavior, and that she experienced his suggestion as a challenge to the validity of her feelings. The therapist countered that he in no way *meant* to devalue her experience, and the session continued to the end with a disagreement between the two about what the therapist had meant to say and what the patient had heard and responded to.

Experiencing Patient Conflicts as Threats to the Therapist's Self-Esteem

A therapist sometimes responds defensively when a patient expresses anger or criticism toward another and the therapist experiences it as implied criticism of her- or himself. In such a situation, the therapist's sensitivity to the "meanings" behind the patient's words and gestures can be more influenced by what is congruent or unthreatening than by what is central to the patient. For example, at a recent psychoanalytic conference a presentation was made of a "live supervision" (Rubinstein, 1979): In order to illustrate and discuss issues of analytic supervision, the candidate presented the contents of an analytic hour to his supervisor in front of an audience, and the supervisor responded much as he would in actual supervision. The candidate and supervisor were men, as were the chair, the secretary of the panel, and the discussant. The patient was a woman. The session under discussion turned on the patient's handling of conflict with others. First she reported a dream, the latent content of which was identified to the audience, but not to the patient, as feelings of criticism toward the analyst. She then continued in the vein of how much she hated complaining, that complaining made her feel "ugly" and "like a witch." The analyst neither responded to her implied criticism of him nor validated this discomfort. Instead he countered her reaction: "What's the matter with complaining? Why should that make you feel ugly?" The patient answered, "What do you mean 'What's the matter with complaining?'" Her associations then led her to relate an incident with some of her fellow male students in an advanced mental health training program in which one student had called her the "class hysteric." She had retorted, "Then you must be the class obsessional," but she felt cowardly and guilty about having such a reaction. The therapist's response did not pick up on the continued theme of her *discomfort* with giving criticism or on the strength of her sense of guilt and "ugliness." He stated instead that he noticed she was smiling as she spoke, and he felt that she must be getting pleasure from criticizing and being criticized. The patient responded that this comment made her feel like the analyst thought that she should just take abuse without returning it, to which he responded, "I'm not telling you what to do." Here the therapist, in a defensive manner, imposed his own reality on their interchange, protecting himself at the expense of exploring her emotions. The consequences here are potentially severe, because the therapist's own formulations suggest that the patient, by criticizing others, is injuring others for the sake of her own selfish pleasure. This notion that one's own wishes and actions can be injurious to others is precisely the precursor of the self-blame that can inhibit women's self-expression and thwart their self-esteem. From the material the analyst presented, this patient was already struggling with issues of fear and guilt associated with being critical of others, and the therapist's remarks seem only too likely to reinforce this area of conflict rather than help the patient toward its resolution.

A CHALLENGE FOR FUTURE TRAINING

Differences in the psychological realities of women and men have created obstacles to learning about women's lives through women's own reports and to empathy with women's affective experiences. The work of both women and men therapists can suffer from these obstacles, but we now can identify them more systematically for members of each sex. That the obstacles exist is not surprising. Traditional psychological theory and the cultural mores within which therapy is embedded strongly support and affirm the male reality. Men have little encouragement in their professional lives to consider the limitations of their own experience, to "suspend" their reality, and to be receptive to and validate the "other" as it is reflected by their women clients. Many women therapists have been encouraged to give greater credence to current theory and the values in which it is embedded than to their own experience, and therefore they have been too ready to "suspend" their reality in the face of ideas that contradict their experience.

Yet, increasingly, women are demanding to be heard. This has implications for the therapy hour, just as it has implications for family and work life and social structure. Male therapists may need to ponder those areas in which they have limited understanding and turn to writings by women and the women in their own lives for guidance and information. But such a stance typically is not encouraged in men. In part, it calls for a measure of humility, a recognition that one has much to learn from others—and that new learning might threaten what one already "knows" or believes. In part, it means developing receptivity to the experience of another along with a suspension of one's own preconceptions. Some argue that this goes against the basic structure of our culture's historical models of thinking. If so, it poses a formidable challenge.

The risk for men is that, as part of the majority culture, they will respond in a defensive, invalidating way to those whose experiences are different from and directly challenge their own. There is some evidence that this pattern does occur with male therapists and female patients, to the detriment of the women's satisfaction with their treatment. The challenge presented to male therapists is great, but the potential gains in personal and professional growth are even greater.

Many women, therapists or not, are not yet accustomed to guiding others and giving information openly. Certainly the culture has not fostered such characteristics. Where theory conflicted with their own intense emotional experience, some women therapists have opted for theory and seeming "safety," attempting to resolve conflict in a way that ultimately is detrimental to themselves as well as their clients. Nonetheless, the research I have cited suggests that in the privacy of their offices some of their basic relational values came through—in spite of their socialization and professional training.

Full and open discussion of these issues in all therapy training would constitute a major stride toward growth among therapists of both sexes. Such discussions would ideally be initiated at the very beginning of therapeutic training and continue throughout its course. Such training would validate self-exploration and lay the groundwork for continued work toward genuine understanding of differences in women's and men's experience. Until such concerns are addressed as a matter of course in major training facilities, it is unlikely that individual practitioners will have the impetus or support to undertake this important and difficult work by themselves.

This paper was presented at a Stone Center Colloquium in December 1982.

17

Empathy, Mutuality, and Therapeutic Change: Clinical Implications of a Relational Model

JUDITH V. JORDAN

Concerns about relationships lead many people, particularly women, into therapy in which a primary goal is to expand the experience of what might be called the sense of "real self," particularly in ongoing relationships. Individuals suffering from all sorts of falsifications and distortions of their experiences of self are looking for ways to be known and understood as well as providing that for others. How can we achieve and maintain a sense of contact and connection in which individuals can experience a sense of wholeness which also contributes to the relational unit? The feelings and behaviors that have been shut down to avoid pain, or amplified in order to gain approval, can begin to unfold anew in the therapy relationship. In its broadest sense, therapy offers an opportunity to expand relational presence, providing a sense of realness and contact with one's own inner experience and with the other's subjective experience. The route to this change is through the enhancement of empathy, both for other and for self. For many women, attention to their own inner experience often feels incompatible with attention to other (it is "selfish,""egocentric," "hurtful"); an ethic of caring for others carries the connotation of self-sacrifice or putting oneself last.

The goal in therapy is not to make women divert their attention from the relational context but to provide an opportunity to develop a new integration of self–other experience in which the validity of one's own experience as well as the other's gets acknowledged. This occurs in current real relationship and in memory organization of relationships. Responsiveness to the other as well as awareness of one's own needs—honoring the self—are enhanced. Attention is paid to empathy for self and other.

The elaboration and development of empathy as a means of interacting is central to my work with women in therapy. Many "modern" women initially see their empathic attunement to others as a burden; they wish they could be "more like men"—singleminded, able to "turn off" feelings in the service of logic; they wish all the important areas of their lives, especially love and work, did not feel so interconnected, entwined. They have unconsciously, sometimes consciously, adopted the broader cultural values of abstraction, linearity, autonomy, compartmentalization. Unfortunately many therapists share this cultural bias and have devalued empathy as less useful or central than intellectual insight or clarification to the process of change. Both empathy and the therapeutic relationship have been seen as the context within which the important and significant work of interpretation and clarification occur. The Stone Center model suggests in fact that relationship, based on empathic attunement, is the key to the process of therapy, not just the backdrop for it. In therapy informed by a relational model of self we begin to see that there is integrity in the interpenetration of affect and cognition, of self–other boundary oscillation; we see that it produces special tensions and dilemmas, but the presence of these conflicts does not indicate a failure on the woman's part.

A part of her problem is living in a world which cannot clearly acknowledge the important contribution of emotional reaction and interpersonal sensitivity to thinking, to work, to all aspects of life. Validation of the special tensions of being a person for whom a sense of identity is closely bound to relational context is a part of what I do as a therapist. I have treated numerous women who were previously in treatment, either in individual or couples' work with therapists who did not appreciate this and I have seen the destructive consequences of the therapist's failure to understand this. A brief vignette will illustrate several of these points: C. is a vivacious, attractive bright 40-year-old divorced lawyer. She came into treatment primarily because of dissatisfaction with an intimate relationship. Her concern with the relationship was pervasive and she had difficulty attending to her professional responsibilities although she was "getting by." She blamed herself for not being able to keep her love life separate from her work life, seeing it as a sign of being "out of control" and "too needy."

She and the man she lived with had consulted a couples' therapist before she came to me, and at the conclusion of a six-week stint of couples' work she met individually with the therapist who reportedly wondered why she was being so "masochistic" in holding on to a relationship which gave her so much pain and so little gratification. She felt devastated by this and found herself agreeing with the therapist. Now, in addition to feeling the pain of the relationship in which her lover was constantly telling her that she asked for too much intimacy, crowded him emotionally and physically, and told her she was suffering from extreme PMS which made her a "raving bitch," she considered herself a failure because somehow, in being "drawn" to all this pain—masochistic. In fact, what she was engaged by in the relationship were the moments of warmth and sharing, the joint venture of building a "we" together; in the face of his dissatisfaction and disappointment with her, she kept trying to make it better, to make the relationship "work" by adjusting to his demands (with understandably an underlying resentment for which she felt quite guilty). Her dedication to the relationship, her identification with the relationship and her willingness to make internal modifications to better the relationship were viewed by her couples' therapist as masochistic and she felt he must be right.

As we worked together in our therapy to seek other explanations for the unsatisfactory state of affairs, which included a real analysis of why she stayed in the relationship, rather than adopt the sense of blame inflicted on her by the couples' therapist, she began to feel some relief and appreciation of her own feelings and wants. Yes, she felt dependent but, yes, she also felt dependable and giving; and, yes, she was willing to expend considerable energy on trying to establish more mutuality. She came to appreciate the importance of her own giving nature but she also began to accept the limitations of this man's real capacity for intimacy and ultimately the relationship ended; instead of feeling she had "thrown four years down the drain," she was able to retrieve a sense of the integrity of her feelings and actions in the relationship as well as truly grieve for the loss of both a real relationship and hoped for growth in the relationship. It was an extraordinarily painful process for her but the pain was no longer exacerbated by the persistent self-blame and sense of total personal responsibility and failure that she had felt following the couples' therapy. In working through this loss and appreciating her own capacity to seek connection and relatedness despite it, she in fact experienced a sense of increasing strength and diminishing vulnerability. Thus, although she lost this specific and valued relationship which caused tremendous grief, she gained an awareness of her very real relational capacities which she could now believe would allow her to eventually move forward into new relationships. She came to know these strengths in the therapy relationship itself.

In part, this example demonstrates an increase of what I have called self-empathy. Using Schafer's (1968) tripartite definition of self as "agent" (knower, doer), "object," and "locus," what self-empathy suggests is that the observing, knowing "agent" focuses on some experience (in which the self is experienced as object) in a new, empathic manner. In a broad sense, I am suggesting that how we relate to or make contact with others is a useful model for relating to parts of internal experience. The observing, often judging self can then make empathic contact with the self as object. This could occur in the form of having a memory of oneself in which the inner state at that time has not been fully integrated because it was not acceptable. To be able to observe and tolerate the affect of that state in a context of understanding becomes a kind of intrapsychic empathy, which actually can lead to lasting structural change in relational images and self-representations. The motivational and attitudinal state of nonjudgment and openness, taking an experience seriously, and readiness to experience affect and understanding may contribute to important shifts in the inner experience of troublesome self images.

As a therapist, I have often been moved by seeing the emergence of self-empathy. One patient identified with her critical, punitive father, and spoke of herself in very derogatory terms; one day she was giving an extremely unfavorable description of herself as she went off for her first day of school. In every comment one could hear her harsh, critical father's voice: "I was such an obnoxious little kid. I wanted everyone to pay attention . No wonder my father got so mad. " A therapeutic intervention indicating that of course she wanted to feel special as she went out into this new, maybe even scary part of the world at first did not seem to have any impact. Later in treatment, when we were looking at this same incident, however, this woman burst into tears and said, " Suddenly I saw myself as the little girl, so scared and uncertain. My heart just went out to her. I feel it now for her . . . the pain. I feel it now for me. I couldn't feel it then. But I understand why I was acting that way. " It was not simply that she became more accepting and less punitive vis-a-vis certain self representations, although that was an important part of it. But she also actually connected with the affect which had been split off in the memory; both the self as object and the experiencing self were modified by this exchange. And the identification with the critical father was altered in the direction of being less punitive and harsh in her self-judgments. Empathy with self, with the memory of the little girl, increased as rejection and judgment of her decreased. Although there was a momentary increase of anger at the father as he came to be seen as harsh and critical, empathically failing the child, that was not the end point of the process. Rather, as it was worked through, the woman also began to experience a deepened empathy with the father. As she put herself emotionally in the place of each figure, an acceptance of their actions and feelings grew.

Self–other representations change. Both her disappointment and anger at father are an important first step but were she to stop the exploration there, she would simply be left with a negative image of father which does not allow for continued relational elaboration. Movement toward ongoing connection, with both father and others as well, is facilitated when, through empathy, movement toward or with, rather than away from or against, is accomplished. Self–other boundaries are importantly altered here; it is not a self endangered by others and defending against others but a sense of "I" that is more permeable to the "we," more available for relationship.

The therapist plays an important role in enhancing the capacity for self-empathy. First, her empathic attitude and response to the experiences being reported allows for a relaxation of some of the engrained patterns of rejection and judgment on the part of the client. There is a kind of "corrective relational experience" in which the unacceptable is accepted and responded to in a caring, affectively present and re-connected manner. Disowned aspects of self are witnessed and allowed. The therapist models an empathic way of being with painful memories and feelings. By bringing some under-standing to bear on the experiencing person from the past (the little girl who was scared, not obnoxious), the therapist assists the patient in both objectifying important value-laden images of the self and paradoxically at the same time, making real affective connections with them. There is room now, however, for new affective-cognitive organization to occur, so old well-worn circuits (obnoxious little kid and disappointed, angry father) give way to new relational organiza-tion of the experience (scared little kid and impatient, unempathic father). The patient gains a new image of self as well as a new understanding of the other. The old relational matrix is freshly understood and there is a reorganization of the relational memory. Empathy for both self and other increase through these therapeutic explorations. In some sense, this involves a growth of compassion—for self and other.

Therapy, as I practice it, exists only in so far as empathic attunement occurs between patient and therapist. Mutuality, or more specifically mutual intersubjectivity, the attunement to and responsiveness to the subjective, inner experience of the other, at both a cognitive and affective level, is what the therapeutic enterprise is about. Therapy occurs through the capacity to share in and comprehend the momentary psychological state of another person (Schafer, 1959); it involves the elaboration of an understanding of the person and the relationship which relies on moment-to-moment cognitive-affective contact between patient and therapist. In therapy there are two active members who are both open to change through their participation in this interaction. The relationship that exists is central to the process, whether we talk about transference, "corrective emotional experience," or empathic attunement. The models of relationship as well as the actual manner of relating of the therapist are crucial to the way the therapeutic context influences individual growth. The therapist's appreciation of the ongoing interdependence of human beings leads the therapist to subtly and sometimes directly encourage the ongoing turning to others for support and assistance rather than emphasizing an ultimate state of self reliance and independence.

A model that acknowledges that therapy is a dialogue also recognizes that therapy is characterized by a process of mutual change and impact. Both therapist and patient are touched emotionally by each other, grow in the relationship, gain something from one another, risk something of themselves in the process—in short, both are affected, changed, part of an open system of feeling and learning. There is significant mutuality. It takes courage on both sides to involve themselves in this interaction. But it is in some respects not a fully mutual relationship. In therapy, one individual discloses more, comes expressly to be helped by the other, to be listened to and understood. The patient's self disclosure and expression of disavowed or split off experiences, in a context of nonjudgmental listening and understanding, is a powerful part of the process. In order to facilitate this, there is a contract which puts the patient's subjective experience at the center and there is an agreement to attend to the therapist's subjective experience only in so far as it might be helpful to the patient. The therapist offers herself to be used for the healing. But within this context there is real caring in both directions and is an important feeling of mutuality, with mutual respect, emotional availability, and openness to change on both sides. And the experience of relationship, of mutuality often grows with the therapy. Some therapists feel uncomfortable with the notion of growing through their work with patients; it feels exploitive or too gratifying. That conforms to an old model which suggests that if I benefit, you do not—a scarcity, power, hierarchy model. This is exactly the model that many of our patients carry in their heads, which makes it so hard for them to attend to their own needs. In practice, very often in giving to another we feel enlarged in expanding the relationship and our understanding of it, both members are enriched. If we honor the notion of a relational self, identity anchored in the world of human connection, interaction, and interdependence, and want to assist patients in expanding their sense of personal aliveness and wholeness in relationships, we must be ready to expand our own awareness and openness in the therapy relationship.

Being defined in, valuing, feeling alive through, and growing into relationship does not alter the reality of one's physical separateness in the world; nor does it deny the experience of solitude. But our culture has overemphasized the agentic, individualistic, competitive, lonely qualities of human life; and women have suffered, as their valuing of relationship, their immersion in caring and open need for connection have been denigrated. Yes, it is important that women learn to deal with anger, but it may be more important that they learn they can stay connected in the presence of anger rather than learn to automatically vent their personal frustrations on others without any attention to the impact of these feelings on others (what some would call a male model of anger discharge). And of course women should enjoy the freedom and be encouraged to develop and exercise their creative, intellectual, and self-expressive abilities for their own pleasure as well as for others' benefit. But here, too, it may be more imporant to find ways to do this which do not necessarily entail the ruthless disregard of others' needs or others' creativity. The reconciliation of self expression and relational enhancement is particularly important for women since so much of our sense of ourselves takes shape in relational contexts. Feeling connected and in contact with another often allows us our most profound sense of personal meaning and reality; at its best, therapy works toward developing and honoring this relational presence.

This paper was presented at a Stone Center Workshop in April 1986.

References

Abelin, E. L. (1971). The role of the father in the separation-individuation process. In J. B. McDevitt & C. F. Settlage (Eds.), *Essays in honor of Margaret Mahler* (pp. 229–252). New York: International Universities Press.

Aberle, D. F., & Naegele, F. D. (1952). Middle class fathers' occupational roles and attitude toward children. *American Journal of Orthopsychiatry, 22,* 336–378.

Alexander, F. (1950). Analysis of the therapeutic factors in psychoanalytic treatment. *Psychoanalytic Quarterly, 19,* 482–500.

Alexander, F. (1963). *Fundamentals of psychoanalysis.* New York: W. W. Norton.

American Psychiatric Association. (1980a). *A psychiatric glossary.* Washington, DC: Author.

American Psychiatric Association. (1980b). *Diagnostic and statistical manual of mental disorders* (3rd ed.). Washington, DC: Author.

American Psychological Association. (1975). Report of the task force on sex bias and sex role stereotyping in psychotherapeutic practice. *American Psychologist, 30,* 1169–1175.

Applegarth, A. (1977). Some observations on work inhibitions in women. In H. P. Blum (Ed.), *Female psychology.* New York: International Universities Press.

Arieti, S., & Bemporad, J. (1978). *Severe and mild depression: The psychotherapeutic approach.* New York: Basic Books.

Atwood, G., & Stolorow, R. (1984). *Structures of subjectivity: Explorations in psychoanalytic phenomenology.* Hillsdale, NJ: The Analytic Press.

Bakan, D. (1966). *The duality of human existence: An essay on psychology and religion.* Boston: Beacon Press.

Bart, P. (1971). Depression in middle-aged women. In V. Gormick & B. K. Moran (Eds.), *Women in a sexist society.* New York: Basic Books.

Basch, M. (1983). The concept of self: An operational definition. In B. Lee & G. Noam (Eds.), *Developmental approaches to the self.* New York: Plenum Press.

Beck, A. T. (1972). *Depression: Causes and treatment.* Philadelphia: University of Pennsylvania Press.

Belenky, M. F., Clinchy, B. M., Goldberger, N. R., & Tarule, J. M. (1986). *Women's ways of knowing: The development of self, voice and mind.* New York: Basic Books.

Belle, D. (Ed.) (1982). *Lives in stress: Women and depression.* Beverly Hills, CA: Sage.

Benedek, E. (1979). Dilemmas in research in female adolescent development. In M. Sugar (Ed.), *Adolescent development* (pp. 3–19). New York: Brunner-Mazel.

Benedek, T. (1959). Parenthood as developmental phase: A contribution to the libido theory. *Journal of the American Psychoanalytic Association, 7,* 339–417.

Bergin, A. E., & Lambert, M. J. (1978). The evaluation of therapeutic outcomes. In S. L. Garfield & A. E. Bergin (Eds.), *Handbook of psychotherapy and behavior change: An empirical analysis* (2nd ed.). New York: Wiley.

Bernard, J. (1971). The paradox of the happy marriage. In V. Gornick & B. K. Moran (Eds.), *Women in sexist society.* New York: Basic Books.

Bernard, J. (1972). *The future of marriage.* New York: World.

Bernardez, T. (1976). Unconscious beliefs about women affecting psychother-apy. *North Carolina Journal of Mental Health, 7*(5), 63–66.

Bernardez, T. (1982). The female therapist in relation to male roles. In K. Solomon & N. Levy (Eds.), *Men in transition.* New York: Plenum Press.

Bernardez-Bonesatti, T. (1978). Women and anger: Conflicts with aggression in contemporary women. *Journal of the American Medical Women's Association, 33*(5), 215–219.

Bettleheim, B. (1954). *Symbolic wounds.* Glencoe, IL: Free Press.

Bibring, E. (1953). The mechanism of depression. In P. Greenacre (Ed.), *Affective disorders.* New York: International Universities Press.

Biller, H. B. (1981). The father and sex role development. In M. E. Lamb (Ed.), *The role of the father in child development* (2nd ed.). New York: Wiley.

Biller, H. B., & Meredith, D. L. (1974). *Father power.* New York: David McKay.

Blanck, G. & R. (1979). *Ego psychology II: Psychoanalytic developmental psychology.* New York: Columbia University Press.

Blatt, S. J., D'Afflitti, J. P., & Quinlan, D. M. (1976). Experience of depression in normal young adults. *Journal of Abnormal Psychology, 85,* 383–389.

Block, J. H. (1978). Another look at sex differentiation in the socialization behaviors of mothers and fathers. In J. A. Sherman & F. L. Denmark (Eds.), *Psychology of women: Future directions of research.* New York: Psychological Dimensions.

Blos, P. (1962). *On adolescence.* New York: The Free Press.

Blos, P. (1979). *The adolescent passage.* New York: International Universities Press.

Blos, P. (1980). Modifications in the traditional psychoanalytic theory of female adolescent development. In S. Feinstein (Ed.), *Adolescent psychiatry VIII.* Chicago: University of Chicago Press.

Blum, H. P. (1971). On the conception and development of the transference neurosis. *Journal of the American Psychoanalytic Association, 19*(1), 41–53.

Blum, H. P. (1977). Masochism, the ego ideal and the psychology of women. In H. Blum (Ed.), *Female psychology: Contemporary psychoanalytic views* (pp. 157–192). New York: International Universities Press.

Bowlby, J. (1969). *Attachment.* Volume 1 of *Attachment and loss.* New York:Basic Books.

Briscoe, C. W., & Smith, J. B. (1973). Depression and marital turmoil. *Archives of General Psychiatry, 29*(6), 811–817.

Brodsky, A. M., & Hare-Mustin, R. T. (Eds). (1980). *Women and psychotherapy*. New York: Guilford Press.

Broverman, I. K., Broverman, D. M., Clarkson, F. E., Rosenkrantz, P. S., & Vogel,S. R. (1970). Sex-role stereotypes and clinical judgments of mental health. *Journal of Consulting and Clinical Psychology, 34*(1), 1–7.

Brown, G. W., & Harris, T. (1978). *Social origins of depression: A study of psychiatric disorders in women*. New York: The Free Press.

Bruch, H. (1973). *Eating disorders*. New York: Basic Books.

Brunswick, R. M. (1940). The pre-Oedipal phase of the libidinal development. *Psychoanalytic Quarterly, 9*, 293–319.

Bryer, J., Nelson, B., Miller, J. B., & Krol, P. (1986). Childhood sexual and physical abuse as factors in adult psychiatric illness. *American Journal of Psychiatry, 144*(11), 1426–1430.

Buber, M. (1958). *I and thou*. New York: Charles Scribner's Sons.

Burlingham, D. (1973). The pre-Oedipal infant–father relationship. *Psychoanalytic Study of the Child, 28*, 23–47.

Caplan, P. (1984). The myth of women's masochism. *American Psychologist, 39*, 130–139.

Carmen, E., Russo, N., & Miller, J. B. (1981). Inequality and women's mental health: An overview. *American Journal of Psychiatry, 138*(10), 1319–1330.

Carson, R. (1971). Sex differences in ego functioning: Exploratory studies of agency and communion. *Journal of Consulting and Clinical Psychology, 37*(2), 267–277.

Chasseguet-Smirgel, J. (1970). Feminine guilt and the Oedipus complex. In J. Chasseguet-Smirgel (Ed.), *Female sexuality* (pp. 94–134). Ann Arbor: University of Michigan Press.

Chernin, K. (1981). *The obsession: Reflections on the tyranny of slenderness*. New York: Harper & Row.

Chesler, P. (1972). *Women and madness*. New York: Doubleday.

Chodoff, P. (1974). The depressive personality. In R. J. Friedman & M. M. Katz (Eds.), *The psychology of depression: Contemporary theory and research*. Washington, DC: Winston.

Chodorow, N. (1978). *The reproduction of mothering*. Berkeley: University of California Press.

Clinchy, B. & Zimmerman, C. (1985). *Growing up intellectually: Issues for college women* (Work in Progress No. 19). Wellesley, MA: Stone Center.

Clower, V. (1977). Theoretical implications in current views of masturbation in latency girls. In H. R. Blum (Ed.), *Female psychology: Contemporary psychoanalytic views* (pp. 109–125). New York: International Universities Press.

Contratto, S. (1986). Fathers presence in women's psychological development. In J. Robow, M. Goldman, & G. Platt, (Eds.), *Studies in psychoanalytic sociology*. Melbourne, FL: Krieger.

Crandall, V. J., Katkovsky, W., & Preston, A. (1962). Motivational and ability determinants of young children's intellectual achievement behaviors. *Child Development, 33*(3), 643–661.

Demos, V. (1982). *Varieties of empathy*. Paper presented at Boston Institute for the Development of Infants and Parents, Chestnut Hill, MA.

Dent, J. K. (1978). *Exploring the psycho-social therapies through the personalities of effective therapists*. DHEW Publication No. (ADM) 77-527. Rockville, MD: National Institute of Mental Health.

Deutsch, H. (1944). *The psychology of women*. New York: Grune & Stratton.

Deutsch, H. (1967). Selected problems of adolescence. *The psychoanalytic study of the child, Monograph 3*. New York: International Universities Press.

Dickinson, E. (1960). Why do they shut me out of heaven? In T. H. Johnson (Ed.), *The complete poems of Emily Dickinson*. Boston: Little, Brown.

Dinnerstein, D. (1976). *The mermaid and the minotaur*. New York: Harper & Row.

Dowling, C. (1981). *The Cinderella complex*. New York: Summit Books.

Dymond, R., Hughes, A., & Raabe, V. (1952). Measurable changes in empathy with age. *Journal of Consulting Psychology, 16*, 202–206.

Easser, B. R. (1976). Womanhood. Reported by E. Galenson in Panel report, Psychology of women: Late adolescence and early adulthood. *Journal of the American Psychoanalytic Association, 24*(3), 634–646.

Edelstein, B. (1977). *The woman doctor's diet for women*. Englewood Cliffs, NJ: Prentice-Hall.

Ehrenberg, D. B. (1974). The intimate edge in therapeutic relatedness. *Contemporary Psychoanalysis, 10*(4), 423–437.

Erikson, E. (1950/1963). *Childhood and society*. New York: W. W. Norton.

Erikson, E. (1968). *Identity, youth and crisis*. New York: W. W. Norton.

Fairbairn, R. (1950/1962). *An object relations theory of personality*. New York: Basic Books.

Fairbairn, W. R. D. (1946/1952). Object relationships and dynamic structure. In *An object relations theory of personality*. New York: Basic Books.

Fairbairn, W. R. D. (1957). Freud, the psychoanalytic method and mental health. *British Journal of Medical Psychology, 30*, 53–62.

Fast, I. (1978). Developments in gender identity: The original matrix. *International Review of Psychoanalysis, 5*, 265–273.

Feifel, H., & Eells, J. (1963). Patients and therapists view the same psychotherapy. *Journal of Consulting Psychology, 27*(4), 310–318.

Fidell, L. S. (1973, May). *Put her on drugs: Prescribed drug usage in women*. Paper presented at the meeting of the Eastern Psychological Association.

Fliegel, Z. O. (1973). Feminine psychosexual development in Freudian theory: A historical reconstruction. *Psychoanalytic Quarterly, 42*, 385–408.

Fliegel, Z. O. (1982). Half a century later: Current status of Freud's controversial views on women. *The Psychoanalytic Review, 69*, 7–28.

Fliess, R. (1942). The metapsychology of the analyst. *Psychoanalytic Quarterly, 11*, 211–227.

Fraiberg, S. (1972). Some characteristics of general arousal and discharge in latency age girls. *Psychoanalytic Study of the Child, 27*, 439–475.

Freeman, T., Cameron, J., & McGhie, A. (1958). *Chronic schizophrenia*. New York: International Universities Press.

Freire, P. (1970). *Pedagogy of the oppressed*. New York: Seabury Press.

Freud, S. (1905). *Three essays on the theory of sexuality. Standard Edition, 7,* 125–243. London: Hogarth.

Freud, S. (1917). Mourning and melancholia. *StandardEdition, Vol. 14.* London: Hogarth.

Freud, S. (1920). Beyond the pleasure principle. *The Standard Edition, 18.* London: Hogarth.

Freud, S. (1924). The dissolution of the Oedipus complex. *Standard Edition, 19,* 173–179. London: Hogarth.

Freud, S. (1925). Some psychical consequences of the anatomical distinction between the sexes. *Standard Edition, 19,* 243–258. London: Hogarth.

Freud, S. (1931). Female sexuality. *Standard Edition, 21,* 223–243. London: Hogarth.

Freud, S. (1933). New Introductory Lectures on Psychoanalysis. *Standard Edition, 21,* 7–182. London: Hogarth.

Freud, S. (1959). *Collected papers,* Vol. *1–5,* New York: Basic Books.

Fulmer, R. H., Nedalie, J., & Lord, D. A. (1982). Life cycles in transition: A family systems perspective on counseling the college student. *Journal of Adolescence, 5,* 195–217.

Galenson, E., & Roiphe, H. (1977). Some suggested revisions concerning early female development. In H. Blum (Ed.), *Female psychology: Contemporary psychoanalytic views* (pp. 29–59). New York: International Universities Press.

Galenson, E. (1976). Panel report, Psychology of women: Late adolescence and early adulthood. *Journal of the American Psychoanalytic Association, 24*(3), 631–645.

Galenson, E., & Roiphe, H. (1982). The pre-Oedipal relationship of a father, mother and daughter. In S. Cath & A. R. Gurwitt (Eds.), *Father, child development and clinical perspectives* (pp. 151–162). Boston: Little Brown.

Gardner, G. G. (1964). The psychotherapeutic relationship. *Psychological Bulletin, 61*(6), 426–437, .

Garner, D. M., & Garfinkel, P. E. (1979). The eating attitudes test: An index of the symptoms of anorexia nervosa. *Psychological Medicine, 9*(2), 273–279.

Garner, D. M., Garfinkel, P. E., Schwartz, D., & Thompson, M. (1980). Cultural expectations of thinness in women. *Psychological Reports, 4*(2), 483–491.

Gearhart, S. M. (1982). The future—if there is one—is female. In P. McAllister (Ed.), *Reweaving the web of life: Feminism and nonviolence.* Philadelphia: New Society Publishers.

Gill, M. M. (1979). The analysis of the transference. *Journal of the American Psychoanalytic Association, 27*(Suppl), 263–288.

Gilligan, C. (1979). Woman's place in man's life cycle. *Harvard Educational Review, 49*(4), 431–444.

Gilligan, C. (1902). *In a different voice: Psychological theory and women's development.* Cambridge: Harvard University Press.

Gilligan, C. (1989). Preface: Teaching Shakespeare's sister. In C. Gilligan, N. Lyons, & T. Hanmer (Eds.), *Making connections: The relational worlds of adolescent girls at Emma Willard School.* Troy, NY: Emma Willard School.

Gilligan, C., Lyons, N., & Hanmer, T. (Eds.). (1989). *Making connections: The relational worlds of adolescent girls at Emma Willard School.* Troy, NY: Emma Willard School.

Gilligan, C., Rogers, A., & Brown, L. (1989). Epilogue: Soundings into development. In C. Gilligan, N. Lyons, & T. Hanmer (Eds.), *Making connections: The relational worlds of adolescent girls at Emma Willard School.* Troy, NY: Emma Willard School.

Giovacchini, P. L. (1976). Symbiosis and intimacy. *International Journal of Psychoanalytic Psychotherapy, 5,* 413–436.

Gleason, J. B. (1975). Fathers and other strangers: Men's speech to young children. In Daniel P. Dato (Ed.), *Georgetown University roundtable on language and linguistics. Developmental psycholinguistics: Theory and applications.* Washington, DC: Georgetown University Press.

Gove, W. R. (1972). The relationship between sex roles, marital status and mental illness. *Social Forces, 51*(1), 34–44.

Greenson, R. (1960). Empathy and its vicissitudes. *International Journal of Psychoanalysis, 41,* 418–424.

Greenson, R. R. (1968). Disidentifying from mother: Its special importance for the boy. *International Journal of Psychoanalysis, 49,* 370–374.

Grinker, R. R., Miller, J., Sabshin, M., Nunn, R., & Nunnally, J. C. (1961). *The phenomena of depression.* New York: Harper.

Guntrip, H. (1973). *Psychoanalytic theory, therapy and the self.* New York: Basic Books.

Gurman, A. S. (1977). The patient's perception of the therapeutic relationship. In A. S. Gurman & A. M. Razin, (Eds.), *Effective psychotherapy: A handbook of research.* New York: Pergamon Press.

Halmi, K. A. (1983). Psychosomatic illness review: Anorexia nervosa and bulimia. *Psychosomatics, 24*(2), 111–127.

Halmi, K. A., Falk, J. R., & Schwartz, E. (1981). Binge-eating and vomiting: A survey of a college population. *Psychological Medicine, 11,* 697–706.

Hammen, C. L., & Padesky, C. A. (1977). Sex differences in the expression of depressive responses on the Beck Depression Inventory. *Journal of Abnormal Psychology, 86,* 609–614.

Heilbrun, C. (1979). *Reinventing womanhood.* New York: W. W. Norton.

Henley, N. M. (1977). *Body politics: Power, sex, and nonverbal communication.* Englewood Cliffs, NJ: Prentice-Hall.

Hennig, M., & Jardim, A. (1977). *The managerial woman.* Garden City, NY: Doubleday.

Herman, J. (1984). *Sexual violence* (Work in Progress No. 83-05). Wellesley, MA: Stone Center.

Herman, J. L. (1981). *Father–daughter incest.* Cambridge, MA: Harvard University Press.

Hillman, J. (1981). Cited in Chernin, Kim. *The obsession: Reflections on the tyranny of slenderness.* New York: Harper & Row.

Hoffman, L. W. (1972). Early childhood experiences and women's achievement motives. *Journal of Social Issues. 28*(2), 129–155.

Hoffman, M. (1977). Sex differences in empathy and related behaviors.

Psychological Bulletin, 84(4), 712–722.

Hoffman, M. (1978). Toward a theory of empathic arousal and development. In M. Lewis & L. Rosenblum (Eds.), *The development of affect.* New York: Plenum Press.

Horner, M. S. (1972). Toward an understanding of achievement-related conflicts in women. *Journal of Social Issues, 28(2),* 157–175.

Horner, M. (1972). The motive to avoid success and changing aspirations of college women In J. Bardwick (Ed.), *Readings in the psychology of women.* New York: Harper & Row.

Horney, K. (1924). On the genesis of the castration complex in women. *International Journal of Psychoanalysis, 5,* 50–65.

Horney, K. (1926). The flight from womanhood: The masculinity complex in women as viewed by men and by women. *International Journal of Psychoanalysis, 7,* 324–339.

Houck, J. H. (1972). The intractable female patient. *American Journal of Psychiatry, 129,* 27–31.

Howard, K. I., & Orlinsky, D. E. (1979). *What effect does therapist gender have on outcome for women in psychotherapy?* Presentation at the conference of the American Psychological Association, New York City.

Jacobson, E. (1964). *The self and the object world.* New York: International Universities Press.

Janeway, E. (1980). *Powers of the weak.* New York: Knopf.

Josselson, R. (1973). Psychodynamic aspects of identity formation in college women. *Journal of Youth and Adolescence, 2(1),* 3–51.

Josselson, R. (1980). Ego development in adolescence. *Handbook of adolescent psychology.* New York: Wiley.

Kagan, J. (1981). *The second year: The emergence of self-awareness.* Cambridge: Harvard University Press.

Kaplan, A. G. (1979). Toward an analysis of sex-role-related issues in the therapeutic relationship. *Psychiatry, 42(1),* 112–120.

Kaplan, M. (1983). A woman's view of DSM III. *American Psychologist, 38,* 786–792.

Kestenberg, J. S., & Buelte, A. (1977). Prevention, infant therapy and the treatment of adults. 1: Toward understanding mutuality. *International Journal of Psychoanalytic Psychotherapy, 6,* 339–367.

Kirshner, L. A., Genak, A., & Hauser, S. T. (1978). Effects of gender on short-term psychotherapy. *Psychotherapy: Theory, Research and Practice, 15(2),* 158–167.

Kleeman, J. (1977). Freud's views on early female sexuality in the light of direct child observation. In H. P. Blum (Ed.), *Female psychology: Contemporary psychoanalytic views* (pp. 3–17). New York: International Universities Press.

Klein, D. (1972). Drug therapy as a means of syndrome identification and nosological revision. In J. Cole, A. Freedman, & A. Friedhoff (Eds.), *Psychopathy and psychopharmacology.* Baltimore: The Johns Hopkins University Press.

Klein, G. (1976). *Psychoanalytic theory: An explanation of essentials.* New York:

International Universities Press.

Klein, M. (1950). A contribution to the psychogenesis of manic-depressive states. In *Contributions to Psychoanalysis 1921–1945*. London: Hogarth.

Klein, M. (1953). *Love, hate and reparation*, with Joan Riviere. London: Hogarth.

Klein, M. (1975). The origins of transference. In *Envy and gratitude and other works 1946–1963*. New York: Delacorte Press.

Kohlberg, L. (1966). A cognitive-developmental analysis of children's sex role concepts and attitudes. In E. Maccoby, (Ed.), *The development of sex differences* (pp. 82–173). Stanford, CA: Stanford University Press.

Kohut, H. (1959). Introspection, empathy and psychoanalysis. *Journal of the American Psychoanalytic Association, 7,* 459–483.

Kohut, H. (1971). *The analysis of the self.* New York: International Universities Press.

Kohut, H. (1978). The psychoanalyst in the community of scholars. In P. Ornstein (Ed.), *The search for the self: Selected writings of Heinz Kohut,* Vol. 2 (pp. 685–724). New York: International Universities Press.

Kohut, H. (1983). Selected problems of self psychological theory. In J. Lichtenberg & S. Kaplan (Eds.), *Reflections on self psychology.* Hillsdale, NJ: Analytic Press.

Kohut, H. (1984). *How does analysis cure?* Chicago: University of Chicago Press.

Lamb, M. (1981). Fathers and child development: An integrated overview. In M. Lamb (Ed.), *The role of the father in child development* (pp. 1–70). New York: Wiley.

Lampl-de Groot, J. (1927). The evolution of the Oedipus complex in women. In R. Fleiss (Ed.), *The psychoanalytic reader* (pp. 180–194). New York: International Universities Press.

Lampl-de Groot, J. (1960). On adolescence. In *The psychoanalytic study of the child,* Vol. 15 (pp. 97–103). New York: International Universities Press.

Landis, B. (1970). *Ego boundaries.* New York: International Universities Press.

Langs, R. (1973). *The technique of psychoanalytic psychotherapy, Vol. 1: The initial contact, theoretical framework, understanding the patient's communications, The therapist's interventions.* New York: Jason Aronson.

Lenrow, P. (1965). Studies of sympathy. In S. S. Tomkins & C. E. Isard (Eds.), *Affect, cognition and personality.* New York: Springer Publishing Co.

Leonard, M. (1966). Fathers and daughters: The significance of "fathering" in the psychosexual development of the girl. *International Journal of Psychoanalysis, 47,* 325–334.

Lerner, H. (1977). The taboos against female anger. *Menninger Perspective,8*(4), 5–11.

Lerner, H. (1983). Female dependency in context: Some theoretical and technical considerations. *American Journal of Orthopsychiatry, 53*(4), 697–705.

Lester, E. P. (1976). On the psychosexual development of the female child. *Journal of the American Academy of Psychoanalysis, 4,* 515–527.

Levinson, D. (1978). *The seasons of a man's life.* New York: Alfred A. Knopf.

Lewis, H. B. (1976). *Psychic war in men and women.* New York: New York University Press.

Lewis, H. B., & Herman, J. L. (1986). Anger in the mother–daughter relationship. In T. Bernay & D. W. Cantor (Eds.), *The psychology of today's woman: New psychoanalytic visions*. Hillside, NJ: Lawrence Erlbaum.

Lifton, R. (1979). *The broken connection*. New York: Simon & Schuster.

Locksley, A. and Douvan, E. (1979). Problem behavior in adolescence. In E. S. Gomberg and V. Franks (Eds.), *Gender and disordered behavior*. New York: Brunner-Mazel.

Loewald, H. (1979). The waning of the Oedipus complex. *Journal of the American Psychiatric Association, 27*, 751–775.

Luria, Z. (1981, October). Presentation at the Dedication Conference, Stone Center, Wellesley College, Wellesley, MA.

Machlinger, V. J. (1981). The father in psychoanalytic theory. In M. E. Lamb, (Ed.), *The role of the father in child development* (pp. 113–153). New York: Wiley.

MacLean, P. (1958). The limbic system with respect to self-preservation and the preservation of the species. *Journal of Nervous and Mental Diseases, 127*, 1–11.

MacLean, P. (1967). The brain in relation to empathy and medical education. *Journal of Nervous and Mental Diseases, 144*, 374–382.

Macy, J. (1983). *Despair and personal power in the nuclear age*. Philadelphia: New Society Publishers.

Mahler, M. (1972). On the first three subphases of the separation-individuation process. *International Journal of Psychoanalysis, 53*, 333–338.

Mahler, M. S., & Goslinger, B. J. (1955). On symbiotic child psychosis: Genetic, dynamic, and restitutive aspects. *The Psychoanalytic Study of the Child, 10*, 195–212.

Mahler, M., Pine F.,& Berman, A. (1975). *The psychological birth of the human infant: Symbiosis and individuation*. New York: Basic Books.

Mahler, M., Pine, F., and Bergman. A. (1975). *The psychological birth of the human infant: Symbiosis and individuation*. New York: Basic Books.

Margolin, G. and Patterson, G. (1975). Differential consequences provided by mothers and fathers for their sons and daughters. *Developmental Psychology, 11*, 537–538.

Maslow, A. (1954). *Motivation and personality*. New York: Harper.

McClelland, D. (1979). *Power: The inner experience*. New York: Irvington.

Melamed, E. (1984). Reclaiming the power to act. *Therapy now*.

Miller, J. (1978). *Living systems*. New York: McGraw-Hill.

Miller, J. B. (1972). Sexuality and inequality: Men's dilemma. (A note on the Oedipus complex, paranoia and other psychological concepts.) *American Journal of Psychoanalysis, 32*, 147–155.

Miller, J. B. (1976). *Toward a new psychology of women*. Boston: Beacon Press

Miller, J. B. (1981). Intimacy: Its relation to work and family. *Journal of Psychiatric Treatment and Evaluation, 3*, 123–129.

Miller, J. B. (Ed.) (1973). *Psychoanalysis and women*. New York: Bruner/Mazel.

Miller, J. B. (1986). *What do we mean by relationships?* (Work in Progress No. 22). Wellesley, MA: Stone Center.

Miller, J. B. (1987). *Toward a new psychology of women* (2nd ed.). Boston: Beacon

Press.

Miller, J. B., Zilbach, J., Notman, M., & Nadelson, C. (1981a). *Aggression: A reconsideration.* Unpublished manuscript.

Miller, J. B., Zilbach, J., Notman, M., & Nadelson, C. (1981b). Aggression in women: A re-examination. In S. Klebanow (Ed.), *Changing concepts in psychoanalysis.* New York: Gardner.

Millman, M. (1980). *Such a pretty face. Being fat in america.* New York: W. W. Norton.

Modell, A. H. (1976). "The holding environment" and the therapeutic action of psychoanalysis. *Journal of the American Psychoanalytic Association, 24*(2), 285–307.

Modell, A. (Chairman) (1985). The Oedipus complex: A re-evaluation. (Panel, presented at Annual Meeting of the American Psychoanalytic Assoc., May 1, 1983). *Journal of the American Psychoanalytic Association, 33,* 201–206.

Mogul, K. M. (1982). Overview: The sex of the therapist. *American Journal of Psychiatry, 139*(1), 1–11.

Moore, B. E., & Fine, B. D. (1968). *A glossary of psychoanalytic terms and concepts.* New York: American Psychoanalytic Association.

Moss, H. (1967). Sex, age and state as determinants of mother–infant interaction. *Merrill-Palmer Quarterly, 13*(1), 19–36.

Moss, H. (1974). Early sex differences in mother–infant interaction. In K. Friedman, R. Reichert, & R. Vandeweile (Eds.), *Sex differences in behavior.* New York: Wiley.

Moulton, R. (1973). A survey and re-evaluation of the concept of penis envy. In J. B. Miller (Ed.), *Psychoanalysis and women* (pp. 207–230). New York: Brunner-Mazel.

Moulton, R. (1977). Some effects of the new feminism. *American Journal of Psychiatry, 134*(1), 1–6, .

Nadelson, C., Notman, M., Miller, J. B., & Zilbach, J. (1982). Aggression in women: Conceptual issues and clinical implications. In M. Notman & C. Nadelson (Eds.), *The woman patient, Vol. 3: Aggressions, adaptations, and psychotherapy.* New York: Plenum.

Nielson Survey. (1978). *Who's dieting and why?* Chicago: A. C. Nielson.

Nylander, I. (1971). The feeling of being fat and dieting in a school population. *Acta Sociomedica Scandinavica, 1,* 17–26.

Oetzel, R. (1966). Annotated bibliography and classified summary of research in sex differences. In E. Maccoby (Ed.), *The development of sex differences* (pp. 223–321; 323–351). Stanford, CA: Stanford University Press.

Olden, C. (1972). On adult empathy with children. *Psychoanalytic Study of the Child, 8,* 11–126.

Orbach, S. (1978). *Fat is a feminist issue.* New York: Paddington Press.

Orlinsky, D. E., & Howard, K. I. (1980). Gender and psychotherapeutic outcome. In A. Brodksy & R. Hare-Mustin (Eds.), *Women and psychotherapy.* New York: Guilford Press.

Orlinsky, D. E., & Howard, K. I. (1978). The relation of process to outcome in psychotherapy. In S. L. Garfield & A. E. Bergin (Eds.), *Handbook of psychotherapy and behavior change: An empirical analysis* (2nd ed.). New York: Wiley.

Oxford English Dictionary, Compact Edition (1976). Oxford University Press.

Padesky, C. A., & Hammen, C. L. (1981). Sex differences in depressive symptom expression and help-seeking among college students. *Sex Roles, 7,* 309-320.

Parens, H., Pollack, L., Stem, J., & Kramer, S. (1977). On the girl's entry into the Oedipus complex. In H. P. Blum (Ed.), *Female psychology: Contemporary psychoanalytic views* (pp. 79–107). New York: International Universities Press.

Pederson, F. A. & Robson, K. S. (1969). Father participation in infancy. *American Journal of Orthopsychiatry, 39,* 466–472.

Piaget, J. (1928). *Judgment and measuring in the child.* New York: Harcourt Brace.

Piaget, J. (1952). *The origins of intelligence in children.* New York: W. W. Norton.

Pleck, Joseph. (1981). *The myth of masculinity.* Cambridge, MA: MIT Press.

Polivy, J., & Herman, C. P. (1983). *Breaking the diet habit: The natural weight alternative.* New York: Basic Books.

Pollack, S., & Gilligan, C. (1982). Images of violence in Thematic Apperception Test stories. *Journal of Personality and Social Psychology, 42*(1), 159–167.

Pollack, W. (1982). *"I"-ness and "we"-ness: Parallel lines of development.* Unpublished doctoral dissertation, Boston University.

Pope, H. G., Hudson, J. I., & Yurgelun-Todd, D. (1984). Anorexia nervosa and bulimia among 300 suburban women shoppers. *American Journal of Psychiatry, 141,* 292–294.

Post, R. D. (1982). Dependency conflicts in high-achieving women: Toward an integration. *Psychotherapy: Theory, Research, and Practice, 19*(1), 82–87.

Racker, H. (1968). *Transference and counter-transference.* New York: International Universities Press.

Radloff, L. S. (1975). Sex differences in depression: The effects of occupation and marital status. *Sex Roles, 1*(3), 249–265.

Radloff, L. S. (1986). Risk factors for depression. What do we learn from them? In M. Guttentag, S. Salasin, & D. Belle (Eds.), *The mental health of women.* New York: Academic Press.

Radloff, S. S. (1975). Sex differences in depression: The effects of occupation and marital status. *Sex Roles, 3,* 249–265.

Rappaport, J. (1984). Studies in empowerment: Introduction to the issue. In J. Rappaport & R. Mess (Eds.), *Studies in empowerment: Steps toward understanding and action.* New York: Haworth Press.

Reik, T. (1986). *Sex in man and woman: Its emotional variations.* New York: Farrar, Strauss & Cudahy.

Rich, A. (1983). Compulsory heterosexuality and lesbian existence. In E. Abel & E. Abel (Eds.), *The signs reader: Women, gender and scholarship.* Chicago: The University of Chicago Press.

Rickles, N. K. (1971). The angry woman syndrome. *Archives of General Psychiatry, 24,* 91–94.

Ritvo, S. (1976). Adolescent to woman. *Journal of the American Psychoanalytic*

Association, 24(5), 127–137.

Rochlin, G. (1980). *The masculine dilemma*. Boston: Little Brown.

Rogers, C. (1975). Empathic: An unappreciated way of being. *The Counseling Psychologist*, 5, (No. 2), 2–10.

Roiphe, H., & Galenson, E. (1972). Early genital activity and the castration complex. *Psychoanalytic Quarterly*, 41, 334–347.

Rosenbaum, M. -B. (1979). The changing body image of the adolescent girl. In M. Sugar (Ed.), *Female adolescent development*. New York: Brunner-Mazel.

Rothenberg, A. (1979). *The emerging goddess: The creative process in art, science, and other fields*. Chicago: University of Chicago Press.

Rubenstein, K. (1979, August). *Sex differences in identification processes in psychotherapy supervision*. Paper presented at the conference of the American Psychological Association, New York City.

Rubin, J., Provenzano, F., & Luria, Z. (1974). The eye of the beholder: Views on sex of newborns. *American Journal of Orthopsychiatry*, 44, 512–519.

Rubin, L. B. (1976). *Worlds of pain*. New York: Basic Books.

Ryan, V. L., & Gizynski, M. N. (1971). Behavior therapy in retrospect:Patients' feelings about their behavior therapies. *Journal of Consulting and Clinical Psychology*. 37(1), 1–9.

Safilios-Rothschild, C. (1976). Dual linkages between the occupational and family systems: A macrosociological analysis. *Signs: Journal of Women in Culture and Society*, 1(3, part 2), 51–60.

Sagi, A., & Hoffman, M. L. (1976). Empathic distress in newborns. *Developmental Psychology*, 12, 175–176.

Salzman, L. (1975). Interpersonal factors in depression. In F. F. Flack & S. C. Droghi (Eds.), *The nature and treatment of depression*. New York: Wiley.

Sander. L. (1980). Investigation of the infant and its caretaking environment as a biological system. In S. Greenspan & G. Pollock (Eds.), *The course of life: Vol. I*. Washington, DC: US Government Printing Office.

Sander. L. W. (1964). Adaptive relationship in early mother–child interaction. *Journal of the American Academy of Child Psychiatry*, 3 231–264.

Sassen, G. (1980). Success anxiety in women: A constructivist interpretation of its sources and its significance. *Harvard Educational Review*, 50, 13–25.

Schafer, R. (1959). Generative empathy in the treatment situation. *Psychoanalytic Quarterly*, 28(3), 342–373.

Schafer, R. (1960). The loving and beloved superego in Freud's structural theory. *Psychoanalytic Study of the Child*, 15, 163–188.

Schafer, R. (1964). The clinical analysis of affects. *Journal of the American Psychoanalytic Association*, 12, 275–299.

Schafer, R. (1968). *Aspects of internalization*. New York: International Universities Press.

Schafer, R. (1974). Problems in Freud's psychology of women. *Journal of the American Psychoanalytic Association*, 22(3), 459–485.

Schaffer, H. R., & Emerson, P. E. (1964). The development of social attachments in infancy. *Monographs of the Society for Research in Child Development*, 29(3).

Scherfey, M. J. (1973). On the nature and evolution of female sexuality. In J. B.

Miller (Ed.), *Psychoanalysis and women* (pp. 115–129). New York: Brunner-Mazel.

Schwarz, J. C., & Zuroff, D. C. (1979). Family structure and depression in female college students: Effects of parental conflict, decision-making power and inconsistency of love. *Journal of Abnormal Psychology, 88,* 398–406.

Searles, H. (1975). The patient as therapist to his analyst. In P. Giovacchini (Ed.), *Tactics and techniques in psychoanalytic therapy: Counter-transference* (Vol. 2). New York: Jason Aronson.

Seligman, M. E. P. (1975). *Helplessness.* San Francisco: W. H. Freeman.

Seligman, M. E. (1974). Depression and learned helplessness. In R. J. Friedman & M. M. Katz (Eds.), *The psychology of depression: Contemporary theory and research.* Washington, DC: Winston.

Shem, S. (1978) *The house of God.* New York: Marek.

Simner, M. D. (1971). Newborn's response to the cry of another infant. *Developmental Psychology,* 136–150.

Slaff, B. (1979). Adolescents. In J. Noshpitz (Ed.), *Basic handbook of child psychiatry.* New York: Basic Books.

Sloane, R. B., Staples, F. R., Cristol, A. H., Yorkston, N., & Whipple, K. (1975). *Psychotherapy versus Behavior Therapy.* Cambridge: Harvard University Press.

Spitzer, R. (1980). *Diagnostic and statistical manual of mental disorders* (third edition). Washington, DC: The American Psychiatric Association.

Stangler, R. S., Printz, A. M. (1980). DSM-III: Psychiatric diagnosis in a university population. *American Journal of Psychiatry, 139,* 937–940.

Staples, F. R., Sloane, R. B., Whipple, K., Cristol, A. H., & Yorkston, N. (1976). Process and outcome in psychotherapy and behavior therapy. *Journal of Consulting and Clinical Psychology, 44*(3), 340–350.

Stechler, G. & Kaplan, S. (1980). The development of the self: A psychoanalytic perspective. *Psychoanalytic Study of the Child, 35,* 85–106.

Steiner-Adair, C. (1986). The body politic: Normal female adolescent development and the development of eating disorders. *Journal of the American Academy of Psychoanalysis, 14*(1), 92–114.

Stern, D. (1980, October). The early differentiation of self and other. In *Reflections on self psychology.* Symposium at the Boston Psychoanalytic Society, Boston, Massachusetts.

Stern, D. (1983). The early development of schemas of self, other and "self with other. " In J. Lichtenberg & S. Kaplan (Eds.), *Reflections on self psychology.* Hillsdale, NJ: Analytic Press.

Stern, D. (1986). *The interpersonal world of the infant.* New York: Basic Books.

Stoller, R. J. (1968). The sense of femaleness. *Psychoanalytic Quarterly, 37,* 42–55.

Stone, L. (1981). Some thoughts on the "Here and Now" in psychoanalytic technique and practice. *Psychoanalytic Quarterly, 50*(4), 709–731.

Strupp, H. H., Fox, R. E., & Lessler, K. (1969). *Patients view their psychotherapy.* Baltimore: Johns Hopkins University Press.

Strupp, H. H., Wallach, M. S., & Wogan, M. (1964). Psychotherapy experience in retrospect: Questionnaire survey of former patients and their therapists. *Psychological Monographs, 78*(11), Whole No. 588.

Sugar, M. (1979). *Female adolescent development.* New York: Brunner-Mazel.

Sullivan, H. S. (1953). *The interpersonal theory of psychiatry.* New York: W. W. Norton.

Sullivan, H. S. (1953). *Conceptions of modern psychiatry.* New York: W. W. Norton.

Surrey, J. (1982). *Survey of eating patterns at Wellesley College.* Unpublished research report, Wellesley College.

Tessman, L. (1982). A note on the father's contribution to the daughter's ways of loving and working. In S. Cath & A. R. Gurwitt (Eds.), *Father–child development and clinical perspectives.* Boston: Little Brown & Co.

Thompson, C. (1942). Cultural pressures in the psychology of women. *Psychiatry, 5,* 331–339. Reprinted in J. B. Niller (Ed.), *Psychoanalysis and women.* New York: Brunner-Mazel and Penguin Books, 1973.

Thompson, C. (1943). "Penis envy" in women. *Psychiatry, 6,* 123–129.

Thompson, M., & Schwartz, D. (1981). Life adjustment of women with anorexia nervosa and anorexic-like behavior. *International Journal of Eating Disorders, 2,* 47–60.

Thorne, B., & Henley, N. (Eds.) (1975). *Language and sex: Difference and dominance.* Rowley, MA: Newbury House.

Ticho, G. (1976). Female autonomy and young adult women. *Journal of the American Psychoanalytic Association, 24*(5), 139–155.

Trevarthan, C. (1979). Communication and cooperation in early infancy: A description of primary intersubjectivity. In J. M. Bullowar (Ed.), *Before speech: The beginning of interpersonal communication.* New York: Cambridge University Press.

Vaillant, G. (1978). *Adaptation to life.* Boston: Little Brown.

Webster's New Collegiate Dictionary. (1971). Springfield, MA: Merriam-Webster

Webster's Ninth New Collegiate Dictionary. (1984). Springfield, MA: Merriam-Webster

Wechsler, H., Rohman, M., & Solomon, L. (1981). Emotional problems and concerns of New England college students. *American Journal of Orthopsychiatry, 51*(4), 719–723.

Weissman, M., & Paykel, E. S. (1974). *The depressed women: A study of social relations.* Chicago: University of Chicago Press.

Weissman, M. D., & Klerman, G. L. (1977). Sex differences and the epidemiology of depression. *Archives of General Psychiatry, 34,* 98–111.

Weissman, M. M., & Klerman, G. L. (1977). Sex differences and the epidemiology of depression. *Archives of General Psychiatry, 34*(1), 98–111.

Willi, Jurg. (1982). *Couples in collusion.* New York: Jason Aronson.

William, J. (1974). *The psychology of women: Behavior in a biosocial context.* New York: W. W. Norton.

Winnicott, D. (1963). The development of the capacity for concern. *Bulletin of the*

Menninger Clinic, 27, 167–176.

Winnicott, D. (1965). The theory of the parent–infant relationship. In *The maturational processes and the facilitating environment.* New York: International Universities Press.

Winnicott, D. W. (1971). *Playing and reality.* New York: Basic Books.

Wooley, S. C., & Wooley, O. W. (1980). Eating Disorders: Obesity and anorexia. In A. Brodsky & R. Hare-Mustin (Eds.), *Women and psychotherapy.* New York: Guilford.

Zeldow, P. B. (1978). Sex differences in psychiatric evaluation and treatment. *Archives of General Psychiatry,* 35(1), 89–93.

Zilbach, J., Notman, M., Nadelson, C., & Miller, J. (1979, August). *Reconsideration of aggression and self-esteem in women.* Paper presented at the meeting of the International Psychoanalytic Association, New York City.

Index

Abandonment, feelings of, 203, 204
  in men, 260
Accommodation, 70, 72, 74, 89
Adolescence, 19–21, 60, 124
  and body weight, 239
  conflict in, 125–127
  discontinuity in, 169
  late, relational self in, 123, 133–140, 170–171, 248
Affective surrender, 29, 69
Agency, 17, 20–21
  as self-control, 246
Agentic ethic, 28,87
Aggressiveness, 189, 190–192, 194
  in games, 191
Anger, 181, 289
  in children, 189–191, 194
  confronting, 24
  cultural structure of, 194–195
  defense against, 70–71
  definition of, 188–189
  expression of, 181, 185, 194, 195, 264
  and "femininity," 5, 155, 184
  inhibition of, 209–210, 214–215
  internalized, 210
  in men, 187–192, 193, 261–262
  in mother–daughter relationship, 110–111
  permitted, 184
  and psychosomatic symptoms, 186
  spiraling phenomena in, 185
  in subordinates, 183, 187
  and unmet needs, 147–148, 155
Anorexia, 239, 244; see also Eating disturbances
Anorexia Aid Society (ANAS), 249
Arieti, S., 206, 219–220
Assimilation, 70, 72, 74
Attunement, empathic, 82, 87, 287, 288

Bakan, David, 17, 28, 162
Basch, M., 79
Being-in-relationship; see Self-in-relation
Belenky, M. F., 3
Bemporad, J., 206, 219–220
Bernardez, T., 259, 262
Blos, P., 124–125
Body weight

obsession with, 238–240
  and "set point" theory, 243–244
Borderline personality disorder, 260, 264–265
Broverman, I. K., 253, 254
Bruch, Hilda, 241, 244
Bulimia, 129; see also Eating disturbances

Caplan, Paula, 265
Career-children conflict, 233
Caretaking, 14–16, 17–18, 41, 49, 146, 186
  vs. "caring about," 250–251, 265–267
  in marriage, 154
  relational, 56–57, 199
  and responsibility, 78
"Carriers," women as, 52, 260
Castration anxiety, 99, 101
  criteria for, 103
  in girls, 101, 103–104, 108
Ceres/Persephone myth, 60
Chassequet-Smirgel, J., 102
Chesler, Phyllis, 253, 254
Childhood, 18–19
  girls' vs. boys' activities in, 18–19
  mother–daughter relationships in, 18, 31
Chodorow, Nancy, 2–3, 97–98
  on mother–daughter relationship, 31, 33, 107, 112
  on mothering, 39
Cinderella Complex, The (Dowling), 226
Cinderella syndrome, 166
Clower, V., 106
College students
  anorexic behavior in, 239–240
  and relational growth, 127–129
Communication
  and expression of emotion, 229–230
  of needs, 157
  styles of, 62
Communal ethic, 28
Competence, 117
Conflict, 125–127, 131
  marital, 145
  in mother–daughter relationship, 108, 110, 117, 125–126, 133, 248
Connected learning, 171
Consciousness raising, 39